12/86

ID0983036

A CALCULUS OF SUFFERING

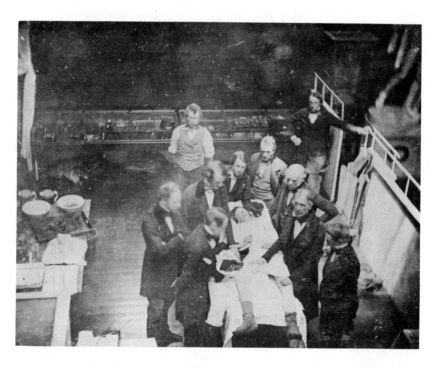

An early operation under anesthesia, circa 1847, Massachusetts General Hospital. Whole plate daguerreotype, attributed to Southworth and Hawes, Boston. Dr. John Collins Warren in foreground, right-center. *Reproduced by permission of Countway Library of Medicine, Boston.*

A CALCULUS OF SUFFERING

Pain, Professionalism, and Anesthesia in Nineteenth-Century America

MARTIN S. PERNICK

Columbia University Press   NEW YORK 1985

Library of Congress Cataloging in Publication Data

Pernick, Martin S.
  A calculus of suffering.

  Bibliography: p.
  Includes index.
    1. Anesthesia—United States—History—19th
century.   2. Medicine—United States—History—19th
century.   3. Surgery—United States—History—19th
century.   4. Pain—Social aspects—United States—
History—19th century. I. Title. [DNLM: 1. Anesthesiology—history—United States.   2. History of Medicine,
19th Cent.—United States.   WO 211 AA1 P4c]
RD80.3.P47 1985   617'.96'0973   84-12664
ISBN 0-231-05186-7 (alk. paper)

Columbia University Press
New York   Guildford, Surrey
Copyright © 1985 Columbia University Press
All rights reserved

Printed in the United States of America

Clothbound editions of Columbia University Press Books are Smyth-sewn and printed on permanent and durable acid-free paper.

For Louis W. Pernick
in loving memory of
Florence P. Pernick

CONTENTS

ILLUSTRATIONS

ACKNOWLEDGMENTS

Professionalism and pain are inherently interdisciplinary topics; without the guidance, comments, and criticisms of colleagues and friends skilled in many different branches of learning, this book could not have come into existence. In particular, my former colleagues at the Department of Humanities of the Pennsylvania State University College of Medicine in Hershey, and at the School of Public Health, Harvard University, created working environments in which valuable interdisciplinary exchange went on daily. At Hershey, Carol Pollard shared an enormous wealth of information on British and American literature. Art Zucker and Dan Clouser introduced me to medical ethics and to philosophical perspectives on penology. Robert Sevensky provided an invaluable entree into the theological literature on suffering and theodicy. Department chairman Al Vastyan made available essential time off for research, and a wide range of support services. Joanne Trautmann helped track down and interpret a number of literary sources. She and Richard Kirby read a portion of an early draft of the manuscript and on several occasions provided important personal support. Jay Gold, a true polymath, eagerly discussed all aspects of the project, never failing to sharpen my ideas and provide valuable additional sources. Barbara Howe (now of West Virginia University) helped locate many hard-to-get sources. Folklorist David Hufford explained the intricacies of the motif-indexes. A particular debt of gratitude is owed to Angelica Thevos-Leskawa and Ruby Smith of the Interlibrary Loan Service. Without their immense expenditure of time and effort, many of the most basic sources for my research would have been unavailable in Hershey.

At Harvard, Marc Roberts contributed both an unquench- able enthusiasm for interdisciplinary thought and many hours of fas- cinating discourse on the political economics of medical utilitarian- ism. Barbara Rosenkrantz shared ideas on all aspects of medical and social history. She provided advice both personal and professional and opened many doors that otherwise would have been closed to me. Harry Marks carefully read several drafts, provided incisive criticisms, and shared his own research unstintingly. John Harley Warner offered many valuable suggestions.

At the University of Michigan, my current colleagues Maris and Mary Vinovskis and Catherine Whitaker spent many hours patiently guiding me through the world of computers. Others who worked on the statistical analysis include Paul Killey and Elaine Wethington. Nick Steneck and Hal Cook (now of Harvard) carefully read and thoughtfully critiqued drafts of several chapters. David Hol- linger, Charles Tilly, Louise Tilly, Robert Berkhofer, Kenneth Lock- ridge, Elizabeth Eisenstein, Peter Railton, and James Bono offered specific and valuable suggestions. The advice and encouragement of Marie Deveney have been especially helpful in surmounting the big- gest hurdle in any project—getting done.

A great many friends and colleagues from other institu- tions also participated in making this book possible. Allan Lichtman and Laura Langbein of The American University aided my stumbling early applications of statistical methods and read a portion of an early draft. Allan also provided the most basic research resource—an un- limited welcome and a place to sleep near the Library of Congress and National Library of Medicine. David Rosner of Baruch College contributed his infectious enthusiasm and thoughtful ideas while pro- viding a home away from home during my many long research trips to New York. Nancy Reed and Sam Perkins carefully and critically read portions of an early draft and offered limitless hospitality during my research in Boston. They gave needed personal support at all the critical times. Morris Vogel of Temple University and Robert Gross of Amherst College provided a combination of colleagueship, advice, and hospitality in the Philadelphia and Boston areas respectively. Many other friends hosted my visits during my research travels; their welcome was deeply appreciated.

Others whose comments and suggestions on portions of early drafts proved especially helpful were Charles E. Rosenberg of the University of Pennsylvania, Cliff Griffin of the University of Kansas, Rosa Lynn Pinkus of the University of Pittsburgh, and Carol Levine of the *Hastings Center Report*.

I owe a special debt of gratitude to Gina Morantz of the University of Kansas: for sharing with me her data, sources, and ideas on the history of women physicians and of medical sectarianism; for her careful reading of the manuscript at several different stages of preparation; and for the concern and advice that helped me over many barriers.

So many archivists and librarians helped in so many ways it would be quite impossible to repay each kindness with an individual acknowledgment, but several whose efforts were vital to the entire project must be mentioned by name. Jim Cassedy of the National Library of Medicine took a deep and understanding interest in my research, generously shared with me sources gathered for his own work on the history of medical statistics, and always made me feel a welcome guest in his office. Caroline Morris spent much time explaining to me the holdings of the Pennsylvania Hospital Historical Library. Nancy Tomes braved the hazards of dust, heat, water, and vermin to guide me to these materials. (Happily these records are now preserved in safe, convenient quarters, thanks to the efforts of these dedicated people.) James Vaccarino of the Massachusetts General Hospital housed me in a corner of his own office for days on end to facilitate my use of his hospital's case records.

Barbara Williams of the Hahnemann University Archives, Adele Lerner and Lisa Hottin of the New York Hospital Archives, Fran Blouin and Mary Jo Pugh of the Bentley Library, Michigan Historical Collections, Carol Fenichel of the Medical College of Pennsylvania Library, Ellen Gartrell of the College of Physicians in Philadelphia, Roger D. Bridges of the Illinois State Historical Library, Peter Parker of the Historical Society of Pennsylvania, and the staff of the Massachusetts Historical Society also went out of their way to provide friendly and helpful assistance. Richard Wolfe of the Countway Medical Library informed me of the existence of the MGH case records and of his impending acquisition of them and thus made these valuable materials available even before they had been catalogued. In addition, he and Barbara Rosenkrantz waded through a blizzard in the middle of one Christmas vacation to make the records of the Boston Lying-In and New England Hospital for Women available.

A number of teachers over the years have had an enormous impact on the content and direction of my research. At Brandeis University, Saul Benison (now of the University of Cincinnati) first showed me how to combine my interests in biology and history; he has been a source of aid and encouragement for the past fifteen years. Marvin Meyers and David Hackett Fischer guided my initial explorations in the history of professionalism and instilled an iconoclastic interdisciplinarity that has remained my ideal of historical scholarship.

At Columbia, the faith, encouragement, and enthusiastic assistance of Stuart Bruchey have been of great importance to me since my first day of graduate school. Walter Metzger sharpened my ideas on the history of professionalism and also made available to me the support of the National Institute of Mental Health Training Program in Social History. David Rothman's provocative critique of my initial venture in the history of anesthesia played a major role in shaping this work, as did Sigmund Diamond's deeply appreciated suggestions and enthusiasm. Above all, Eric L. McKitrick proved a wise and judicious counselor in guiding the dissertation on which this book is based.

National Institute of Mental Health grant number 1-To1-MH-12221-01 provided financial support for my initial years of graduate training. National Endowment for the Humanities grant number EO-4579-71-197 and United States Public Health Service grant number 417-04 HY helped defray some of my research expenses during my employment at Penn State. The University of Michigan provided computer time.

Many other scholars generously provided specific source materials and/or shared with me their unpublished manuscripts. I have tried to acknowledge each such contribution in the notes. Finally, my parents, Louis W. and Florence Pernick, played an active role in the creation of this work by providing a careful critique of an early draft, by serving as a full-fledged private clipping service, and by maintaining just the right mixture of faith and impatience.

An earlier version of part of chapter 5 appeared in the *Hastings Center Report,* April 1983. Portions of chapter 2 and the afterword are extensive revisions of "Medical Professionalism," *Encyclopedia of Bioethics* (New York: Macmillan, 1978), 3: 1028–34, Warren T. Reich, Editor in Chief, reprinted by permission of The Free Press, a Division of Macmillan, Inc. and the Kennedy Institute of Ethics, Georgetown University, copyright © 1978 by Georgetown University.

ABBREVIATIONS

AJMS	American Journal of the Medical Sciences
AMA	American Medical Association
B Med Surg J	Boston Medical and Surgical Journal
ed.	edited, edition, editor
MGH	Massachusetts General Hospital
NYJ Med	New York Journal of Medicine and the Collateral Sciences
NYH	New York Hospital
OED	Oxford English Dictionary
Pa. H.	Pennsylvania Hospital
Phil Med Ex	Medical Examiner of Philadelphia
rev.	revised
S.D.	surgical division
Trans AMA	Transactions of the American Medical Association

PART ONE: Anesthesia and Medicine in Nineteenth-Century America

CHAPTER ONE

THE CASE OF McGONIGLE'S FOOT: NONANESTHETIC SURGERY IN POSTANESTHETIC AMERICA

On October 16, 1846, a Boston dentist named William T. G. Morton first demonstrated that the vapor of sulphuric or diethyl ether could prevent the pain of surgery. In the steep-walled, bleacher-seated, domed amphitheater of the Massachusetts General Hospital, Morton administered his ''Letheon Gas'' to a young printer about to have a large tumor cut from his face. The operation, performed by Boston's preeminent surgeon, John Collins Warren, failed to fully remove the massive growth, but the ether succeeded in rendering the patient largely insensible to pain.[1]

Use of the new discovery spread with unprecedented speed. Within three months of Morton's demonstration, the leading hospitals of New York, London, and Paris began employing ether anesthesia. In Vienna, St. Petersburg, even far-off Canton, surgeons rapidly adopted the new discovery. By 1848, nitrous oxide (laughing gas), chloroform, and other compounds had been added to the list of known anesthetics. The new painkillers found employment in dentistry, obstetrics, and therapeutics, in addition to surgery. Some enthusiastic prophets predicted the imminent end of all human suffering.[2]

The use of anesthesia spread far more rapidly than had such earlier innovations as smallpox vaccination or would such later discoveries as antisepsis. Vaccination remained controversial for over a century after Jenner's initial experiment; antisepsis aroused bitter opposition for more than three decades following Lister's first demonstration.[3] Anesthetics won acceptance at most major world medical institutions within a few months of Morton's exhibition. With the introduction of ether at the Pennsylvania Hospital in July 1853, the new discovery gained the approval of virtually the last of its opponents—all within seven years.[4]

Yet the rapid diffusion of anesthetic use did *not* mean the end of painful surgery for all patients. There was, for example, a man named McGonigle, an immigrant laborer living in Philadelphia. On July 15, 1862, he fell while intoxicated, severely fracturing his ankle. He was rushed to the Pennsylvania Hospital, where his foot was immediately amputated. Although it was almost sixteen years after the discovery of anesthesia and nearly a decade after ether had been adopted at the Pennsylvania Hospital, McGonigle received no anesthetic at any time during the operation. Two days later, he died of shock.[5]

McGonigle's case was not very unusual. Over the years 1853 to 1862, about 32 percent of all major limb amputations for fractures at the Pennsylvania Hospital took place on conscious patients.[6] Even at the Massachusetts General Hospital, one of every three potentially painful operations in 1847 was performed without anesthesia.[7] In the five years following their first use of ether, the surgeons of the New York Hospital may have done as many as one-third of their amputations on nonanesthetized people.[8]

Private surgery seemingly followed the same pattern, though the statistical evidence is more limited. Most operations in antebellum America took place, not in hospitals, but in individual homes or medical offices.[9] Unfortunately, without the discipline of institutional regulations, surgeons rarely kept detailed records of their private practices. One exception was Dr. Frank Hamilton of New York, a pioneer in the use of medical statistics, who kept case records covering his thirty-five years of experience as America's foremost expert on fractures. Hamilton first used ether in August 1847 and had tried chloroform by July 1849. Yet, over the next quarter century, more than one-sixth of the nonmilitary amputations he performed were done on conscious patients. In June 1873, for example, an anonymous twenty-three-year-old Irishman was run over by a railroad train in New York. Hamilton amputated the man's leg, without administering any anesthetic. Despite his gruesome ordeal, the patient recovered.[10]

In addition to the available statistics, anecdotal accounts from a wide variety of sources confirm that instances of nonanesthetic surgery remained common occurrences long after most surgeons had adopted the use of anesthesia. Physicians and laypeople, easterners and westerners, in tones ranging from acceptance to outrage, recorded numerous cases of surgery without anesthesia performed in the 1850s and 1860s. As late as 1876, the respected *Cincinnati Lancet* published an article on "Alcohol as an Anaesthetic." The author advocated replacing chloroform with a stiff drink, in at least some cases of surgery, and reported three successful case histories. In short, many if not most mid-nineteenth-century practitioners who recorded their views or practices anesthetized some of their patients and not others.[11] The issue for them was not whether to use anesthetics but when and on whom.

This study attempts to explain why mid-nineteenth-century physicians followed such a pattern of selective anesthetic use and which patients were most likely to be given the new painkillers. But the answers to these questions go beyond the history of anesthesia itself, to explore many larger issues. How did such a startling innovation win acceptance into routine medical practice? How did the medical profession's view of suffering affect the introduction of the new painkillers; and how did anesthesia change physicians' attitudes toward pain? What did the development of anesthesia derive from or contribute to mid-nineteenth-century humanitarian reform movements? And how did these developments affect and reflect the changing place of the profession in a democratic society?

Pain and Professionalism: An Overview

Even its most ardent advocates agreed anesthesia had drawbacks. Such criticisms derived from rational and humane concerns, including the belief that anesthesia could be dangerous, that pain could be valuable, that the power over others conferred by anesthesia could be abused, and that its use violated professional norms. And the alleged advantages were as varied as the drawbacks; they too included issues of power and status in addition to benevolence. The introduction of anesthesia was not a simple triumph of progress over reaction, humanitarianism over sadism. Most practitioners saw anesthesia as neither all good nor all bad but as a mixed blessing to be used selectively.

This discretionary nineteenth-century use of anesthesia drew upon a new utilitarian approach to professional decisionmaking, dubbed by its proponents "conservative medicine." "Conservative" doctrine cautioned that every drug had both good and bad effects; that the damage done by drugs and the damage done by disease were equally undesirable; and that professional duty required measuring the benefit-harm balance before employing any therapy. Conservative professionalism constituted a dramatic new departure in medical ethics, in its use of a utilitarian calculus to circumvent the ancient distinctions between acts of omission and of commission; between the effects of "Nature" and the results of human "Art." Medical conservatives adopted this approach in the hope it would provide a moderate synthesis, capable of reuniting a profession torn by scientific and ideological civil war.

Furthermore, conservative physicians held that their calculus of risks and benefits would vary widely from patient to patient. Thus nineteenth-century medical literature urged doctors to consider a patient's sex, race, age, ethnicity, economic class, personal habits, and temperament, as well as a wide range of technical factors, before using anesthetics. Women and children supposedly required painkillers more often than did men; the rich and educated more often than the poor and ignorant; etc. The operations considered too "minor" for anesthesia included many procedures that today are considered quite painful. And case statistics show that surgeons who kept records seemingly did follow the advice of this professional literature when actually prescribing anesthetics.

Selective anesthetization often derived from the widely shared belief that different types of people differed in their sensitivity to pain, a doctrine whose implications reached far beyond anesthesia. The notion that women, children, whites, the rich, and the educated were more sensitive than were their social opposites played an important, previously unrecognized role in such diverse areas as feminism, imperialism, abolition, penology, pedagogy, and poetry. This tailoring of prescriptions to fit the patient, as well as the disease, provoked explicitly political controversy, because it required confronting the conflicting demands of individuality and equality.

Anesthetic usage spread more rapidly than any other medical innovation before the twentieth century. But whereas most physicians almost immediately adopted some uses of anesthesia, the frequency with which any given practitioner employed the new painkillers increased only gradually between 1846 and the 1870s. A doctor's age, sex, location, professional network, and therapeutic sect all influenced how often that physician prescribed anesthetics at any point in time; and the relationships sometimes proved surprising. Thus homeopaths and hydropaths, alternative healers who generally prided themselves on their mild, painless therapies, tended to employ anesthetics less frequently than did other, more orthodox practitioners.

By the 1880s a profusion of new anesthetic techniques, and a bacteriologically inspired revival of medical interventionism, marked the end of the era of selective anesthetization. Instead of choosing which patients were suitable for anesthesia, physicians could now select which anesthetic was best adapted to each operation.[12] At the same time, new concepts of disease causality revolutionized both the technical and the ethical standards of surgical professionalism.[13] But by then, anesthesia had already permanently changed both medicine and society.

Anesthesia deeply altered the practice of surgery. Case records indicate that, where anesthesia was introduced rapidly, it led to a dramatic increase in surgery; that these new operations were mostly necessary, not experimental; that the death rate following anesthetic surgery actually was much lower than most nineteenth-century physicians thought; and that industrialization, not anesthesia, caused the shocking midcentury increase in postoperative mortality. Anesthesia increased the power of surgeons over their patients; promoted the entry of women into surgery; fostered the bureaucratization of military and urban hospitals; and contributed to the "medicalization" of human suffering.

Though I have used a fairly large number of British and French sources, I have limited myself to those non-American authors whose works demonstrably penetrated American thinking (or at least were published in American editions). Though the ideas are European, I treat only of their use in the United States, not of their meaning in their own world. This is also not a complete history of American anesthesia but only of how one generation of mostly eastern urban professional leaders used it and why.

This work began as an attempt to compare how several different professions decreased the amount of pain they inflicted in nineteenth-century America. The introduction of surgical anesthesia bears close comparison with the decline of other painful therapies in medicine and with the lessening use of whipping in education and criminal justice. Several such examples are presented in this study; I hope someday to be able to develop them further.

This study is, in other words, much more and somewhat less than another history of anesthesia. My concern has been to use the introduction of anesthesia as a case study, to illuminate links that united elements of nineteenth-century American culture whose integral connections have not previously been noticed. This book is intended as a study of the relation between ideology and action, between the values in professional textbooks and ethics codes, and the way people actually practiced their jobs. It is a study of professionalism, how and why it changes, and how it influences such things as the reception of innovations, the emotions of practitioners, and the role of the expert in an egalitarian society.

CHAPTER TWO

A HOUSE DIVIDED: AN INTERPRETIVE OVERVIEW OF NINETEENTH-CENTURY AMERICAN MEDICINE

William T. G. Morton introduced anesthesia to a medical profession battered by brutal internal dissension and external assaults. Every aspect of medicine, its theory and practice, its structure and ideology, provoked vitriolic controversy, both within and beyond the profession. To understand nineteenth-century America's response to Morton's discovery, it is necessary to comprehend these bitter disputes, over the causes and cure of disease, the ethical obligations of a physician, and the purpose of an organized profession.

Disease and Environment

In the fall of 1793, an epidemic of yellow fever wiped out 10 percent of the people in Philadelphia, then the capital of the new United States. From that time until early in this century, virtually every summer produced another yellow fever outbreak in at least one American city. The arrival of cholera in 1832 added another new killer to the roster of epidemics—a roll that already included smallpox, typhoid, and diphtheria. Cholera too would be back, in 1849–54, 1866, and 1877–78.[1]

Such epidemics panicked the population and seriously disrupted society, but as causes of death and suffering they paled before the less dramatic, ever-present tuberculosis, malaria, and infant diarrheas. Tuberculosis alone carried off almost half a percent of the population each year, while 15 percent of the babies born in 1880 did not live to celebrate their birthdays in 1881. The life expectancy of an American born in 1860 was only approximately 40 years.[2]

Today medicine recognizes the leading killers of the nineteenth century as having been infections—invasions of the body by pathogenic microorganisms. But before the 1870s, few physicians conceived of disease in such terms. Instead, like their predecessors for millennia, nineteenth-century American doctors attributed disease either to "contagion" or to noncontagious factors in the victim's living conditions and environment. "Contagion" meant a specific disease-causing substance transmitted by touching a sick person. Noncontagious causes included diet, exercise, emotions, and other aspects of personal regimen.[3] They also included factors beyond the control of individuals, such as pollution of the environment by "miasma": the noxious products of decay, fermentation, human crowding, and filth.[4]

Virtually all physicians regarded "poxes," including smallpox, syphilis, and measles, as contagious. But they divided over the relative role of contagion and environment in most other illnesses. Impressive evidence and glaring discrepancies marked both viewpoints. Diseases like malaria, cholera, yellow fever, and typhoid spread from place to place just like the "contagion" of smallpox, yet direct contact with the sick was neither necessary nor sufficient to spread them from person to person. These diseases struck hardest at those who lived in poverty and filth, yet grossly unsanitary environments often existed without spawning epidemics.

Conflict over what caused disease led to divisions over how to prevent it. Contagious diseases could be warded off by quarantining travelers and the sick in isolation hospitals; diseases spawned by unhealthy living conditions required better personal hygiene and community sanitation. Each approach had complex social and ethical implications. Quarantine placed the social stigma, moral blame, and economic costs of disease on merchants, travelers, immigrants, and seamen. On the other hand, sanitation projects, such as sewers, waterworks, smoke abatement, and housing inspection, disproportionately burdened manufacturers, city landowners, and municipal taxpayers.[5]

Today, medical science regards both theories as having been half-right. Most infectious diseases require *both* a contagious microorganism and specific environmental vectors; furthermore a wide range of social conditions and personal habits may raise or lower individual resistance to the germ. But lacking this modern synthesis, physicians before the 1870s could not fully reconcile the evidence for and against the contagious origin of most diseases.

Over the century from 1770 to 1870, in America and Europe, however, most physicians came to regard contagion as less important than personal hygiene and community sanitation in explaining and preventing the great majority of serious illnesses. The political and medical problems caused by quarantines, plus scientific optimism about the controllability of natural phenomena, helped speed the decline of contagionism. Most important, the unprecedented population migrations and unplanned urbanization of nineteenth-century society provided powerful evidence of the dramatic correlation between poor health and bad living conditions. A growing public health reform movement gathered volumes of statistics implicating inadequately ventilated and overcrowded housing, nonexistent municipal sanitation, faulty diet, restrictive dress, lack of exercise, overwork, mental stress, alcohol, immorality, and poverty as likely causal factors in disease.[6]

Belief in the environmental causation of disease led reformers to demand and win creation of municipal water, sanitation, and sewage systems, and state and local boards of health. Concern over the health effects of personal habits and living conditions also deeply influenced many other nineteenth-century social movements, from temperance to poor-relief, public schooling to feminism.[7]

Nineteenth-century medical theories implicated both an individual's personal hygiene and the sanitary conditions of the community as causes of disease; however, the relative importance of each remained controversial. Thus, while most physicians agreed that filth caused illness, some stressed teaching the immigrants to wash, while others emphasized creating municipal sewage systems, sanitation departments, and housing codes. An emphasis on personal hygiene could encourage self-reliance and individualism but could also obscure those obstacles to health over which individuals have no control. Like other antebellum American reformers, the public health movement was thus torn between those who sought to alter individual behavior and those who sought to change the social structure, between those who blamed society for causing disease and those who blamed the sick.[8]

Theory and Therapy

A complex succession of schools, systems, and theories has marked the history of medical therapy, from classical Greece through much of the nineteenth century. Yet, despite these repeated changes in theory, much of the nineteenth-century *materia medica* consisted of centuries-old techniques and agents. Bloodletting; blistering the skin; drugs to induce vomiting, diarrhea, or perspiration— all were ancient remedies by the second century A.D., when Galen systematized their use for restoring a harmonious balance among the four elemental body fluids ("humors").[9] These and other time-tested remedies remained cornerstones of therapy well into the nineteenth century, long after the demise of the particular medical systems from which they had emerged. In fact, new theoretical systems of pathology often began by claiming to offer a better explanation of how old remedies worked; only rarely did a new theory introduce a totally new form of treatment.[10]

Nineteenth-century therapies did not usually employ specific drugs to cure specific diseases. The goal of these treatments was rather to produce a given effect on the body, either to directly counter an observed symptom or to offset an hypothesized disease mechanism. Thus mercury in various forms was used both to stimulate bowel movements in diseases that produced actual constipation and to purge the body of excess "bile," by inducing diarrhea and profuse salivation, in diseases where the symptoms indicated a "bilious" pathology (usually gastrointestinal and nervous disorders).[11]

Nineteenth-century physicians did have available a few

drugs that modern medicine regards as effective in specific diseases, such as chinchona bark, the source of quinine, for malaria; and foxglove, the source of digitalis, for congestive heart failure. Yet even these drugs were usually used, not as specifics for one disease, but for their supposed general effects on the body. Quinine was thus used as a stimulating "tonic" and antifever drug in all depletive fevers; foxglove was prescribed to reduce all accumulation of fluid in the tissues ("dropsy"), regardless of the specific disease.[12]

Physicians rarely prescribed numerically measured doses of drugs; a drug was administered until it "worked"—until the desired effect was produced. And in their own terms, these remedies did "work." They usually did produce the desired effect on the body— vomiting, perspiration, diarrhea, constipation, etc. Thus, they were capable of producing symptomatic relief when administered to combat specific symptoms, while their often dramatic and visible impact on the body served powerfully to reassure both doctor and patient that something was being done.[13]

Medical theory did play a key role in actual therapy, even though theories tended to change much more rapidly than practice. Between 1800 and 1830, American medicine was deeply influenced by the therapeutic system of Philadelphia's Dr. Benjamin Rush. Rush, a signer of the Declaration of Independence and a founder of America's first medical school, based his practice on two innovations: universal employment of harsh "depletive" remedies and "heroic" administration of massive doses. Most previous medical systems taught that disease could result from either an excess or a deficiency of some bodily elements; thus most doctors employed both "depletive" remedies—bloodletting, mercury, emetics—and such restorative "tonics" as chinchona, opium, and alcohol.[14] Rush held, however, that all fevers, perhaps all diseases, resulted from excess tension in the blood vessels—thus all required only "depletive" remedies.[15]

Furthermore, Rush believed that the efficacy of a remedy was proportional to its impact on the body. The more dangerous the disease, the more powerful the effect necessary to dislodge it. Rush therefore prescribed his depletive remedies until they produced "heroic" results: repeated massive bloodlettings, to or beyond a state of collapse; calomel till the gums hemorrhaged. Whereas mercury and bloodletting had been part of medicine for centuries, Rush pioneered their use as virtual panaceas, in dangerously heroic doses.[16]

Rush's system dominated American medicine only briefly and was largely discredited by the 1830s. Yet his stern legacy still influenced his successors, whether they attempted to adapt or repudiate his ideas, in much the same way that the shade of orthodox Calvinism continued to haunt nineteenth-century American theology.

Rush's system declined for many reasons. The new science of clinical statistics, developed in Paris by Pierre Louis, enabled doctors to measure the survival rates of patients with and without medical therapy. The results revealed most existing remedies as impotent at best. Louis attracted many American disciples, who spread both his quantitative techniques and his resulting therapeutic skepticism.[17]

The growing popularity of rival healing "sects"[18] also helped turn physicians away from heroic therapy. Partly in reaction to the excesses of Rush's system, many mid-nineteenth-century Americans began to patronize botanics, homeopaths, hydropaths, Eclectics, and other healers beyond the pale of "orthodox" medicine. Homeopathy, the creation of a German physician, Samuel Hahnemann, won the largest and most influential following. Hahnemann taught that a drug that produced a given symptom in a healthy person would cure a similar symptom in the sick and that the potency of a drug increased the more it was diluted.[19]

Hydropathy, another product of Germanic romanticism, banned the use of all drugs and surgery as "artificial" human meddling with nature. Hydropaths used only water, steam, and ice to assist natural healing. The key to hydropathic therapy was rigid obedience to the "natural laws of physiology": exercise, rest, temperance, and hygiene. With such "natural" living, drugs would be totally unnecessary; without it they were utterly futile.

Hydropaths demanded the sacrifice of too many of life's unhealthy pleasures to ever win the mass following attracted by homeopathy. But hydropathy deeply influenced vegetarian health reformers such as wheat-cracker pioneer Sylvester Graham and John Harvey Kellogg, the developer of flaked cereal. Its radically perfectionist call for total obedience to nature, and its promise of perfect health, also made hydropathy very influential among the most extreme immediatist advocates of other social causes, from abolition to women's rights, as well as among millennarian religious sects such as the Millerites and Adventists.[20]

While most of these medical sects rejected bleeding, purging, and heroic dosing, the botanic physicians, disciples of American folkhealer Samuel Thomson, outdid Benjamin Rush himself in the use of purges, blisters, and violent emetics. Thomson believed his system simply popularized and simplified Rush's therapies, so that they could be used without professional assistance. His therapies differed from Rush's mainly in his exclusive reliance on "natural" home-grown herbs to produce his pharmaceuticals. Likewise, the so-called Eclectics, followers of Cincinnati's Dr. Wooster Beach, often employed heroic remedies borrowed from both Rush and Thomson.[21]

From Environmental Causes to Environmental Cures

The repudiation of Rush's system did not mean that orthodox physicians suddenly abandoned bleeding and purging. These remedies had outlived millennia of systems by 1830, and no new drugs had been discovered to replace them. But gradually, through the mid-nineteenth century, most American physicians substituted for Rush's heroic doses a more conservative and cautious use of these ancient remedies. Likewise, Rush's unvarying reliance on depleting therapies gave way to a more individualized and balanced pharmacopia, including "tonics" like opium, wine, and quinine, for many patients judged to be already overly depleted by disease or by poor living conditions.[22]

Furthermore, physicians increasingly supplemented their drugs with attempts to cure disease by correcting the conditions believed to cause illness, an approach I label "environmental-moral therapy." If poor personal habits and unsanitary living conditions could produce sickness, perhaps well-ordered and hygienic surroundings could help to cure it. Thus, mid-nineteenth-century physicians began looking to living conditions, not only to explain the origins of disease and prevent its outbreak, but also to actually cure the sick. Midcentury doctors might prescribe a change in ventilation, diet, bathing, dress, exercise, habits, occupation, residence, even politics or religion, to supplement their continued reliance on drugs and surgery.[23]

For most patients, the best therapeutic environment remained the home. Frequent house calls by the doctor were not simply for the comfort and convenience of the patient; they allowed the physician to observe and modify the home environment as an integral part of therapy.[24] But environmental-moral therapy also played a major role in promoting the growth of hospital care, especially for those patients judged to be medically, economically, or morally incapable of improving their living conditions themselves.

Before the nineteenth century, the handful of English and colonial hospitals existed almost solely to provide surrogate "home care" for the homeless or enforced isolation for the dangerous. Some hospitals originated as private charities; most grew as annexes to municipal almshouses or jails. There were no known medical services that could not be provided more effectively and safely in the poorest home than in a hospital. Eighteenth-century hospitals were not simply death houses; they provided medical treatment with the hope of curing the patients. However, the hospital environment itself was hardly expected to contribute to the process of cure or the chances of recovery.[25]

With the mid-nineteenth-century rise of environmental-moral therapy, however, many physicians concluded that, for some patients, hospitalization itself could indeed be curative. By removing the sick from the conditions that caused disease, providing wholesome and hygienic influences to speed recovery, and teaching the skills and virtues necessary to avoid a relapse on release, hospitalization could be a kind of therapy. The work of Florence Nightingale in the Crimea and of the U.S. Sanitary Commission in the Civil War convinced many doctors that a well-regulated hospital environment itself could be a powerful form of medicine.[26]

Thus, while home care remained the preferred alternative, the nineteenth century witnessed a substantial increase in hospitalization. Much of this growth resulted from immigration and urbanization, forces that rapidly swelled the ranks of the homeless sick. But by midcentury, American hospitals also attracted a growing number of paying patients, individuals not poverty stricken, but whose lodgings were too small, noisy, crowded, dirty, or lonely to provide a curative milieu.[27]

Medical faith in the therapeutic powers of the environment extended beyond the hospital, to help shape many other "curative" institutions. The nineteenth-century founders of such diverse organizations as Utopian communes, insane asylums, and public schools all believed that changing a person's physical and spiritual surroundings could cure a wide variety of medical and social ills.[28]

Scientific doctrines that linked social conditions to the cause and cure of disease also led physicians to participate in such reform movements as free public education and temperance.[29] And the creation of hospitals and health boards in turn owed much to the support of social and political reformers.[30] One leading midcentury physician called medicine ''the link that unites Science and Philanthropy.''[31]

The medical profession had often played a leadership role in society before. But now, instead of basing such involvement on their social status and duties of stewardship, physicians justified their reform activities on the narrower technical grounds that social and moral conditions could prevent and cure disease.[32]

Environmental-moral therapy supplemented rather than supplanted the use of drugs and surgery. Medication remained central to most medical practice. Yet, mid-nineteenth-century physicians placed much greater emphasis on environmental-moral treatments than had practitioners before or since. In that sense, such regimens were the hallmark of midcentury medicine.

How are we today to assess the meaning and results of nineteenth-century environmental-moral therapy? No question in current medical history is as complex or controversial.

On the one hand, belief in the curative power of proper living conditions both drew upon and helped promote recognizably scientific study of real correlations between environment and health. Such therapies also provided a safe substitute for the excruciating and lethal remedies of earlier medical systems, while holding out new hope of recovery to those whose diseases had previously been seen as hopeless. And hospitals offered at least the poorest of the sick a cleaner and safer niche than they could have obtained anywhere else in nineteenth-century America.[33]

However, by making every aspect of life into a technical concern of medical science, the new therapeutics inevitably fostered invasive and paternalistic doctor-patient relations. As one French physician wrote, in 1806,

It is important for the happiness of all that man be placed under the sacred power of the physician. That he be brought up, nourished, clothed after his counsel and that the systems according to which he should be governed, educated, punished, etc., be designed by him . . . . Who is better qualified to play this role than the physician who has made a profound study of his physical and moral nature?[34]

   In addition, a physician's judgments about what constituted healthy, natural living were inevitably influenced by his personal values, cultural norms, and biases. Environmental-moral therapy thus either openly or subtly made middle-class Protestant virtue an active ingredient in medical prescriptions. The New York Hospital in 1846 combined painful active therapy with a ''moral lecture'' from the chief resident to cure a young boatman who was diagnosed as ''addicted to masturbation.'' Ethnic prejudice too could easily influence environmental therapy. Massachusetts General Hospital surgeons recorded that one Irish patient

is importunate for delicacies; declaring that he was always accustomed to them. This last is hard to believe, he being an undoubted bogtrotter.—May have as an addition to his bill of fare, a potatoe.[35]

   Nineteenth-century hospital builders and health reformers also clearly overestimated the therapeutic powers of environmental change. Good food, regular habits, and clean air did help heal the sick, but not as rapidly, as often, nor as cheaply as they had hoped. Given these very visible failures modern observers like Erving Goffman and Christopher Lasch have concluded that such failure was inevitable—that paternalism and confinement can never really cure, because the loss of autonomy is itself pathogenic.[36] Yet such an assessment may be somewhat more pessimistic than the historical data warrant. Like any other therapy, nineteenth-century institutionalization did inevitably produce damaging social and physical ''side effects.'' But showing that institutions inevitably do harm is hardly the same as proving that they never produce cures.[37]

   Environmental-moral therapy could also provide a convenient pretext for those who wanted greater professional power and those who sought to remove unwanted or threatening deviants from society. Therapeutic regimens tend to become therapeutic regimentation, especially when applied en masse. The extent to which such motives actually promoted social acceptance of environmental-moral medical theories remains bitterly controversial; a full examination would go far beyond the scope of this book.[38]

But at bottom, the current debate over environmental therapy reflects a deep-seated conflict of values, rather than simply a question of historical facts. Nineteenth-century hospitals tried to regulate and regiment every aspect of their patients' lives, based on the claim that the habits and environment they imposed were essential components of medical treatment. Even if environmental-moral medicine had delivered its promised quota of cures, historians would still disagree over whether these health benefits were *worth* the surrender of individual autonomy that institutionalization so often required. We do not yet all agree on the relative value of life and of liberty when the two seem to conflict.[39]

Art vs. Nature: In Therapy and Ethics

The shift from the heroic drugging of much early-nineteenth-century practice to a greater emphasis on environmental-moral cures by midcentury reflected the fundamental dichotomy between "Art" and "Nature."[40] Benjamin Rush had insisted that, without the intervention of medical art, most illnesses would naturally worsen, terminating in death. The advocates of environmental and regimen-based therapies, both orthodox and sectarian, appealed instead to what they termed "natural healing" as an essential accompaniment of, or even a replacement for, the physician's art.

Nineteenth-century Americans used "nature" in two different ways. "Natural" could mean the opposite of "supernatural"—those forces that man could learn to predict and control. Or "natural" could be used as the opposite of "artificial"—those forces that operated free of human interference.[41]

Nineteenth-century American "natural healing" conflated both meanings of the word. Used in the first sense, the "laws of nature" comprised scientifically predictable causal relations such as the links between bad living conditions and bad health. Used in the second sense, the "healing power of nature" *(vis medicatrix naturae)* constituted a beneficent vital force, one that promoted recovery and preserved health without any active human intervention. Boston's eminent Dr. Jacob Bigelow concluded that this natural healing force alone was sufficient to cure most common diseases; as early as 1835 he introduced the term "self-limiting" to describe such ailments.[42]

In short, "natural healing" meant avoiding the known environmental-moral causes of disease ("obeying natural law") and allowing the body to heal itself without the "artificial" interference of manmade drugs or surgery.[43] The distinction between Nature and Art thus played a central role in the conflict between heroic and environmental-moral methods of therapy.

However, the Art-Nature dichotomy went far beyond a disagreement over the best methods of treatment. Heroic and natural healing represented not simply two rival methods of cure but two competing visions of the doctor's professional role and ethical duties. For Benjamin Rush, heroic practice was as much an ethical obligation as an efficacious therapy. In Rush's estimation, the first duty of a doctor was action—"heroic" action—to fight disease. Rush regarded a physician who killed a patient through overdosing as perhaps overzealous, but one who allowed a patient to die through insufficiently vigorous therapy was both a murderer and a quack. "To permit a curable disease to terminate in death," Rush insisted, constituted a far graver professional sin than to overdose a patient with drugs.[44]

Likewise, "natural healing" constituted an ethical role model, as well as a technique of therapy. The natural healers' version of professional duty (denounced by critics as "medical nihilism") portrayed the doctor's role as simply to help the patient avoid anything that might interfere with nature's healing power. Nineteenth-century physicians traced the roots of this philosophy to the Hippocratic injunction to "do no harm," often rendering this credo, *"primum non nocere"*—*"first of all,* do no harm."[45] In addition to such classical roots, natural healing drew upon a peculiarly nineteenth-century vision of nature as beneficent. The scientific claim that nature heals shaded easily into the ethical fallacy that nature is good. Advocates of natural healing revealingly denounced unhealthy living conditions as "violations of natural law"; the more radical hydropaths excoriated poor hygiene as a "sin" against nature.[46] In this view, medical interference with nature was not simply harmful, it was immoral. Natural healing held a physician ethically responsible only for the damage done by medicine; the ravages of untreated disease were blamed on nature. In 1849, the eminent Dr. Worthington Hooker, of Connecticut, eloquently captured the change:

Heretofore the great object of the physician has been to do *positive good* to the patient—to overcome disease by a well-directed onset of *heroic* remedies—and it has been a secondary object altogether to guard against doing him harm. But medical practice is becoming reversed in this respect. It may at the present time be said of quite a large proportion of the profession, that it is the principal object of the physician to avoid doing harm to the patient . . . .[47]

The Art-Nature dichotomy thus overlapped with the ancient theological distinction between sins of "omission" and "commission." Heroic professionalism regarded inaction as morally worse than wrong action; natural healing taught that allowing evil to occur was preferable to directly causing it.[48]

"Heroic" and "nihilistic" versions of professional duty comprised the theoretical end points of a continuum; only a handful of the most doctrinaire extremists actually attempted to follow one to the complete exclusion of the other. In practice, most nineteenth-century healers, orthodox and sectarian, adopted some intermediary position, giving *primacy* to one value without negating the claims of the other. Those who regarded action as a doctor's primary obligation included most early-nineteenth-century orthodox practitioners, as well as the Thomsonians, botanics, and to a lesser degree, the Eclectics. The most antiinterventionist healers were the hydropaths, though critics charged that homeopathy's minuscule doses were equally nonactive. Yet these were differences of degree; the conflict between Art and Nature affected every medical sect. Some homeopaths practiced quite heroically; a few orthodox physicians verged on medical nihilism; even hydropathic steam baths were sometimes carried to heroic extremes by overzealous practitioners. And over the first half of the century the shift from a predominantly heroic to a less interventionist professional role cut across virtually every school of healing.[49]

Conservative Medicine: Art and Nature Reconciled

In a self-consciously moderate attempt to synthesize the competing demands of Art and Nature, many leading midcentury physicians promulgated a new vision of professional duty they labeled "conservative" medicine. Physicians like Austin Flint, Oliver Wendell Holmes, and Worthington Hooker and surgeons like Frank H. Hamilton sought an exact midpoint between extremes. In therapy they continued to employ bleeding and purging but deplored the abuses in heroic dosing. They likewise touted the body's natural recuperative powers and endorsed environmental-moral therapies, while repudiating the nihilistic demand that these be the only measures in the medical arsenal.[50]

But conservative medicine was far more than just a pragmatic mix of heroic and natural therapies. Conservative treatments derived from a new and distinctive approach to professional ethics, a new definition of a doctor's duties, not dependent on the primacy of either Art or Nature. The core of conservative ideology was the belief that neither action nor inaction was inherently preferable to the other. Neither the duty to fight disease nor the obligation to avoid doing harm held priority among the moral obligations of a physician. Rather, a conservative doctor's duty was to select whatever combination of active and passive measures was most likely to minimize the overall damage from either the treatment or the disease. The conservative synthesis of Art and Nature drew upon a variety of precedents, from the classical concept of the Golden Mean, to the highly influential late eighteenth-century British handbook of medical ethics by Thomas Percival.[51] But despite such antecedents, the mid-nineteenth-century conservative approach to professional decisionmaking represented a new approach to medical duty. Its utilitarian approach to ethics and its statistical effort to quantify a precise balance between helping and avoiding harm distinguished conservative professionalism from its predecessors. And conservative professionalism won an unprecedented degree of acceptance among both orthodox and sectarian practitioners in mid-nineteenth-century America; it thus played a key role in shaping the professional reaction to such innovations as anesthesia.[52]

Professionalism in Crisis: Ideology and Organization

Divisions over therapy and ethics paralleled the institutional disarray of the organized medical profession. Unprecedented public hostility and internal dissension made the mid-nineteenth century an age of crisis for all American professions. The roots of this upheaval extended deep into the colonial past.

American professionalism originated in the traditions and practices of seventeenth- and eighteenth-century England, though the colonial environment produced important new adaptations. The English recognized three learned professions: law, medicine, and divinity. While any occupation might be termed a "profession" these were the "liberal professions," requiring a collegiate education.

In eighteenth-century Britain, professional standing was integrally linked to status as a gentleman. Training in the classics and liberal arts provided the breadth of mind and personal character deemed essential for a gentleman. Vocational skills and techniques were not ignored, but they were considered items any liberally educated gentleman could acquire on his own, through apprenticeship or literally by practice.

A gentleman's income proved indispensable to most physicians, since poor transportation and limited demand made it difficult to subsist solely on earnings. In addition, a practitioner whose income derived from fees would never have the gentleman's leisure for the pursuit of truth. Most importantly, someone whose livelihood depended on practice would lack the independence to administer needed but unpopular therapy or advice.[53] For class-conscious Britons, gentility served to support professional authority. As a gentleman, the professional expected deference to his opinions on all aspects of community life. In turn, the physician, clergyman, and barrister incurred a professional duty to play a leadership role in society and government.

Very few people had access to the services of a professional gentleman; most ordinary citizens relied on members of other occupations or on kin for medical assistance. Other healing occupations included surgeons and apothecaries, who belonged to distinct, nonprofessional vocational groups. They did not face the need to reconcile academic and technical values, since they were not expected to have a gentleman's liberal education. Surgeons were craftsmen, apothecaries were tradesmen.[54]

A shared identity based on gentlemanly values gave the medical fraternity a high tolerance for technical disputes and personal rivalries. The liberal ethos allowed great latitude for conflict among individual practitioners without posing a serious threat to the profession's sense of corporate unity. Acrimonious personal feuds and competing schools of practice flourished, all more or less within the confines of eighteenth-century professional acceptability.[55]

The American colonies did not offer an attractive field for most professionals until well into the eighteenth century, and few came. The resulting shortage of gentleman-practitioners in the colonies broke down the English distinctions among physicians, surgeons, and druggists. And with the creation of vocationally oriented medical schools in Edinburgh, Philadelphia, and New York, colonial and provincial practice strayed even further from the basic London ideal.[56]

Whereas colonial practitioners had always deviated from the London model, the American Revolution marked a self-conscious repudiation of the institutions and ideals of professional gentility. The earliest plan to replace the gentleman-professional with a distinctly American role model was formulated by Benjamin Rush. Rush urged the adoption of national, republican professional ideals, liberated from dependence on Old World class values. In his remarkable 1789 lecture on the "Duties of a Physician," he even suggested that Americans replace the gentleman-physician with the more republican farmer-physician.[57]

Rush's professional values and his medical practice were both highly influenced by his politics. They reflected his Enlightenment faith in the simplicity and rationality of the universe and his Jeffersonian hostility toward mystery and artificial privilege. For Rush, a truly professional medical system had to be simple enough for almost anyone to comprehend and administer. Mystery and monopoly he regarded as antithetical to professionalism, because such impediments to the diffusion of medical knowledge left the people ready victims of quackery. Rush repudiated neither academic training nor professional distinctions. Rather, he felt that the way to ensure the victory of professionals over quacks was to permit everyone to learn and practice legitimate medicine. Removing artificial barriers to medical knowledge and practice would not result in simple leveling but would deepen popular appreciation of the professional elite.[58]

Rush's stand against restricting medicine to doctors reflected a division within the profession over the proper function of licensing laws. In eighteenth-century London, licensing by the Royal College of Physicians had served a dual function—primarily to distinguish professional gentlemen from other lower status healing practitioners and only secondarily to restrict the practice of healing to professionals. By the eve of the American Revolution, several large colonial cities had adopted some form of medical licensing, sometimes administered by local medical societies. But in opposition to Rush, many leading early American physicians, such as John and Samuel Bard of New York, favored using licenses to restrict the practice of healing to physicians. All but three states passed some form of medical licensing legislation by 1830, though the extent of monopolistic restriction varied widely from jurisdiction to jurisdiction. Although Rush's therapies enjoyed wide acceptance between 1810 and 1830, his radically republican version of professionalism won few medical followers.[59]

The gentleman-professional had never been more than a useful fiction in colonial America, but as an ideal type of what a doctor should be, the model had served reasonably well to define, unify, and justify the colonial profession. By the 1830s, the failure to find an acceptable American replacement for the gentleman ideal helped plunge all American professions into a crisis of self-definition. The existence of professionalism in any form came under increasingly sharp attack, from within and outside the ranks of practitioners, as part of a general hostility to all forms of distinction in a professedly egalitarian society. First raised as a partisan issue by radical free-trade Democrats, hostility to all professional distinctions soon entered the mainstream of American political rhetoric. By the 1850s, no more than three states retained any form of medical licensing legislation.[60]

The attack on medical professionalism sprang in part from the growth of the alternative healing sects. The most extreme sectarian opponents of professional distinctions were the botanical healers, disciples of folkdoctor Samuel Thomson. In both his heroic therapies and his hostility toward professional monopoly, Thomson closely followed the views of Benjamin Rush. But while Rush saw himself as creating a new republican form of professionalism, Thomson touted his self-cure system as an egalitarian assault against professionalism in any form.[61]

However most nineteenth-century medical sects were divided between lay practitioners who opposed all professional distinctions and full-time healers who sought to expand the definition of a professional to include themselves. Homeopathy in particular featured both an inexpensive mail-order self-cure kit and a network of homeopathic medical schools, professional associations, and scholarly journals. In fact, the homeopaths founded their national professional association in 1844, three years before the creation of the orthodox American Medical Association. No other medical sect shared Thomson's radical antiprofessionalism; even most botanical practitioners soon abandoned it. Yet a strong emphasis on lay self-help remained a central ingredient in the appeal of most sectarian systems.[62]

Estimates of the numerical strength of nineteenth-century medical sects are approximations at best, since little is known about the actual remedies and less about the professional values of the rank-and-file practitioners. The graduates of orthodox medical schools far outnumbered the graduates of sectarian schools throughout the century. However, many sects depended heavily on lay practitioners, and apprenticeship was still a viable alternative to medical school even for the orthodox. Furthermore, many students of orthodox schools "converted" to other sects or practiced pansectarian empirical healing after graduation. On paper, the orthodox maintained numerical superiority, but sectarian practice was clearly an important minority influence.[63]

In an attempt to reorganize and defend their beleaguered profession a small elite of leading orthodox physicians initiated a series of "medical reform conventions" in the mid 1840s. These meetings culminated in the formation of the American Medical Association (AMA) in 1847, as well as of such influential new local organizations as the New York Academy of Medicine.[64]

One major goal of these organizations was to mold institutional solidarity in the face of ideological disarray. The decline of the gentleman ideal and the increasingly competitive spirit of the national economy had completely upset the tenuous professional balance between the interests of the individual physician and the unity of the profession. In an attempt to reestablish a workable solution, these new associations on the local and national level promulgated increasingly detailed rules of etiquette, fee scales, consultation rules, and ethics codes. This impulse toward increasing formal organization was also made possible by the communications revolution. The steamboat, railroad, and telegraph made national and regional associations truly practical for the first time.[65]

As a replacement for the repudiated gentleman-professional role model, many of the founders of the AMA seized on the new definition of professional duties provided by "conservative" medicine. The conservatives' consistently middle-of-the-road synthesis provided a way of reconciling the profession's divisions over both professional duty and practical therapy. Their even-handed moderation seemed ideally well suited for rebuilding internal consensus and unity. And the "practical," calculating utilitarianism that characterized conservative medical ethics accorded harmoniously with the values of the new middle class, whose members had displaced the eighteenth-century gentleman as both the practitioners and clients of professional medicine.

While not all AMA members espoused the new conservatism in either ideology or therapy, the leading conservative spokesmen all played major roles in the new association. And the AMA's first code of ethics read like a treatise on the new conservative ideology.[66]

However, the new conservative synthesis could not reconcile all the differences dividing the midcentury profession. Medical education proved the most divisive issue for the AMA. Between 1830 and 1845, the number of orthodox medical schools in the United States had doubled. This expansion resulted both from local boosterism in growing western communities and from economic competition among physicians who found tuition fees an attractive source of income. The large number of graduates produced by these proprietary institutions competed with established practitioners for patients, while the growing competition for students among the schools forced a gradual reduction in academic requirements.[67]

A minority of AMA leaders, represented by Worthington Hooker of Yale, advocated a laissez-faire response, based on the belief that open competition among practitioners was the best way to ensure the triumph of professional medicine. He denied that professionalism required any form of legal privilege or legislative recognition. Unlike Benjamin Rush, Hooker did not go so far as to argue that the average citizen could practice good medicine, but he did believe that most people were capable of learning to choose a good doctor. Organizations like the AMA could help, Hooker declared, by providing a seal of approval by which the public could recognize a well-trained professional physician. But he regarded monopolistic licensing by the state as impractical and unnecessary. Such views within orthodox medicine probably contributed as much as sectarian opposition to the midcentury repeal of license laws.[68]

A competing vision of professional education gradually came to predominate within the AMA, under the leadership of Nathan Smith Davis. Davis advocated strict control of medical education by the medical societies, in order to raise educational requirements, cut the supply of new graduates, and reduce competition. However, the schools, dependent on student fees for faculty salaries, successfully resisted all such regulation until the present century.

Although AMA attempts to control the medical schools sprang from a clear difference of economic interest, these economic issues also subsumed an ideological conflict between apprenticeship and academic professional values. Apprenticeship to a preceptor remained the major source of practical, technical training for most nineteenth-century doctors, despite the growth of medical schools. The resulting conflict of ideals between "school" and "shop" professional cultures was not fully resolved until the twentieth century. Conservative medicine long remained torn between these two overlapping yet distinct models of medical education.[69]

Uncertainty and change in nineteenth-century concepts of professionalism also helped alter the status of women practitioners. So long as a professional physician was by definition a gentle*man*, the large number and variety of women healers could never achieve *professional* status, no matter how skillful or how successful they might be in *practice*. But with the decline in professional importance of the gentleman ideal and the replacement of "heroic" by more "natural" therapies, a surprisingly large elite of midcentury women healers first began to win recognition as *professional* physicians, despite continued male hostility.[70] Black healers also sought professional status in this period. Excluded from the AMA, they formed the National Medical Association in 1870.[71]

Specialization provided still another source of discord within conservative medicine. For the founders of the AMA, as for their liberal genteel predecessors, "specialist" remained a term largely synonymous with "quack"; it often served as a code word for the ubiquitous peddlers of phony venereal disease cures.[72] This hostility to specialization was based on technical factors, as well as on ideological preferences. With the exception of vaccination and a few other practices, midcentury medicine still depended on general systemic treatments, rather than the disease-specific therapies characteristic of modern medical specialties. Medical knowledge consisted of information about how the body as a whole reacted to drugs, diseases, and environment, not about specific organs or ailments.

However, the growth of separate hospitals to provide specialized environmental needs for the insane, the blind, the retarded, the deaf, and other classes of patients produced a form of de facto specialization in the practitioners who staffed these institutions. And unlike general medicine, surgery in the mid-nineteenth century experienced an increase in the technical complexity and specificity of its procedures, with a resulting growth in specialization, especially in gynecology and ophthalmology. Older technical specialties such as dentistry and pharmacy also found it possible to achieve a degree of professional recognition unthinkable by eighteenth-century standards. With its formation of specialty sections in 1859, the AMA legitimated the activities of physicians who had begun to develop specialized areas of interest within general practice, but the full-time practice of any one specialty still remained unacceptable.[73]

Surgery and Medicine

The relatively high level of surgical specialization reflected another important difference between nineteenth-century medicine and surgery—the surgeon's necessarily more specific and localized concept of disease. While nineteenth-century physicians favored general remedies for whole-body symptoms, operative surgery assumed that correcting local lesions in specific organs could cure specific diseases.[74]

Nineteenth-century surgery differed from medicine in other important ways as well. Surgery inevitably requires manual labor and technical proficiency. In eighteenth-century Britain, these features usually relegated surgeons to skilled craft status, separate from and subordinate to the gentleman physician. But in nineteenth-century America, the utilitarian, outcome-based ethic of conservative medicine turned these previous liabilities into virtues. By midcentury, physicians and patients alike held surgery in high regard, for its practicality, virtuosity, and its unambiguously measurable results.[75]

Surgery also appeared to be inevitably more heroic than medicine. Operative surgery seemed the epitome of heroic art, totally out of step with the midcentury medical emphasis on nature's healing powers. Surgery was a destructive, active interference with nature. Pre-anesthetic surgery was also synonymous with excruciating pain. And with antisepsis virtually unknown until the 1870s, surgery often meant infection and death as well. Because of its heroic image, hydropaths initially renounced surgery completely, while homeopaths and Eclectics believed that, in almost all cases, their therapeutic systems would eliminate the need for such unnatural mutilations.[76]

Yet despite its heroic elements, midcentury surgery shared fully in the growth of professional conservatism. In fact, Austin Flint credited surgeons like Frank Hamilton with having been the first to adopt the label "conservative." While heroic surgeons had emphasized operations to destroy or remove diseased organs, conservatives pioneered procedures to rebuild and "conserve" damaged parts of the body. Surgery to reposition and wire together shattered bones began to replace immediate amputation as the preferred treatment for compound fractures. Conservative surgeons saw themselves as combining Art and Nature, as assisting rather than eliminating natural healing. Furthermore, conservative surgeons now demanded that the risks of their procedures be weighed against the benefits before undertaking any operation.[77]

By the 1860s, American surgery had moved so far from its heroic origins that even the most ardently nihilistic sects sometimes welcomed operative surgeons to their ranks. Surgeons who joined such natural healing sects claimed that their sectarian treatments minimized the need for operations and that they provided more natural preoperative and postoperative regimens. But their operating techniques increasingly followed the methods of midcentury orthodox surgeons.[78]

Morton's demonstration of anesthesia in 1846 introduced a radically new remedy to a profession undergoing massive changes. The eighteenth-century ideal of the liberal gentleman was dead; the twentieth-century technocratic specialist was only an uneasily anticipated vision of the future. For mid-nineteenth-century Americans, the new conservative synthesis provided the best available role model of the professional physician in an age of unprecedented professional discord. These challenges to the profession, and the new conservative response, markedly influenced the medical reception of Morton's remarkable innovation.

PART TWO: Why Not Everyone? The Meaning of Selective Anesthetization

CHAPTER THREE

THE DRAWBACKS
OF ANESTHESIA

O ur twentieth-century sensibilities recoil at the thought that sane, responsible physicians could ever have opposed the use of anesthetics. Today, the concept of operating on a fully sentient patient conjures up only hellish images of concentration camp doctors. Yet in mid-nineteenth-century America, humane, conscientious, highly reputable practitioners and ordinary lay people held many misgivings about the new discovery. Neither sadists nor fools, these critics alleged a variety of rational drawbacks to the use of anesthesia.[1]

No single social or professional ideology lay behind these criticisms; they represented the full range of differing, often conflicting nineteenth-century medical, social, and moral beliefs. And allegations against anesthesia came not merely from the handful of individuals opposed to using the new drugs but also from the vast majority of practitioners, who employed anesthetics with varying degrees of misgivings.

Although we discuss alleged disadvantages here, and consider the benefits claimed for the new painkillers in chapter 4, the two sets of ideas did not come from two mutually exclusive groups of people. The debate over anesthesia was hardly a simple confrontation between distinct groups of advocates and opponents. Few people in midcentury America believed anesthesia was worthless, but even fewer believed it totally faultless. Almost every group in society found both advantages and drawbacks to the new discovery.

"A Practice Fraught With Danger"

Any previously untested innovation in medicine poses an unknown degree of potential risk to human life. Concern that the introduction of anesthesia would endanger the lives of patients led many physicians and nonphysicians alike to fear the results of its use. The *New York Journal of Medicine and the Collateral Sciences* warned of ether in 1847, "It is not safe even when administered in a skilful manner." "Serious and almost fatal consequences have followed the inhalation of it." The Philadelphia *Medical Examiner* similarly declared the use of ether to be a practice "fraught with danger." For seven years, Philadelphia's venerable Pennsylvania Hospital barred all use of anesthesia, it "being considered by the judicious surgeons of that institution as a remedy of doubtful safety."[2]

Aside from the simple fact of its newness, critics raised a variety of specific separate concerns over the safety of anesthesia. One set of fears centered on the dangerous properties of the drugs themselves. Although ether had been used without serious side effects long before 1846, both as a medicine and as an intoxicant, it had been administered only in small doses. In the quantities required to produce surgical anesthesia, however, the standard pharmacopoeias of the day declared it to be "poisonous."[3]

The first decade's reports of anesthesia's harmful effects were truly fearsome. In an 1852 series of articles in the prestigious *American Journal of the Medical Sciences*, Army surgeon John B. Porter stated flatly, "By the inhalation of ether, in the most cautious manner, in sufficient quantity to produce insensibility to pain, the blood is poisoned, the nervous influence and muscular contractility is destroyed or diminished, and the wound is put in an unfavourable state for recovery." "Anaesthetics poison the blood and depress the nervous system; and, in consequence," he concluded, "hemorrhage is

Ether → Chloroform

much more apt to occur, and union by adhesion is prevented."[4] The Committee on Surgery of the AMA listed reports of: "convulsions more or less severe and protracted, prolonged stupor, high cerebral excitement, alarming and long continued depression of the vital powers, and asphyxia. As secondary effects, bronchitis, pneumonia, and inflammation of the brain," as a result of anesthesia.[5] Other specific dangers cited in the medical literature included: dissolving the red blood cells,[6] thickening of the blood,[7] delayed healing,[8] suffocation,[9] tuberculosis,[10] abortion or poisoning of the fetus,[11] depression,[12] insanity,[13] and death.[14] "The use of ether," summarized one critic, "has caused great suffering."[15]

One of the most frightening possibilities concerned the danger that anesthesia might not "really" remove pain at all but only cause partial paralysis followed by amnesia. The real effect of anesthetics might be to create a torment worthy of Poe, in which the patient felt all the pain but was unable to scream and afterward could not consciously recall the horror. "Can it be maintained that because patients on awaking express no recollection of that suffering, there was therefore no painful impression conveyed to the sensorium?" asked British physician Robert Barnes, quoted in the *American Journal of the Medical Sciences*.[16]

The fear of anesthetic poisoning heightened following James Simpson's introduction of chloroform in 1848. Because this new anesthetic did not cause the irritation produced by ether, and because it was not flammable, its advocates claimed it to be safer than ether. But soon after its introduction, case reports of sudden death from cardiac arrest began to fill the medical and popular press. Such reports did not always increase confidence in ether; rather the growing number of "Anaesthetic Death" headlines often lent credence to the belief that both gases were highly toxic chemicals. According to John Collins Warren, "The use of Chloroform instead of the Ethers seems to have afforded more grounds of objection to etherization than existed before the introduction of the latter." Philadelphia dentist-surgeon John Foster Brewster Flagg complained, "Deaths, and less serious injuries, resulting from the use of other agents, particularly chloroform, have been freely attributed to sulphuric ether." "Chloroform was proved to possess the power to kill"; he concluded, "and ether, as a matter of course, shared largely in its disgrace."[17]

Many of these supposed dangers were disproved or minimized in the 1850s, as surgical experience with anesthesia increased. However, serious side effects continued to be reported throughout the nineteenth century. The most frequently cited dangers were: lung, heart, and nervous diseases, including insanity;[18] delayed healing and increased mortality from infection;[19] increased shock;[20] and, especially with chloroform, sudden death from syncope and cardiac arrest.[21]

Case histories reveal that patients, as well as doctors, worried about the danger. In 1869, a woman objected to being anesthetized, "fearing for her lungs." In addition to lung irritation, the most common side effects worrying patients seemed to have been vomiting and intoxication.[22]

Physicians disagreed about how anesthetics produced their harmful effects. According to one theory, anesthetics interfered with the oxygen-carrying functions of the blood and thus caused loss of consciousness, circulatory disease, shock, brain damage, and slow healing. A larger number of physicians felt that anesthetics produced their effects by directly suspending the functions of the nerves and brain.[23] Others, especially temperance advocates, regarded anesthesia as a form of intoxication.[24] Those physicians who shared a more romantic, less mechanistic philosophy believed anesthesia depressed the "vital spirit."[25] And, for such natural healing sects as the hydropaths, the fact that anesthetics were artificial chemicals was enough to explain their poisonous effects.[26]

From our modern viewpoint, some of the charges against anesthesia seem more valid than is generally realized. Chloroform does produce unpredictable, sometimes fatal disruptions of heart rhythm. Pneumonia after surgery or circulatory failure on the operating table can be caused by any prolonged anesthesia. Anesthesia-induced vomiting can cause suffocation or tear delicate tissues. Additional long-term side effects are still being investigated, including liver and brain damage and cancer.[27] Even the possibility that anesthesia might suspend motion and memory without affecting sensation finds some modern support. The introduction of curare as an "anesthetic" in the late nineteenth century created exactly this situation. Occasionally the same effects still occur with ether today. The impossibility of regulating dosage in most early techniques of anesthetization may well have made the abolition of memory, but not sensation, a real if infrequent occurrence.[28]

Since the introduction of antisepsis, physicians no longer

attribute surgical wound infections to any direct effect of anesthesia, but the indirect infection-promoting role of anesthetics in the dirty, crowded operating rooms of the mid-nineteenth century is still a subject of debate. Likewise, while anesthetics probably do not promote shock today, they do not eliminate it and under nineteenth-century conditions could well have increased it. Today, general anesthesia has come to be regarded as the most dangerous part of many operations; in 1970 it was estimated to kill about one in every 2,000 patients.[29]

But the strength and longevity of nineteenth-century fears about the safety of anesthesia cannot be explained simply by the fact that modern medicine shares some of these concerns. Nineteenth-century allegations against anesthetics also proved especially persistent because of the institutional disarray of the American medical profession. For one thing, American physicians of 1846 lacked the organizational facilities to minimize and regulate the risks involved in human medical experimentation. American medicine lagged far behind Europe in developing effective means of legitimating experimental results. The use of medical statistics was still new and controversial; in fact, the debate over anesthesia provoked some of the earliest systematic American efforts to develop statistical techniques for measuring the risks of a new drug.[30]

More important than such technical problems were the personal rivalries, regional jealousies, and sectarian divisions among American physicians, which precluded rapid general acceptance of any experimental results. There was no Royal College, no FDA, no central authority in American medicine with the power to confer legitimacy on any new drug. Army surgeon Porter explained, "Fifty or one hundred years ago, some acknowledged leader might have dictated to the whole body of the profession; but those days have fortunately gone by." "In the present age the profession acknowledges no leader,"[31] he concluded. Fledgling organizations like the AMA and the New York Academy refused to take a stand on such controversies, tabling even noncommittal resolutions concerning anesthetic safety. The AMA preferred to act only as a clearinghouse, passing along whatever experimental data were submitted to it. Likewise the New York Academy in 1847 refused even to vote on the report of its own committee to investigate anesthetic safety; members instead were instructed to consult European practice. In fact, the official medical bodies of London, Edinburgh, and Paris provided the only generally ac-

cepted authority to which the divided American profession would turn
to validate the results of experiments on such innovations as anesthetics. "The successful employment of sulphuric ether by eminent
surgeons in Europe has served to moderate the vehemence of tone
with which the early experiments with this novelty had been denounced," noted the *Boston Medical and Surgical Journal* in 1847.[32]
The only research-legitimating institutions in American medicine were
the handful of urban public hospitals, where operations were open to
spectators, records were kept, and patients were generally powerless
charity cases.[33]

In America the safety of ether thus had to be tested mostly
by individual physicians willing to introduce it uncontrolled into their
general practices.[34] Such a course involved danger not only to the patient but also to the practitioner and to the profession. And the medical profession in nineteenth-century America was particularly appre-
hensive about incurring such risks. Whereas medical experimentation
has always raised serious moral and ethical issues,[35] the nineteenth-
century experimenter faced a number of unique problems. American
public opinion was exceptionally and vociferously hostile to research
performed on living human subjects. This antipathy, very similar in
spirit to the popular revulsion against autopsies, even led to occasional mob violence against such medical experimenters as the pioneer ovariotomist Dr. Ephriam McDowell.[36] Morton himself encountered threats of physical violence when he attempted to hire
subjects for his early ether experiments.[37]

Furthermore, nineteenth-century American law offered few
safeguards to medical researchers; physicians who did prescribe new
drugs faced a real threat of prosecution.[38] The hapless Morton was
sued for "poisoning" one of his patients as a result of his early experiments with ether. The Philadelphia *Medical Examiner* warned
practitioners to consider "if fatal results should happen to one of their
patients, what would be the effect upon their conscience, their reputation and business, and how the practice would be likely to be viewed
by a Philadelphia court and jury."[39]

Experimentation was a threat not only to the individual
researcher but also to the reputation of the entire profession. In a classic
version of Alphonse and Gaston, the New York *Annalist* conceded
the value of having ether tested on the public, so long as only dentists
were implicated. An association of Boston dentists, on the other hand,

warned its members to let physicians have the dubious honor of testing the disreputable and perhaps lethal novelty.[40] Perhaps, too, some of the opposition to experimentation with anesthesia was derived from a lingering eighteenth-century association between such research and "empiricism."[41]

But, while some medical publications attacked anesthesia because it involved experimentation, professional organizations like the AMA avoided endorsing such innovations for the opposite reason—an alleged lack of empirical data. The 1848 convention of the AMA refused to either pass or defeat a resolution, "That considering the present limited amount of authenticated facts in relation to the danger or safety of anaesthetic agents in Medicine, Surgery, and Obstetrics, this Association is not now prepared to determine upon their value or the propriety of their use." Instead, they adopted a separate committee report clarifying their general approach to medical innovations.

It is rare that any signal improvements in practical medicine are introduced and established in the brief space of a year. Improvements in the treatment of individual diseases are effected only, or, for the most part, by careful and reiterated observation and experiment, and cautious and rigorous induction. The medical journals and periodical retrospects are replete with announcements of novel methods of managing various diseases. Many of these methods disclose in their narratives, evidence of their hypothetical origin; while others seem to betray a disregard of well established principles and rules of practice, and are mere crude substitutes for accredited plans of treatment.[42]

Innovation often stirred up controversy, personal rivalries, and internal disunity, luxuries the divided and beleaguered profession of 1846 could ill afford. As a result, such new professional organizations as the AMA attempted to develop standards of professional duty that gave clear priority to clinical practice over research and experimentation, to corporate unity over individual innovation. A radically new technique always poses some threat to professional unity, but physicians of the 1840s seemed less willing and less able to take such risks than they had been in the confident, free-wheeling days of Benjamin Rush.[43]

The Massachusetts General Hospital records provide an illustration of just how seriously physicians may have taken such professional suspicion of innovation. The original case reports of the first patients to be etherized carefully omitted any mention of anesthesia, the presence of Dr. Morton, the test of "Letheon," or the performance of any unusual procedure. Only later, after the innovation had gained general acceptance, were the records altered to preserve for posterity any evidence that such innovation had ever taken place.[44] Anesthesia was a possibly dangerous new procedure introduced at a time when the corporate medical profession seemed particularly cautious about sanctioning innovation.

To Suffer Is To Live: The Benefits of Pain

The hardest to comprehend and easiest to caricature of the arguments against anesthesia is the claim that pain might be necessary or even good. Such opinions usually get dismissed as stoic fatalism or as penitential masochism, when they have been noted at all.[45] Yet a surprisingly broad segment of nineteenth-century opinion throughout the Western world held some version of the belief that physical pain had important benefits and that these benefits would be lost by the use of anesthesia. Such views were not limited to any one ideology or social group, nor did they constitute a unitary or even consistent set of arguments. They sometimes drew upon religious philosophies, ranging from the most radical perfectionism to the most rigid predestinarianism; yet others depended on no particular theological presuppositions. Some critics saw pain as a just and deserved punishment of human misdeeds; others saw it not as punishment at all, but as a functional aspect of normal human physiology. Such objections to anesthesia shed light on the wide range of nineteenth-century attitudes toward pain and suffering and on the complex interrelations of medicine, theology, and philosophy in the Western world.

PAIN AS FUNCTIONAL

By far the largest number of alleged drawbacks to anesthetic painlessness dealt with the supposed biological and psychological functions of pain, apart from any explicitly stated punitive function. On this view, pain was "natural" in the sense of "normal"; not a punishment for violation of divine or natural laws, but an essential part of the process of life.

DRAWBACKS

Nineteenth-century physicians and laypeople had good reason to suspect that pain was integral to life, since the loss of sensation so often indicated conditions verging on death. The depth of insensibility achieved through anesthesia had previously been seen only in cases of coma or shock, following massive brain damage, severe poisoning, extensive blood loss, and similar portents of an impending demise.[46] "The man seeming to suffer comparatively little during the operation—a circumstance which is generally considered rather unfavorable," recorded the attending physician at the New York Hospital, describing an amputation performed in about 1830.[47] Conversely, pain was a sign of vitality, indicating a prompt recovery. "Painful . . . sensations all require sound and healthy organs," declared Felix Pascalis in 1826. "It is, therefore, our axiom, that the greater the pain, the greater must be our confidence in the power and energy of life."[48]

Because of this long-observed association between insensibility and death, some physicians came to suspect that pain was integral to life. Any technique to suspend sensibility would therefore constitute a monstrous and foolhardy suspension of life itself. For the eminent French physiologist, François Magendie, pain was so basic to living that to be anesthetized was literally to be a "corpse." For Magendie, pain was "one of the prime movers of life."[49] "It is not the particular agent, it is the condition of insensibility, however produced, that puts the patient into such peril," declared the *British Medical Journal* in 1858. A popular anesthesia textbook of 1865 quoted approvingly New York surgeon Frank H. Hamilton's observation, "The very annihilation of sensation itself impairs the health of the organs of the body."[50] "The danger lies in the anesthesia rather than in the anesthetic," agreed another New York physician in 1870. "It has been well said that anaesthesia, whatever its form, is an assault upon the vital functions."[51] As one pithy dentist summarized, "Anesthesia is death!"[52]

Pain was equated not only with life in general but with healing and recovery in particular. The word "anesthesia" itself reflects an almost automatic association between the loss of sensibility and the lack of healing power. Since ancient times, the medical term "anesthesia" has designated a potentially very serious pathological numbness in some or all parts of the body, such as might be caused by hereditary disease, nerve damage, or gangrene. Nineteenth-century physicians knew that the appearance of this type of anesthesia following a wound usually portended an injury that would heal poorly, if at all.[53]

From this observed correlation between insensibility and poor healing, it was only a short step to the assumption that insensibility *caused* poor recovery and thus that pain must play a vital role in the healing process. As one worried dentist wrote to John Collins Warren, "If freedom from pain should continue the wound would not get well." "Pain is curative," declared AMA Vice President John P. Harrison in 1849; "—the actions of life are maintained by it—were it not for the stimulation induced by pain, surgical operations would more frequently be followed by dissolution."[54] Because they believed the absence of pain indicated deficient healing power, many nineteenth-century surgeons refused to operate on patients who were in a coma or in shock until the subjects regained consciousness.[55]

According to the common vitalist explanation, pain triggered the "system" to "react," that is, to revitalize and begin recuperation, in much the same way a slap on the rump supposedly got the "system" started at birth. An alternative explanation of the mechanism by which pain aided healing was based on the medical theory that one patient could not have two diseases simultaneously. Since pain was in one sense a disease and wound sepsis was also a disease, the presence of one drove out the other. As developed by the British surgeon John Hunter, this theory of "counterirritation" meant that therapy had to be painful in order to work.[56] Benjamin Rush explained:

> All evils cured by evil. Diseases cure each other, as gout and mania, dropsy, consumption, &c. Even remedies are nothing but the means of exciting new diseases. Whipping a dog prevents the effect of Nux Vomica. . . . What would be the effect of hot iron after swallowing poison?[57]

Blistering the skin with chemical burns was a favorite technique of medical counterirritation; likewise the agony of surgery was thought essential to the proper healing of operative wounds. Several midcentury believers in this doctrine even attempted to use ether and chloroform, applied to the skin, in order to produce painful therapeutic burns.[58]

Belief in the curative power of pain was not confined to the medically orthodox but was shared by the Thomsonian and Eclectic sects as well. Eclectic obstetrician John King recommended, as a substitute for anesthesia in controlling childbed convulsions, *"basti-nadoing the soles of the feet."* "It may, at first sight, appear a rough measure, but the life of a human being is at stake."[59]

The theory that pain is therapeutic reflected overtones of older beliefs—medicine must be painful to be effective because nothing of value can be attained without suffering. Pain constitutes one of the oldest measures of value, a connection still expressed by the dual connotations of words like "labor" and "painstaking." The word "indolent" now usually means "lazy," but in medical terminology it retains its original meaning, "painless." The doctrine of counter-irritation thus built upon a pervasive cultural tradition that anything which may be obtained without suffering is worthless.[60]

Patients too, it was claimed, preferred painful remedies because they could *feel* them working. A medicine whose effects were immediately perceived inspired much more confidence than a remedy which did not produce any perceptible changes.[61] "One who really desires to be cured of a disease, prefers an active nauseous dose to a more agreeable but ineffective one," explained Frederick Adolphus Packard in 1849.[62]

Whatever mechanism they thought was involved, surgeons who viewed pain as essential to healing considered anesthetics a threat to recovery. Sir John Hall, inspector-general of hospitals and chief medical officer in the Crimea, "disparages chloroform, and lauds the lusty bawling of the wounded from the smart of the knife, as a powerful stimulant," according to a Confederate Virginia manual of military surgery. "Some of the older surgeons characterize the cries of the patient as music to the ear, and speak of it as an advantage to be courted, and not to be suppressed," the same handbook continued. A student at the University of Pennsylvania College of Medicine quoted another British authority for the view that "pain during surgical operations, is, in the majority of cases, . . . desirable; and, its prevention is for the most part, hazardous to the patient." The *New York Journal of Medicine* declared pain "an *essential* attendant on surgical operations" and "the natural incentive to reparative action." The author concluded that anesthesia could seriously retard or completely prevent proper healing by removing the pain essential to recovery.[63]

Just as some surgeons concluded pain to be essential in

the healing process, some obstetricians determined pain to be necessary in the process of giving birth. The association between the physical process of labor and the perceptual experience of suffering was so ingrained that the same word, "pains," was used for both the actual muscular contractions and their accompanying sensations.[64] Not surprisingly, a few doctors concluded that both types of pains were equally necessary for delivery. "Pain—the psychical perception of pain—has its use. The abolition of pain has its danger," according to an article on obstetrics by Robert Barnes reprinted from the *Lancet* in the *American Journal of the Medical Sciences*.[65]

According to Barnes' theory, the sensation of pain was caused by the pressure of the baby in the birth canal. This pain sensation in turn triggered the contractions. Thus, without the feeling of pain, there could be no contractions, and therefore normal delivery would be retarded. At the same time, obstetrical pain supposedly might also act as a safety valve—if the contractions became too forceful, the woman would scream, allowing air to escape, thus "reduc[ing] the pressure" and averting lacerations. "Pain," Samuel Gregory of Boston quoted the *Edinburgh Medical Journal*, "is the mother's safety, its absence her destruction."[66]

In addition to physiological processes such as wound healing and birth contractions, pain allegedly played a vital role in emotional health, especially in the formation of appropriate sexual characteristics. For men, pain was necessary to the development of healthy masculine endurance. The most extreme advocates of this viewpoint, military surgeons, tended to lump painless surgery in the same category with the work of Dorothea Dix, Florence Nightingale, and Clara Barton, as products of misguided effeminate sentimentalism. Grizzled veteran medical officers on both sides of the Atlantic, men like Dr. Hall and Dr. Porter, scoffed at surgical anesthesia as a "mistaken philanthropy."[67] A deep-rooted hostility toward "enthusiasm," "zeal," reformers, sentimentalism, and philanthropy pervaded their arguments. The military traditionally argued that philanthropic attempts to relieve suffering would only deprive the troops of a vital opportunity to become inured to the pains of battle and would thus actually worsen their suffering by causing the men to think about their miseries.[68] Such opinions were not limited entirely to bullet-biting combat physicians. Perhaps the most extreme example was Benjamin Hill, a surgeon of the Eclectic sect. Hill encouraged his patients to submit to cauterization of cancers without anesthetics, in favor of the "moral medication" provided by pain:

I have not unfrequently had patients, after submitting, perhaps for an hour, to this "burning alive," without flinching or groaning, open their mouths for the first time, after I had got through, to express their fears that the operation had not been carried far enough, because they had felt it so much less than I had given them reason to expect. I have told them beforehand that, unless they had fortitude enough to bear to have their arm chopped off, inch by inch, on a block, or to hold it out like the Roman youth of old, while it burnt off on the altar, they need not expect to have their cancer cured—that its moral "final cause" was to develop such heroism in them![69]

Even confirmed sentimentalists like Samuel Gregory, the patriarch of the Boston Female Medical College, scorned surgical anesthesia, scoffing that "this suffocating one's self to avoid a trifling pain is no mark of prudence or courage."[70]

If pain could anneal manly hardness, it could also refine womanly tenderness. The close and complex connection between pain and love was a preoccupation of midcentury sentimentalists. Suffering was "interesting"—a wonderful word meaning "capable of inspiring sublime emotions." Physician-poet Josiah Gilbert Holland wrote,

> Hearts, like apples, are hard and sour,
> Till crushed by Pain's resistless power.

As formulated by Emerson, the doctrine of "compensation" seemed to guarantee that all bodily pains carried with them their own spiritual rewards. Thus, Dr. Augustus K. Gardner, a prominent New York gynecologist, rhapsodized about the sufferings of his women patients, "I feel that these compensations are not limited to the mere physical strengthening of other . . . facilities; . . . this baptism of pain and privation has regenerated the individual's whole nature . . . by the chastening made but a little lower than the angels."[71]

In particular many nineteenth-century obstetricians suspected that the pain of delivery was essential to promote normal and healthy maternal emotions. "The very suffering which a woman undergoes in labor is one of the strongest elements in the love she bears for her offspring," explained one such critic.[72] In the effusive words of Dr. Edward R. Mordecai, a young Southern medical student at the University of Pennsylvania,

[T]he associations connected with the pangs of parturition may play an important part in framing the indissoluble link which binds a parent to its offspring; in rearing the foundation upon which rests no inconsiderable share of the social happiness of this world. From such a source springs, no doubt in part, that exhultation with which a mother beholds for the "first time her new-born babe," that soul-stirring sympathy which weeps with it in sorrow, which smiles with it in prosperity; that unremitted affection which follows it from the cradle to the grave.[73]

In the mouth of young Dr. Mordecai, such sentiments seem patronizing, but some Victorian feminists used the same argument to prove that the pain of childbirth made women morally superior to men.[74]

Some of the physicians who believed pain to be an integral part of life did not attempt to spell out the precise vital functions that suffering might serve. After cataloging all the detailed physical and spiritual mechanisms by which bodily torment benefited the sufferer, there remained a strong residual feeling that pain was something more elemental—something simply inherent in the essential nature of human flesh. To lose the ability to feel pain was to become less than human, to be literally a vegetable or a brute.[75]

Whereas most physiological explanations of the value of pain depended on no particular theological assumptions, Philadelphia obstetrician Dr. Charles D. Meigs in 1856 cautioned against both surgical and obstetric anesthesia by noting the morally "doubtful nature of any process that the physicians set up to contravene the operations of those natural and physiological forces that the Divinity has ordained us to enjoy or to suffer."[76] Unlike the perfectionist belief that God created nature so that only those who violated natural laws would suffer, Meigs' Divinity created suffering itself as a natural law.

Although such criticism of anesthesia was grounded for the most part in careful and intelligent argumentation, it would be wrong to overlook the influence of superstition, fear of change, and an uneasy feeling that what had always been was always meant to be. The belief that it was "natural" to feel pain when cut with a scalpel paralleled the belief that obstetric pain was "natural"—both drew upon the ethical fallacy that everything "natural" was both good and necessary. "The pain attendant upon human parturition is a physiological one, and is probably imposed upon this particular function for a specific object, the nature of which may to us be yet unknown," explained Dr. Edward H. Horner, a University of Pennsylvania medical student.[77] In one international example of the romantic era's penchant for the naturalistic fallacy, Samuel Gregory quoted a German report to the Royal Scientific Association, on obstetric etherization: "These pains are natural phenomena . . . and are therefore endured without detriment." The British obstetrician Francis Ramsbotham summed up that argument as well as anyone by declaring that women should be "contented to have children as it would seem, Nature intended they should."[78]

Belief in a physiological function for surgical or obstetric pain is an empirically testable hypothesis, one that we might assume would have been disproved by the rapidly accumulated evidence of successful anesthetic procedures. Yet the same institutional problems that impeded the precise assessment of anesthesia's side effects kept alive well into the 1880s the debate over the physical functions of pain.[79] The spiritual and psychological functions of pain are even harder to test. Belief in these emotional benefits of suffering has remained strong to the present day, especially in regard to childbirth.[80]

PAIN AS PUNISHMENT

While some saw pain as biologically and emotionally functional, other critics of anesthesia portrayed physical suffering as punishment; in their view anesthesia constituted an attempt to circumvent the chastisements inflicted by some Higher Power. Today, such opinions are usually dismissed as the product of fundamentalist objections to the use of anesthesia in childbirth.[81] Yet in actuality these attacks were leveled against dental and surgical anesthetics too and came from a diverse assortment of theological and scientific viewpoints. Many nineteenth-century Americans agreed that pain was a just and beneficial discipline, but they disagreed over every detail of which pains were punishment, who or what was being punished, and by Whom.

Nineteenth-century Americans generally distinguished between physical pains whose immediate cause was a visible human agent, such as the agonies of dental or surgical operations, and those pains whose cause did not visibly involve human infliction, such as the throes of childbirth and disease. Both were seen as deserved punishments, but the arguments are best considered separately. Since birth and disease pains did not seem to depend directly on human infliction, they were easy candidates for attribution to the judgment of some higher purpose. But who was punishing whom for what? Was the infliction divine or natural? Did the guilt lie with the particular individual afflicted, the sufferer's entire community, the individual's immediate ancestors, or humanity's original ancestors? On these questions there was sharp debate.

The most familiar such argument pictured the pangs of childbirth as God's judgment on womankind for tempting Adam's Fall.[82] Biblical literalism underlay a number of attacks on obstetric anesthesia throughout the nineteenth century, everywhere in the Western world. "I consider that *mothers* would consult their own happiness, to say nothing of health, by fulfilling the edict of bringing forth children 'in sorrow,' " warned a New York dentist in 1848. An American summary of a leading British textbook cited "the morality of pain" as one reason for the "impropriety of etherization" in childbirth. Biblical literalism in fact underlay many of the supposedly naturalistic functional explanations of birth pain. Thus the English obstetrician Ramsbotham believed labor pains to be functional but blamed this state of affairs on "an ordinance of the Deity" as punishment for the Fall.[83]

But biblical literalists had no monopoly on the claim that obstetric anesthesia was an attempt to escape from a deserved punishment. Rather, it was the advocates of "natural healing," especially those inclined toward a perfectionist theology, such as hydropaths and vegetarians, who most loudly proclaimed that the pains of labor (and disease) were righteous chastisements. In this view, Nature, not God, was wielding the lash; and individual sins against natural law, not a universally shared original sin, was the provocation. Hydropath Dr. T. L. Nichols, for example scorned the literalist dogma that God intended for womankind to suffer, declaring it "an insult to Providence." "This world is the work of infinite power and benevolence,"[84] he continued. Perfect freedom from pain was both possible and intended for us in this world. "In a state of health no natural process is painful." "There is no more certain fact in physiology, than that the nerves of organic life, in a healthy condition, are not susceptible of pain,"[85] he concluded.

But if God is both benevolent and omnipotent, where do

pain and disease come from?[86] Pain for Nichols was unnatural, abnormal, pathological—the result of human free will contending against the beneficent laws of nature. Pains, declared the *Water Cure Journal*, "follow the sinner legitimately and unavoidably, the sure sumpenalty of violated laws, as universal in their application and precise in their reference as any laws of nature." Physical suffering existed only because sinful humanity used its free will to violate natural law, but pain could be totally eradicated simply by following these laws—by adopting a pattern of life based on exercise, fresh air, cleanliness, virtue, and temperance.[87] Childbirth was painful only to the precise extent that women lived unnatural lives.

Hydropaths therefore denounced obstetric anesthesia as an attempt to suspend the wise judgments of nature. For them, anesthesia was both an immoral escape from the retributive side of nature's punishment and also an unhealthy suspension of the deterrent and reformatory aspects of such penalties. Pain was nature's warning to change one's ways. If mothers used anesthesia to remove the pangs of childbirth without making fundamental changes in the unnatural habits that caused the pain, the result would be more serious pain and injury later on.[88]

Hydropaths believed that human pain could be totally vanquished but only through adopting a way of life rigidly governed by the dictates of natural law. Their goal was not simply to eradicate pain but to revolutionize society according to nature's blueprint. Anesthesia threatened to subvert this revolution by deluding people into trying to eliminate pain without making any fundamental changes in their underlying unnatural behavior; it was a new opiate for the masses. Dr. Ellen Snow advised students at the New York Hydropathic Physiological School not to let the discovery of artificial painkillers divert them from their larger purpose. "By teaching mankind how to live, we can be far more serviceable to the world than we can by bending all our energies to invent some mode of subverting nature's laws, so as to relieve ourselves from suffering the penalty attached thereto." Orthodox medicine had discovered a way to make burning yourself painless, she told her audience; hydropathy taught you not to put your hand in the fire.[89]

Compared to the biblical view that pain was an inescapable curse, the perfectionism of hydropathy offered unbounded hope. Contrary to strict Reformed theology, hydropaths taught that total freedom from pain was both moral and achievable. Pain could and should be eradicated—by the eradication of wrongdoing. But despite their differences, both perfectionists and predestinarians taught that pain was a righteous and deserved punishment for the existence of evil and therefore should not be anesthetized away.

Biblical literalism at least had offered the victim the solace of resignation and companionship—all were sinners, all would suffer. Strict Calvinists did not tantalize themselves with hopes of escape this side of heaven, nor did they impute particular individual guilt to the sufferer. Most early Reformed churches in colonial America, from Congregationalists to Quakers, viewed God's punishments as falling upon entire communities rather than simply upon the guilty individuals. Such theology accorded well with actual social conditions in pioneer New England and Pennsylvania. Accidents, diseases, famines, and disasters clearly did punish everyone, not merely those directly stricken. In small, isolated, highly interdependent communal societies, the incapacitation of a few individuals could easily threaten the well-being of all. Thus, breaking a leg or catching the ague did not necessarily imply that the victim was any more guilty or sinful than his or her neighbors. A member of the community of saints did not ask for whom the bell tolled.[90]

But in the Erewhonian utopia of the hydropaths, where freedom from suffering was freely available to everyone, simply being in pain constituted *prima facie* evidence of individual moral guilt. "Sin, or violation of physical law, is the cause; and pain, sickness, and death in their largest signification, are its effects. To be sick, then, is sinful," proclaimed the *Water-Cure Journal*.[91] Dr. Samuel Gridley Howe explained that mental retardation "*must* be the consequence of some violation of the *natural laws*,—that where there was so much suffering, there must have been sin."[92] The victim was always to blame. If a mother suffered in labor, it proved her to be a moral and physiological failure.

Furthermore, these natural healers defined "natural" according to their own preferences. Those perverse, depraved beings who obstinately clung to different tastes in food, sex, clothing, religion, ethnic traditions, or politics would be stricken, and it served them right.[93]

The major point of difference between biblical literalists

like Ramsbotham or Charles Meigs and perfectionists like the hydro-paths concerned whether birth pain was a universal or an individual punishment. For the literalists, birth pain was a universal law, built by God into the natural structure of female physiology, to punish all women. Hydropaths and other cosmic optimists rejected obstetric anesthesia on opposite grounds, that birth pain was an individual pun-ishment, totally unnatural, nonnormal, hence pathological. Birth pain should be eliminated, but the only way to do it was through moral hygiene, not through drugs. Thus, although they were at opposite poles of nineteenth-century theology, both radical perfectionists and bibli-cal literalists rejected obstetric anesthesia as an evil interference with a righteous punishment.

Although hydropathy claimed only a tiny handful of doc-trinaire believers, many of its basic ideas were simply radical exten-sions of very widely held concepts. Their extreme perfectionism and individualism, their belief that every individual was independently capable of *total* obedience to natural law, won few adherents. But the concept that at least some pains were nature's punishment for poor hygiene and intemperate habits enjoyed the support of physicians, health reformers, educators, and other advocates of "natural healing," rep-resenting a broad segment of both sectarian and orthodox medical opinion. And their judgment that what is "natural" is "right" was shared by nineteenth-century romantics of all varieties.[94]

Homeopaths declared, "Pain is the penalty we suffer for violating a physical law," according to an 1883 student at Hahne-mann Medical College.[95] "If you suffer," the homeopathically in-clined Elizabeth Cady Stanton told mothers, "it is not because you are cursed of God, but because you violate his laws."[96] Like the hy-dropaths too, homeopaths attacked all chemical pain relievers as ar-tificial interference with nature's beneficial punishments. Long before anesthesia, Hahnemann himself had denounced opium and morphine. His views remained dogma to pure homeopaths through the end of the century.

Pain is the . . . true physician's best guide to the seat and character of the cause of the pain. Deadening the nervous system by Morphine or any of its equivalents is virtually choking off Nature's voice . . . , thus leaving us to work in the dark.

Better let the patient suffer a while than complicate the troubles and retard the final recovery, or risk the patient's life by paralyzing the . . . nervous system with Morphia.[97]

Many homeopaths applied the same logic against anesthetics, when they were used for such "natural" pains as childbirth or disease. An 1868 student at Hahnemann declared obstetric etherization to be "one use of Anaesthetics by the Allopathic School, which we as Homoeopaths, most certainly should condemn."

We as students of Hahnemann, have been taught that all natural diseases (if I may call them such) can be so treated by the means of [homeopathic] remedies, properly given . . . . When therefore we are called upon to attend a case of labor, we do not expect to carry with us a bottle of Ether to make the patient insensible.[98]

Both sects shared a commitment to natural healing; both held a deep suspicion that obstetric anesthesia constituted an immoral escape from nature's wise correction.

However, there were important differences between the two sects. Few homeopaths endorsed the hydropathic claim that perfect painlessness came exclusively through natural living. They regarded (homeopathic) drugs as invaluable aids to nature in eliminating pain. And most homeopaths doubted that a perfectly painless life was either possible or desirable.[99]

To the extent that they shared a belief in natural healing, orthodox practitioners, as well as sectarians, criticized anesthesia as an immoral or unwise interference with nature's punishments. One young University of Michigan medical student unequivocally endorsed the most radical perfectionist position. "By leading a life in strict conformity with the requirements of physical laws man will live a life of absolute immunity from pain or suffering of any kind whatsoever."[100]

Other advocates of natural healing rejected such perfectionism, regarding some pains as naturally avoidable and others as naturally necessary and beneficial. Samuel Gregory of Boston's Female Medical College reasoned that, if some birth pain was normal and some not, then those pains that were pathological should be prevented through hygiene and those pains that were natural should be endured as nature intended. "If women would, by activity and a proper course of life, preserve their health and vigor, and follow the dictates of reason in conception, pregnancy, and parturition, ether would be unnecessary, for they would experience no more pain than is actually favorable . . . no more suffering than is salutory."[101]

Conservative physicians carefully balanced their commitments to Art and to Nature, avoiding an exclusive reliance on either. But to the extent they endorsed the basic concept of natural healing, they shared its critique of anesthesia. Influential conservatives such as New York surgeon Frank H. Hamilton portrayed pain as the proper penalty for defiance of nature and regarded obstetric anesthesia as an unnatural form of interference.[102] An anonymous newspaper clipping included in Dr. Hamilton's lecture notes (apparently by Hamilton himself) illustrates the influence of natural healing on the medical conservatives' view of pain.

THE USE OF PAIN—The power which rules the universe, this great tender power, uses pain as a signal of danger. Just, generous, beautiful Nature never strikes a foul blow; . . . Patiently she teaches us her laws, plainly she writes her warnings, tenderly she graduates their force. . . .

And what do we do for ourselves? We ply whip and spur on the jaded brain as though it were a jibing horse. . . . We drug the rebellious body with stimulants, we hide the signal and think we have escaped the danger . . . .

At last, having broken Nature's laws, and disregarded her warnings, forth she comes . . . to punish us. Then we go down on our knees and whimper about it having pleased God Almighty to send this affliction upon us, and we pray him to work a miracle in order to reverse the natural consequences of our disobedience, or save us from the trouble of doing our duty. In other words, we put our finger in the fire and beg that it may not be hurt.[103]

In summary, a wide variety of nineteenth-century healers concluded that the pains of childbirth and disease were deserved punishments, chastisements that it might be immoral and unhealthy to anesthetize away. A literal reading of the Bible did play a role in such opinion. However such arguments were derived more from the doctrines of natural healing than from the book of Genesis. And the most extreme exponents of such views were not strict predestinarians but such radical perfectionists as the hydropaths and Grahamites.

That the pains inflicted by surgery, dentistry, and similar professional ministrations might also be viewed as righteous chastisements seems hard to believe; yet a few nineteenth-century Americans apparently considered the *doctor* as much a part of their punishments as the *disease*. For a handful of the most rigid predestinarians, all the miseries of this life, including those medically inflicted, were punishments from God and could be taken away only by God. Infinitely depraved mankind deserved all the pain and more. As reported by *Harper's Magazine,* the city of Zurich (a wellspring of Reformed theology) banned *all* use of anesthetics, on the grounds that "pain was the natural and intended curse of the primal sin; therefore any attempt to do away with it must be wrong." In America, too, these extreme doctrines of predestination and human depravity may occasionally have lurked behind opposition to all forms of anesthesia, at least according to pro-anesthetic observers. Several Philadelphia surgeons reportedly called the use of ether "damnable." [104]

Dr. William Henry Atkinson, an M.D. and first president of the American Dental Association, reportedly declared,

> I think anesthesia is of the devil, and I cannot give my sanction to any Satanic influence which deprives a man of the capacity to recognize the law! I wish there were no such thing as anesthesia! I do not think men should be prevented from passing through what God intended them to endure.

Occasionally, physicians recorded cases in which patients refused surgical or dental anesthesia for reasons of religious belief. [105]

Predestinarian denominations like the Hard Shell Baptists and Old School Presbyterians believed pain to be God's punishment of human depravity. Fallen mankind could not be saved without God's discipline; thus pain was a manifestation of God's love, evidence of His paternal concern for the proper upbringing of His children. "He who spares the rod hates his son" applied to the Heavenly Father, as well as to His earthly counterparts. [106] However, even with proper punishments, true repentance was impossible without the aid of grace, a divine gift that most Reformed churches believed was sparingly bestowed. Thus, some portion of humanity would be subjected to God's chastisements, even though God had withheld from them the means of benefiting from their punishment. These miserable creatures existed for a higher purpose than simply to suffer. Their pains provided the fortunate with an opportunity to exercise benevolence. If the Lord caused some to suffer less than others, He expected the recipients of His favor to act as benevolent stewards on behalf of those less fortunate. Charity was a duty. However, there was no expectation that this benevolence could or should *cure* the pains of the afflicted. Despite all human efforts, the tormented, like the poor, would always be among us.[107]

But in surgery, as in obstetrics, more opposition to anesthesia came from natural healers than from predestinarians.[108] Many hydropaths and homeopaths denounced surgical anesthesia because they rejected surgery itself as an attempt to shortcut nature's punishments through human art. Surgery offered the illusion of cure without the necessary hygienic reforms; anesthesia only made the illusion more seductive.[109] Even medically orthodox physicians and surgeons agreed that, by making cure seemingly painless, surgical anesthetics might tempt people to stray from the straight and narrow road of natural law.

Another common punitive justification of surgical pain derived from the medical theory of "counterirritation." Although overtly a purely scientific explanation of the natural function of pain, the doctrine that medicine must be painful to work was often expounded in frankly punitive metaphors. Such rhetoric reveals the extent to which many nineteenth-century Americans still saw the surgeon as God's enforcer, and regarded the doctor as part of their deserved punishment for sin.[110] In this view, medical therapy was part of the retribution for getting sick, just as sickness itself was a punishment. Painful medical treatment was simply substituting a controlled form of chastisement for a less controlled one. By punishing one's self with medicine, the necessity for punishment by disease might be eliminated. Only by doing medical penance could one expunge the sin that caused the illness. The same train of thought that led Rush to theorize that whipping might cure poisoning, led him to declare, "Punishment, therefore, of all kinds [is] benevolent."[111] The physician to the Massachusetts State Prison in 1827 saw his job as the administration of "the severe, but needful physic, for the body and the soul." Such punishment could also be deterrent as well as retributive. By making the cure dreadful enough, maybe people would be discouraged from the sins that caused the disease. The Massachusetts prison physician used the specific example of venereal disease, which he claimed afflicted more than one-fifth of all his patients, to illustrate the utility of painful therapy as a deterrent.[112] Thus, while only a minority of nineteenth-century Americans overtly criticized surgical anesthesia as sacrilegious, a wide variety of religious and medical viewpoints each led to the conclusion that surgical pains could have positive punitive value.

The Control of Anesthesia: Power and Its Abuse

Knowledge is power, noted Horace Mann, but power can be a force for evil as well as for good. Without the self-control and internalized discipline of a moral education, Mann warned, nineteenth-century scientific advances would produce only stronger and more ingenious knaves. In his summary report as superintendent of the common schools of Massachusetts, Mann repeatedly declared the need to keep technological prowess under moral restraint. He illustrated his point with the example of anesthesia. ''A benefactor of the race discovers an agent which has the marvelous power to suspend consciousness, and take away the susceptibility of pain; a villain uses it to rob men or pollute women.''[113] Anesthetics conferred vast new power over pleasure and pain, and thus over rewards and punishments, even over consciousness itself. How and by whom would such awesome capabilities be controlled? While Mann believed moral self-discipline could prevent abuse, others feared the temptations might be too great.

THE MISUSE OF MEDICAL POWER

One fundamental anxiety of critics was that anesthetics gave physicians too much power over their patients. The new discovery threatened to overturn the vital checks and balances governing professional authority—restraints that had been built into the doctor-patient relationship since antiquity. One possible evil was the loss of the patient's supervisory power over the operation. The ability of the unanesthetized patient to observe the proceedings had a number of advantages. In many common operations, such as those for scrotal tumors, cataract, crossed-eyes, and bladder stones, doctors had come to depend on help from the subject to oversee the progress of the procedure and to prevent the operator from cutting too much. As late as 1862, it was not uncommon to find surgeons who "expected the patient to assist in small operations," such as probing wounds and removing bone fragments.[114] But with an insensible client, complained A. C. Castle, a New York dentist, "the operator obtains no assistance whatever from the patient."[115] In childbirth, too, a conscious patient could both assist the obstetrician and minimize medical mistakes.[116]

Unanesthetized patients had the power to protect themselves against all sorts of medical carelessness, including the ability to make sure the right tooth, growth, or limb was being removed. "By rendering the patient insensible to pain, it [anesthesia] may throw the practitioner off his guard, and prevent that thorough examination . . . that would otherwise be made," a correspondent warned the AMA Committee on Obstetrics.[117] Ether "presents an excellent cover for bungling mutilations in dentistical operations," declared Dr. Castle.[118] A French cartoonist in 1847 gave voice to popular anxiety on this score in a drawing that depicted a patient awakening to find all his teeth had been pulled by mistake.[119]

Even when there was little likelihood of medical error a few patients found satisfaction in knowing they had the authority to participate in what was being done to their bodies, especially (though not exclusively) in obstetrics. Until quite recently in Western history, many people seemingly preferred to be conscious when facing death, in order to prepare their temporal and spiritual affairs.[120] The French physiologist Magendie thought it brutally dehumanizing to deprive someone of consciousness at such a critical hour; to carve a human being like so much meat. "I do not use any anesthetic of any kind," an Iowa physician declared bluntly, as late as 1887. "I want the patient to know what is going on."[121]

The powerlessness of the anesthetized subject would lead not merely to carelessness and disrespect but also to involuntary surgery and to unnecessary and experimental operations, according to advocates of the cautious conservative approach to surgery, including even such anesthesia pioneers as Henry J. Bigelow. Bigelow worried that the availability of ether might provide an irresistible temptation for hack surgeons to perform unnecessary operations.[122] The artist who portrayed "Furor Operativus" had no doubt that anesthesia left patients the helpless victims of knife-happy butchers (plate 1).[123]

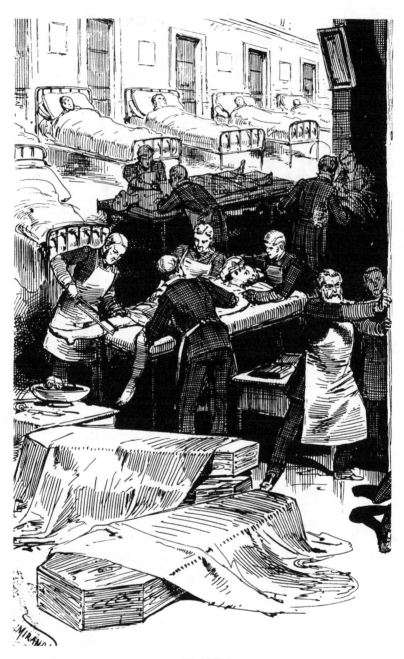

PLATE I

"Furor Operativus"
Bettmann Archive

Anesthesia eliminated the ability of patients to refuse unwanted medical procedures. It also sometimes made rational patient consent impossible to obtain, by producing not unconsciousness but intoxication and even violent drunken behavior. The *American Journal of the Medical Sciences* felt it necessary to warn doctors against physically forcing troublesome patients to be anesthetized and to "deprecate violence of any kind."[124]

Concern that anesthesia would stimulate unnecessary and unwanted operations was especially strong in regard to childbirth. There were a variety of reasons for such objections, based on differing medical, political, and moral viewpoints. Advocates of natural healing saw obstetrics as the prime example of excessive medical meddling with nature. They denounced anesthesia for encouraging "ignorant unnecessary manipulations in parturition." In addition to sharing such naturalistic views, radical feminists like Elizabeth Cady Stanton added a political concern. Stanton objected to surrendering her consciousness and body to a male doctor, particularly during the uniquely feminine experience of birth. "Dear me, how much cruel bondage of mind and suffering of body poor woman will escape when she takes the liberty of being her own physician . . . !" she exulted on refusing anesthesia and delivering her own infant.[125]

Less radical feminists feared the moral rather than the political dangers anesthesia posed for parturient patients. Samuel Gregory, who founded the Boston Female Medical College largely to preserve the virtue of women patients from the effects of exposure to male obstetricians declared,

> On a careful and candid perusal of these reports of cases of inhalation of ether in labor, its greatest benefit would seem to be that it puts women's modest sensibilities asleep, so that Nature . . . can perform her office in the presence and under the diligent attentions of gentlemen.[126]

The anesthetization of women patients by male doctors posed a moral threat that went beyond mere obstetric voyeurism, however. As Horace Mann frankly warned, anesthesia could be used to "pollute women." Fears that ether would enable doctors to rape their female patients began to be expressed almost immediately after the announcement of the discovery itself. Within a year the Philadelphia *Medical Examiner* was able to gloat, "That which had been suspected as a probable result of the introduction of a new narcotizing agent, has . . . occurred,'' an ''Alleged rape, perpetrated on a Female while under the influence of Ether.''[127] Similar cases multiplied rapidly. Following one well-publicized incident in 1854, Dr. Edward Hartshorne of Philadelphia reported that large numbers of women patients now refused to undergo anesthesia. Throughout the century, textbooks of surgery and anesthesia devoted considerable space to the problem of rape. Many feared that the extreme vulnerability of the anesthetized patient created an inherently explosive situation.[128]

Rape was only the most extreme example of the crimes into which practitioners might be led by the excessive power of anesthesia, according to critics. ''Should itinerant tooth-drawers take to ether, and the public foolishly take to them, we advise the unhappy victims to look to their pockets, and leave all their personal movables, of any value, at home,'' warned Littell's Living Age.[129]

Perhaps, too, there was a deeper link between the belief that anesthesia was an excessive surrender of the patient's autonomy and a belief in the value of suffering. Freedom from pain can conflict with other freedoms. As we have seen, hydropaths and other natural healers regarded suffering as the direct consequence of human free will. Conversely, the influential eighteenth-century Scottish Common Sense philosophers regarded the ability to suffer as a necessary condition for individual freedom. In this view, the freedom to choose implies the freedom to choose wrongly and the freedom to bear the natural consequences of these errors. Thus, one can only purchase exemption from suffering by surrendering one's freedom. To eliminate human pain inevitably diminishes human autonomy by robbing people's choices of meaning, of consequences. Such doctrines were common explanations of theodicy in nineteenth-century America. ''Power is only Pain—,'' wrote Emily Dickinson in 1861. ''Give Balm—to Giants/—And they'll wilt, like Men—.'' The Philadelphia Presbyterian warned, ''Let every one who values free agency beware of the slavery of etherization.''[130]

PUBLIC ABUSES AND PROFESSIONAL WEAKNESS

While some Americans feared that anesthesia enhanced professional power, others worried for exactly the opposite reason. Some physicians denounced anesthetics for undermining professional authority and opening opportunities for abuse by the public. One problem with ether and chloroform was that they were readily available and could be administered by anyone without having to rely on a doctor.

Every montebank, who digs out a corn, and dignifies himself with the title of chiropodist; every itinerating dentist, who gouges out a tooth or fills a cavity with amalgam; or anything that can creep, or crawl or sneak into any of the unguarded sanctuaries of medicine, can arm himself with an inhaling apparatus, and a bottle of an anesthetic material, with which he expects to prey on the public,

according to a special committee of the American Society of Dental Surgeons in 1848.[131] The availability of anesthesia weakened professional authority because patients were in effect able to prescribe for themselves. A New York dentist whose professional advice ran counter to his clients' incessant demand for painkillers complained, ''My patients hear my advice, thank me for my frankness, and go elsewhere and *have it applied*.'' This general availability of anesthetics weakened the authority of all practitioners, but because their profession was more open and competitive than surgery, dentists found their power particularly threatened.[132] The difficulty in maintaining professional control over the use of anesthesia was compounded by advertising and newspaper reports. The press both excited public demand and encouraged assertion of the public's right to judge medical issues for itself.[133]

The accessibility of anesthetics meant that the public shared with the profession many of the same opportunities to pervert the power of the new painkillers for immoral or criminal purposes. Concern over criminal abuse of anesthetics by nonphysicians dealt mainly with robbery and rape, although chloroform eventually graduated to a starring role in dime-novel murders.[134]

But many moralists considered anesthetic intoxication the main threat. The use of anesthetics for pleasure predated their use in surgery by at least a decade. Well before 1846, ether and laughing gas ''exhibitions'' had become a staple popular amusement (see plate 2). Private ether-sniffing parties also reportedly were quite common, especially among students and the young.[135] The standard pharmacology texts used terms like ''narcotic'' and ''intoxication'' to describe the effects of inhaling ether.[136]

A GRAND

EXHIBITION

OF THE EFFECTS PRODUCED BY INHALING

NITROUS OXIDE, EXHILERATING, OR

LAUGHING GAS!

WILL BE GIVEN AT *The Mason ic Hall*

Saturday **EVENING,** *15th*

30 GALLONS OF GAS

will be
prepared and administered
to all in the audience
who desire to inhale it.

MEN will be invited from the audience, to protect those under the influence of the Gas from injuring themselves or others. This course is adopted that no apprehension of danger may be entertained. Probably no one will attempt to fight.

THE EFFECT OF THE GAS is to make those who inhale it, either

LAUGH, SING, DANCE, SPEAK OR FIGHT, &c. &c.

according to the leading trait of their character. They seem to retain consciousness enough not to say or do that which they would have occasion to regret.

N. B. The Gas will be administered only to gentlemen of the first respectability. The object is to make the entertainment in every respect, a genteel affair.

Those who inhale the Gas once, are always anxious to inhale it the second time. There is not an exception to this rule.

No language can describe the delightful sensation produced. Robert Southey, (poet) once said that " the atmosphere of the highest of all possible heavens must be composed of this Gas."

For a full account of the effect produced upon some of the most distinguished men of Europe, see Hooper's Medical Dictionary, under the head of Nitrogen.

Date: 1845   #403, Buck Hill Associates, Johnsburg, N.Y.

PLATE II

"A Grand Exhibition of . . . Laughing Gas!"
Buck Hill Associates

The discovery of anesthesia coincided with a period of growing militance in the American temperance movement, a movement that had always attracted a share of medical support.[137] Thus many physicians came to fear that Demon Anesthesia constituted a real threat to public morality and to individual self-control. "Does not this subject come under the jurisdiction of the temperance people, and will they sanction one's getting dead drunk with ether?" asked the *Annalist.*[138]

The specific alleged dangers of anesthetic intoxication varied. For hydropaths, vegetarians, and other healers whose doctrines demanded total abstinence, the belief that ether and chloroform were "both preparations of alcohol" was sufficient evidence to reject their use.[139] Anesthetic intoxication also posed a special threat to the virtue and self-control of female patients. Not only were they liable to be raped, but, under the influence of the drug, genteel Victorian ladies actually attempted to seduce their physicians. Drunk on ether, normally respectable women supposedly said, felt, and did the most shocking things and experienced explicitly erotic fantasies. A few physicians also feared the masochistic perversity of a drug that could turn medical pain into sexual pleasure. The *American Journal of the Medical Sciences* cited an internationally renowned obstetrician who "insist[ed] upon the impropriety of etherization, . . . in consequence of the sexual orgasm under its use being substituted for the natural throes of parturition."[140] Anesthetic intoxication during labor posed another serious threat, because according to nineteenth-century theory, impressions received at birth were very likely to become hereditary—a mother who gave birth while drunk on ether would probably beget a race of congenital inebriates.[141]

Most doctors, however, did not consider the infrequent use of anesthesia in *medicine* a very serious direct threat to their patients' morals. What concerned them more was that the legitimate professional use of anesthetics might unintentionally encourage or sanction *public* abuse of anesthetics as intoxicants. "The inhalation of an intoxicating drug has produced disastrous effects in China, and if a habit more pernicious than that of the use of alcohol should be here introduced, it is to be feared it might spread," warned a correspondent of the *Boston Medical and Surgical Journal.* Even ether pioneer Dr. John Collins Warren (president of the Massachusetts Temperance Society), feared the new potential for intemperance created by unlimited public access to anesthetics. His brother, Dr. Edward

Warren, also acknowledged that "ether and chloroform may be used as means of intoxication or for the mere purpose of amusement, and may thus produce injurious effects."[142] These effects included such dangers as insanity, idiocy, addiction, and of course, hangover.[143]

Turnbull's respected anesthesia textbook of 1885 published the DeQuinceyesque "Confessions of an Ether Inhaler."

He was originally temperate, and had been a university student, passing all his examinations with credit; he was, however, of a mystical turn of mind. . . . Becoming gradually more and more addicted to his habit, he no longer confined himself to indulging himself in his own room, but with his etherized handkerchief before his face, he wandered through the streets, purchasing small quantities of ether at the druggists' shops, until, at last, he became . . . . a houseless wanderer, reduced in means and in health.

When finally hospitalized, he could be cured of his ether habit only by substituting large doses of marijuana.[144]

Public abuse of anesthetics not only undermined the health and moral fabric of society, it also cast disrepute on the otherwise legitimate professional use of the new painkillers. When Horace Wells, a former partner of Morton's, used chloroform to commit suicide while in jail for a series of crimes committed under the influence of anesthetic intoxication, the most lurid fears of critics seemed confirmed. The American Society of Dental Surgeons wanted it "distinctly understood" that its objections to the use of ether and chloroform rested squarely "on the abuse of anesthetic agents, and the consequent disgrace brought on the profession generally."[145]

Nineteenth-century Americans were not sure who would abuse the power of anesthesia, nor did they agree on what constituted "abuse," but many were troubled that such great power created the potential for vast misuse by someone.

"The Quagmire of Quackery": Anesthesia and Professional Respectability

Much early opposition to the use of ether was based on the belief that William T. G. Morton was a quack. Morton's actions clearly violated several long-established professional taboos and flew in the face of traditional gentlemanly professional standards of conduct. First, Morton and a partner, Dr. Charles T. Jackson, patented their "Letheon Gas." The intent was purely commercial. Even before the first public demonstration, Morton had been industriously hawking franchises and licenses for the use of his discovery. Such vigorous entrepreneurial activity directly violated traditional norms of professional gentility. Refusal to use a patented medicine long symbolized the gentleman's repugnance toward the crasser aspects of unrestrained profit seeking.[146] Thus, the Philadelphia College of Physicians, America's oldest and, in 1847, most prestigious medical organization, condemned the use of ether as an example of the spirit of commercialism infiltrating medicine. The *New York Journal of Medicine* denounced the commercialization of ether as "quackery." The editor blasted the use of anesthesia as an action "certainly contrary to the ethics of the profession [that] should not be tolerated for a moment in anyone."[147] The Massachusetts Medical Society agreed, chiding its members for unprofessional conduct in using Morton's patented preparation. The medical press rang with denunciations of any physician who would lower himself into the "quagmire of quackery" by using Letheon.[148]

Like the patent, Morton's vigorous advertising campaign clearly violated the limits of a professional gentleman's restraint in trade. In a series of broadsides, Morton publicly extolled the virtues of Letheon and promoted his personal fame as its discoverer. By the fifth edition (1847) *Morton's Letheon Circular* boasted nearly one hundred pages of testimonials and endorsements. In format and content, the *Circular* was indistinguishable from the promotional advertising pioneered by other patent medicine manufacturers. Critics denounced such crass commercialism. "The eye of the honorable dental surgeon was dimmed by honest indignation, at the injury done the profession, as his gaze met in the public prints, *fulsome* advertisements, headed, 'Dentistry without pain,' " reported the outraged American Society of Dental Surgeons.[149] "Everything now a-days must be introduced to the public, as well as to the profession," grumbled the *Annalist*.[150]

Morton's employment as a dentist constituted further ground for professional mistrust. Traditionally, dentists were mere toothpullers whose narrow specialization, empirical training, and mechanical employment clearly violated the old ideals of genteel profes-sionalism. "The practice of dentistry is not sufficient to entitle a gentleman to membership in this body, although he be a licensed physician," sniffed the New York Academy of Medicine. Doctors denounced ether as just one more example of the dental penchant for empirical dodges and technical tricks. According to one aggrieved practitioner, *"Physicians* have opposed it for the very cogent reason, that it was the discovery of a dentist!"[151]

An additional factor that contributed to the unprofes-sional image of anesthesia was the notorious, bitter, and interminable debate over priority in the discovery. At one time or another through the rest of the nineteenth century a dozen or more persons, including Jackson, Morton, and Wells, each claimed that he alone deserved credit for the discovery. Each of the participants in this controversy went to extraordinary lengths to brand the others as frauds and quacks—the one endeavor in which they all succeeded. In the course of the vi-cious mudslinging, most of the claimants lost all professional repu-tation, Jackson lost his mind, and Wells and Morton lost their lives.[152]

While the activities of ether's discoverers thus violated many old norms of professional behavior, the intensity with which anesthesia was attacked derived more from the state of uncertainty within medicine over what the appropriate standards were than from any consensus that Morton had violated universally accepted rules. The discovery of anesthesia came at a time of bitter controversy con-cerning the hallmarks of professional status. Whereas the use of ether clearly violated older standards of gentlemanly respectability and lib-eral professionalism, the relevance of such eighteenth-century norms to mid-nineteenth-century Americans had become a subject of violent dispute, even before Morton's discovery. By 1846, the concept of the professional as a "liberal gentleman" no longer provided clear, meaningful, or reliable criteria by which to distinguish the reputable practitioner from the quack. The old genteel distinctions were in-creasingly hard to apply, yet no new consensus existed on what was to replace them.

True, Morton's patent and advertising violated the liberal gentleman's sensibilities concerning the crassness of individual profit seeking. But in "venturesome" Jacksonian America, the profit mo-tive no longer provided a very workable distinction between profes-sionals and quacks. Although medical societies still routinely condemned blatant professional commercialism, many eminent physicians, including the first president of the AMA, prescribed, promoted, and even manufactured patent remedies. The eighteenth-century concept of a patent medicine as a backyard brew peddled door to door by elderly women and disreputable hucksters no longer provided much guidance in dealing with an industry that now included reputable businessmen who used the latest distribution, advertising, and production techniques to develop national and international markets. By 1846, even highly prestigious orthodox medical journals like the *Boston Medical and Surgical Journal* had become economically dependent on patent medicine advertising.[153]

Advertising also implied recognition of the public's right and ability to judge medical issues for itself, another subject on which mid-nineteenth-century American physicians lacked clear and consensual values. Worthington Hooker argued strongly that the gentlemanly distaste for publicity was outdated, that the repeal of licensing had given the public the legal right to choose their own medical beliefs, and that careful publicity efforts by regular physicians were essential if the public was to choose wisely.[154]

Anesthesia was also undoubtedly an empirical remedy, discovered by serendipity and incapable of explanation by existing medical theory. But in the "practical" America of 1846, empiricism no longer constituted a very clear standard of quackery either. In fact, "theorizer" had become almost as great a slur as "empiric" had been a generation before. "Do not *think* but try," one young Pennsylvania medical student began his dissertation on ether. "When any thing new is discovered in medicine," he concluded, "almost invariably, those who theorize upon its 'modus operandi,' will be found its opponents." "To the everlasting disgrace of science," J. F. B. Flagg noted (tongue-in-cheek), "this discovery, as such, can never take rank above a simple *Yankee guess.*" Flagg insisted that "pioneers" had to resort to "empiricism, to a certain extent." "Among this class," he boasted, "it has been my lot to be placed, even at the risk of being denominated 'quack.' " New York physician David M. Reese dismissed the critics of anesthesia, "for the most part mere theorists," and claimed "the extensive experience and success of practical men," provided the best authority for its use.[155]

Anesthetics were the discovery of dentists, and according to older professional standards, dentistry was an occupation beyond the bounds of respectability. But here, too, nineteenth-century realities had rendered the old distinctions less and less functional. Dentists themselves had begun to professionalize. In 1839, Dr. Thomas E. Bond Jr. and a few other dentists launched a drive to restructure their craft according to the ideals of medical professionalism. By the time of Morton's discovery, the new profession boasted an academically affiliated training institution, a national organization, and several journals. By 1846 it was not uncommon for big city dentists (including Morton) to have had formal medical school training. Bond, H. Willis Baxley, and other dental leaders held degrees from and taught at orthodox medical colleges. The once axiomatic identification of dentistry and quackery simply did not hold true by 1846.[156]

In fact, while physicians may have scoffed at anesthesia for its humble origins in dentistry, professional dentists, with both the zeal and the insecurities of new converts, outdid the doctors in denouncing ether as quackery. Dental spokesmen like Bond feared that Morton's violations of professional etiquette would undermine the entire struggle of ''dental surgeons'' to win professional respectability. Furthermore, dental status anxieties coincided with economic fears of the expense to dentists if Morton's patent should actually be enforced.[157]

The public brawling of Morton and his associates clearly went beyond the gentleman's code of professionalism, but once again, the violation itself does not fully explain the extent of the criticism it aroused. In the eighteenth century, the profession, confident and secure in its standards of legitimacy and identity, had tolerated repeated instances of personal mudslinging and internal rivalry without reading the participants out of the fraternity. But in the uncertain, hostile environment of midcentury America, such individual disputes came to be seen as more serious threats to the public respectability and internal unity of the entire profession. The combination of growing public intolerance for conflicting medical advice,[158] and a siege mentality within medicine itself, led organizations like the AMA and the New York Academy to restrict internal dissension in the name of preserving corporate unity. As a result, even John Collins Warren considered the debate over the title of discoverer to be a blow to the respectability of the profession and a serious threat to his own professional reputation.[159]

For a few physicians, the sense of uncertainty and threat

caused by this blurring of once-clear professional distinctions made defense of the old values imperative at all costs. The extremity of this position was derived, not from a feeling that using anesthesia was itself an unprecedented or uniquely heinous form of quackery, but from the sense of confusion and despair caused by the steadily growing difficulty of distinguishing doctors from quacks at all. The Philadelphia *Medical Examiner* made the stakes perfectly clear. If ether were "to be sanctioned by the profession, there is little need for reform conventions or any other efforts to elevate the professional character; physicians and quacks will soon constitute one fraternity." Holding the line against anesthesia involved, not an attack on the legitimacy of one drug, but the final act of resistance in the fall of a long-beleaguered professional civilization. "The Goths are in the Capitol; alas! for medicine!" mourned Dr. Bond upon seeing a Letheon advertisement in the *Boston Medical and Surgical Journal*. According to the editor of the New York *Annalist*,

> These gentlemen should have remembered, that these are no times for trifling with the strictness of professional observances; that the profession is now bleeding at every pore, from the wounds inflicted on her by so many of her own degenerate votaries—that conduct which involves the loss of professional honour, should *not* be undertaken unadvisedly . . . . They mutilate the fair form of their chosen science by abetting quackery in any shape, by swerving but the "turning of one poor hair" from the straight path of professional rectitude.

Such remarks captured well the mood of siege in which desperate defenders of traditional gentlemanly professional ideals were driven to denounce anesthesia.[160]

Factors beyond the questionable behavior of Morton and his rivals also fueled suspicion that anesthetics were professionally disreputable drugs. By 1846, physicians had seen so many pain preventives come and go that many considered the whole subject of pain inherently suspect. Bleeding, burning, drinking, freezing, even mesmerism, all had been tried; each produced a few remarkable successes, some highly embarrassing failures, a great deal of dangerously divisive intraprofessional hostility, and a mood of increasingly surly impatience on the part of a public whose expectations had been repeatedly raised and disappointed.[161] By 1846, leading surgeons such as Valentine Mott of New York had declared the search for painless surgery to be "a chimera that we can no longer pursue in our times."[162]

As reputable physicians became disillusioned with the subject, however, less fastidious entrepreneurs moved in to fill the void. The year before the discovery of anesthesia, another almost forgotten breakthrough occurred—the discovery by America's patent medicine industry of the lucrative national market for general pain cures. In 1845, Morton's fellow New Englander Perry Davis registered his "Celebrated Pain Killer" trademark and thereby christened an entirely new concept in patent drugs. Unlike most previous nostrums, supposedly good for a variety of *diseases,* Davis' Pain Killer seems to have been the first nationally advertised remedy specifically for *pain.* It enjoyed almost instantaneous, worldwide success, surviving both the outlawing of its main ingredients and the discovery of aspirin.

Unlike Letheon, Davis' Pain Killer was not primarily for surgical pain; however advertisements clearly recommended it for domestic surgical procedures (see plate 3). By 1848, the booming business of patent pain remedies included nationally marketed competitors such as "Herculean Embrocation" and "Pond's Extract, the Universal Pain Extractor." Pond's in particular adopted a populist, antiprofessional, "vegetable cure" stance reminiscent of Samuel Thomson (see plate 4). Homebrewed products for local markets also proliferated.[163]

Pain, like tuberculosis, venereal disease, and cancer, had been pronounced incurable by official medicine; thus "painkillers," like "consumption drops," "clap cures," and "cancer plasters," had become almost synonymous with quackery. Any new patented pain remedy introduced in 1846 would have encountered more than the usual degree of professional skepticism.[164]

At the same time, those few practitioners who had already staked their reputations on endorsing mesmerism, freezing, or one of the patent painkillers were not pleased at having Morton steal their thunder. The *New-Orleans Medical and Surgical Journal* declared that, compared to ether, mesmerism could perform "a thousand times greater wonders, and without any of the dangers," an assessment with which the embattled British pioneer of surgical mesmerism John Elliotson wholly agreed.[165]

Claims that anesthesia was quackery played an extremely

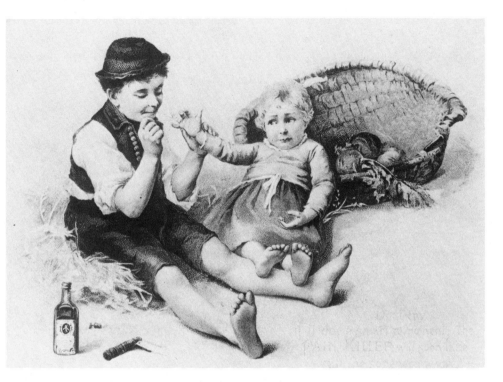

PLATE III

"Don't cry if it does smart a moment, the PAIN-KILLER will
soon take all the soreness away."

New York Hospital Archives

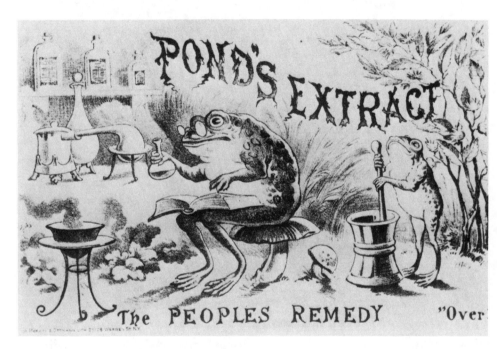

PLATE IV A

"Pond's Extract—The People's Remedy"

New York Hospital Archives

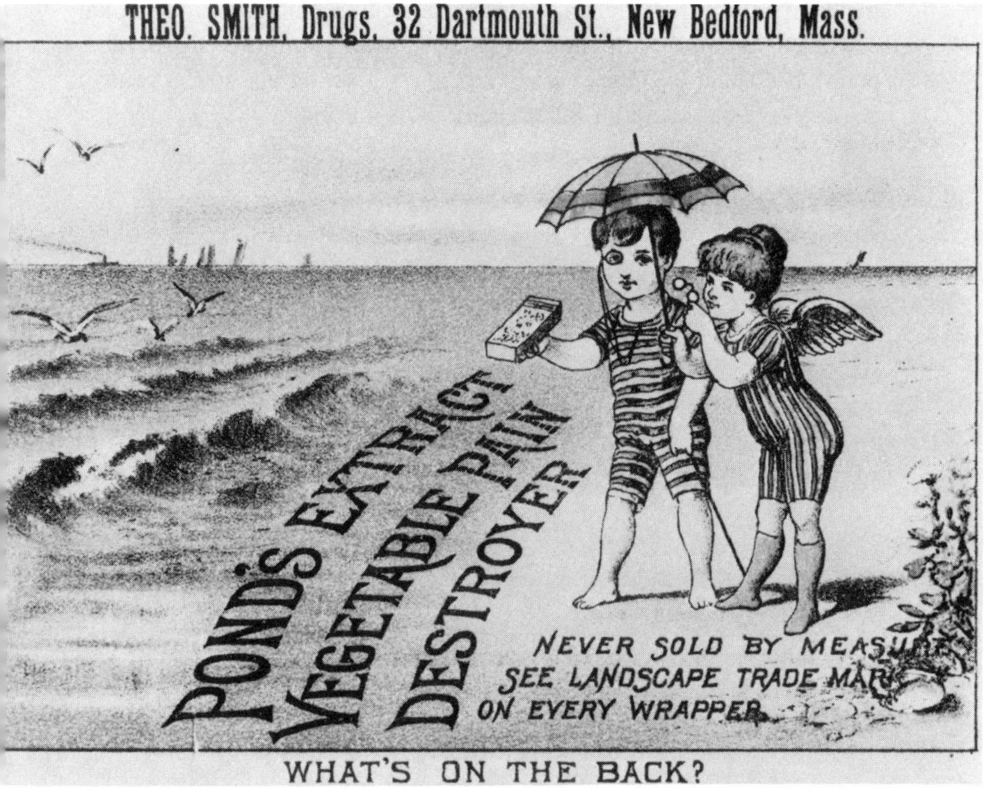

PLATE IV B

"Pond's Extract Vegetable Pain Destroyer"

New York Hospital Archives

important role in its early reception and were kept in the public mind to some extent by the long controversy over the title to its discovery. But these charges did not have the same lasting impact on anesthetic usage as the other objections to the new painkillers did. The short-lived fury of such criticism represented, not an outraged professional consensus against the heinousness of Morton's crimes, but the desperate last stand of those few physicians still committed to the genteel professional standards of a past age.

CHAPTER FOUR

THE BENEFITS
OF ANESTHESIA

The use of anesthesia clearly had disadvantages, but it also offered benefits—far more different kinds of benefits than might readily be apparent. The alleged advantages of anesthesia went beyond simple painlessness; in fact, the variety of suggested uses almost rivaled the diversity of supposed drawbacks. Praise, like criticism, sprang from no one ideology, but drew upon a wide range of often incompatible biological, ethical, and professional ideas and values. Many of the same people who pointed out the drawbacks also tabulated the advantages. In addition, many of the same facts that some people regarded as costs, other people valued as benefits.

The Advantages of Painlessness

Of course, the most basic thing to be said in favor of anesthesia was that it prevented pain. Yet, as we have seen, a wide range of nineteenth-century opinion held that painlessness had drawbacks. Thus, users of anesthesia were forced to specify what particular benefits might result from the removal of pain.

While pain might serve some useful ends, in itself it was the very essence of evil; at least as defined by physicians like New York's eminent Dr. Valentine Mott. "Pain is only evil, and that continually," Mott declared without reservation.[1] By defining pain as evil, its elimination became a categorical imperative. That we should seek to combat evil is not a proposition capable of demonstration or argument; it is a fundamental axiom of almost any ethical system. Painless surgery thus constituted a victory in the struggle against evil, a moral as well as a technical breakthrough.[2]

But is pain always evil? Many nineteenth-century Americans rejected such a hedonistic equation. The evil nature of pain could not be assumed; it had to be explained and defended. To do so, many physicians turned to concepts of sympathy, benevolence, and humanitarianism. "To prevent pain is humane," Mott continued. With heartfelt sentiment, nineteenth-century writers again and again dubbed anesthesia "a boon to suffering humanity."[3] John Collins Warren saw the use of anesthetics as primarily an act of benevolent humanitarianism: "As philanthropists we may well rejoice that we have had an agency . . . in conferring on poor suffering humanity so precious a gift." Other physicians praised Warren for his "warmth and enthusiasm of benevolent feeling." Eliza L. S. Thomas, a Philadelphia medical student, declared anesthesia "A subject which should interest every philanthropic heart . . . . those devoted hearts that beat in sorrowing sympathy for the afflicted."[4]

James Simpson went further, portraying his discovery of chloroform anesthesia as part of a larger mid-Victorian humanitarian movement for the relief of all human suffering. He explicitly compared painless surgery and pain-free childbirth with such causes as feminism, antislavery, and the melioration of conditions for criminals and soldiers. Simpson wrote to Ramsbotham,

Yesterday I was reading a letter from Dr. [Samuel Gridley] Howe describing a public slave-whipping scene in New Orleans where a poor shrieking girl had a series of horrid lashes inflicted on her to serve merely the temper and prejudices of the master; and while the Dr. gives a most heart-rending account of her agonies, he adds that what struck him as *worst* of all was all the other masters maintaining that this inhuman and cruel practice of theirs was the only *safe* practice with slaves—just as on equally untenable grounds you still . . . maintain that the shrieking of patients in labour is the only *safe* practice for them.[5]

Just as there were religious arguments against painlessness, there were also religious arguments in favor of it. Simpson worked his concordance to the marrow, matching precept against precept, line against line, to prove that God clearly intended humankind henceforth and forevermore to escape the pangs of birth and surgery.[6] Although most Reformed denominations believed God inflicted pain to punish human misdeeds, all but the most extreme predestinarians also believed God had given man the power of reason as a means of avoiding unnecessary pains. Though reason remained a frail and uncertain guide, the use of this God-given talent was a theologically accepted way of avoiding the avoidable—from the child's discovery that fire burns to Rev. Cotton Mather's 1721 introduction of smallpox inoculation. Thus, Dr. Mary Seelye, a late-nineteenth-century physician, saw no conflict between her belief that pain was God's literal punishment for the Fall and her intention to prescribe God's gift of anesthesia.[7] The more romantically inclined Dr. Eliza L. S. Thomas saw anesthesia as a second dispensation—a gift from God to forgive us our sins against nature; "one of Heaven's best gifts bestowed on erring mortals as if in relenting forgiveness of their disobeyance of Nature's laws."[8]

Such sentiments grew more common with the increasing romanticism of midcentury theology. "Our every idea of a God of love and mercy constrains us to believe that He does not delight in the sufferings of His creatures," affirmed a young Michigan doctor in 1871.[9]

While some physicians used their Bibles to prove that anesthesia was God's gift to humanity, they also saw an immense advantage in the existence of theological opposition. Many nineteenth-century doctors had grown increasingly uncomfortable with the presumption of clergymen who ministered to bodies as well as souls. "Why is it that clergymen are so frequently found abetting quackery?" the *Western Lancet* began an 1848 editorial.[10] The shortage of doctors in colonial America, combined with broad eighteenth-century criteria of gentlemanly competence in all professions, had given the clergy a large role in early American medicine, a position many nineteenth-century physicians were eager to eliminate. If the clergy as a group could be branded as antianesthesia, perhaps their medical authority could be broken once and for all. Physicians like Mott and Warren were certainly not irreligious, but they were strongly against clerical doctoring. Thus, they magnified every instance of clerical opposition to ether as evidence of "stupid fanaticism" by "madm[e]n."[11] For some physicians, anesthesia provided a longed-for excuse to go parson-skinning.

Many physicians believed that pain was a just punishment for violating nature's laws but simply refused to apply that doctrine to the use of anesthetics. Thus John Collins Warren disingenuously presented obstetric anesthesia as a man-made "exception" to nature's laws.[12] Boston's pioneer health statistician Lemuel Shattuck believed,

"Pain, suffering, and the various physical evils to which we are exposed, . . . result from the violations of [nature's] laws; and are permitted for wise purposes, perhaps for the discipline and development of our physical and moral powers. . . . [S]ome innocent may suffer; but they are individual exceptions to the general rule; . . .

"The fountain of the evil is in ourselves," Shattuck concluded. Yet, despite this belief that pain was a deserved punishment, Shattuck laughed at those who opposed the use of anesthesia. Attracted by the perfectionist goal of a naturally pain-free world, Shattuck was less doctrinaire than the hydropaths about restricting mankind to "natural" means of achieving painlessness.[13]

In addition, such midcentury diseases of the poor as cholera and typhus led a growing number of physicians to conclude that violations of natural law were not solely the result of individual guilt. Ignorance or compulsion, as well as vice, could produce violations of nature's rules. Economic and social injustice could force people to live in slums and work at jobs where obedience to the natural laws of physiology and hygiene was impossible; society sometimes held the fingers of the disadvantaged in nature's relentless fire. The pains of these worthy sufferers, the "deserving poor," occurred because nature mechanically punished all infractions of its laws, regardless of whether or not the offender was morally responsible for the violation.[14] Surely there could be nothing wrong in helping the innocent avert such natural punishments, through anesthesia for example, while in the meantime working for the needed social reforms.

But most nineteenth-century physicians shied away from claiming a direct connection among anesthesia, social reform, and humanitarianism. Many doctors seemed distinctly uneasy about the reformist image anesthesia was acquiring. Edward Warren noted that Dr. Walter Channing's pioneer work on obstetric anesthesia had been attacked on the ground

that our author writes with the zeal of an advocate, rather than the coolness of an impartial investigator. Dr. Channing is well known for his zeal in the various benevolent enterprises of the day, and for his exertions for the amelioration and reform of social evils. The eagerness of his desire to extend the use of this remedy for pain might be supposed to carry him too far.[15]

To emphasize that anesthesia was not simply a matter of philanthropy, many physicians stressed the physical rather than the humanitarian advantages of painlessness. Doctors repeatedly asserted that pain was not only painful but dangerous, that preventing pain could be lifesaving, as well as simply benevolent. The *Western Lancet* insisted "that the object in employing ether is not merely to avoid the temporary pain incident to a severe surgical operation; but it is rather to obviate the *secondary* results—the *shock* which follows extensive and painful operations." "So much has been said of etherization as a remedy for pain, that too little attention has been paid to its more important but remote effect in preserving life and health," Edward Warren agreed. "There is a much higher advantage in the use of these agents; by preventing pain, life will often be saved, and lingering and dangerous disease be avoided."[16]

The belief that pain could kill was an ancient, if controversial, doctrine,[17] controversial because it was hard to explain exactly how pain—presumably a purely mental phenomenon—might influence the physical health and life of the body.[18] The most common mechanism suggested by defenders of anesthesia was that pain killed by causing the disease "shock."[19] Others explained that pain kills by expending the body's fixed stock of vital energy. "Pain is always injurious to the animal economy, and if excessive or long continued may so prostrate the system as to produce death," according to young Dr. Edward H. Horner. Pain "exhausts the powers of life, and may

even produce death! hence . . . every rational means for its prevention [is] worthy of the attention of the Surgeon,'' one Philadelphia
practitioner explained to the College of Physicians.[20]

Not only could pain kill directly; it could also cause poor
healing and inflammation. ''If pain be the initiatory step to inflammation and the prevention of one arrests the other, then we may begin to estimate the value and importance of these new anaesthetic
agents,'' declared Dr. Paul F. Eve, perhaps the best known surgeon
of the antebellum South.[21] Even the natural pains of childbirth could
kill.[22] In addition, reducing the pains of labor might save lives indirectly, by discouraging the increasingly controversial practice of
abortion. ''The wife of a Christian physician'' explained in the *Boston Medical and Surgical Journal* in 1866, ''One great reason for the
aversion to child-bearing is the . . . certain agony at the end . . . .
If the blessed, benevolent suggestion of the use of chloroform could
be adopted, the world would hear less of abortions.''[23]

The prevention of pain could also save lives by encouraging a more prompt and more frequent resort to surgery. According
to Valentine Mott, ''The dread of suffering has prevented thousands
of human beings from submitting to necessary operations, and their
lives have been the forfeit.'' Surgeons too would be less hesitant in
performing needed operations. ''Severe and formidable operations may
be performed under the influence of those agents, which the most bold
and adventurous surgeon would not have had the temerity to touch,''
Mott concluded. Thus, anesthesia would both save lives, and benefit
surgeons by increasing their business.[24]

The elimination of pain was expected to benefit doctors
in other ways as well. Operating on screaming, pain-ravaged people
took its toll on surgeons, as well as on their clients. The cliché that
''this hurts me more than you'' can be traced in innumerable variations back to the maxims of Hippocrates.[25] In the powerful metaphors
of Walt Whitman, the tired adage leaps to life: ''I do not ask the
wounded person how he feels, I myself become the wounded person.''

> I am firm with each, the pangs are sharp yet
>   unavoidable,
> . . . .
> Yet I think I could not refuse this moment to die
>   for you, if that would save you.[26]

Anesthesia, it was hoped, would spare physicians the need to die for their patients' sins. Practitioners repeatedly praised ether as "a great relief to both patient and surgeon." Anesthesia "to the surgeon brings pleasure from the knowledge that he inflicts no pain," declared Dr. Jonathan Frederick May of Washington, D.C.[27]

The benefits to the surgeon went beyond empathetic relief. With the elimination of the coarser and more violent aspects of the art, the professional respectability of surgery and dentistry also increased.[28] Furthermore, with the elimination of suffering, the effort formerly expended in empathizing with the patient could be devoted to the technical aspects of the operation. Surgeons found anesthesia advantageous, not only out of consideration for the patient's feelings but also because it allowed them to bypass such feelings altogether and to focus exclusively on the mechanical procedures at hand. FitzWilliam Sargent declared it "very gratifying to the operator and to the spectators that the patient lies a tranquil, passive subject, instead of struggling and perhaps uttering pitious cries and moans, while the knife is at work; and this facilitates, undoubtedly, in many instances, the performance of the operation."[29]

Initially, surgeons believed the main technical advantage would be to allow faster and more efficient procedures. However, most soon came to agree with Robert Druitt that anesthesia "enables the surgeon to proceed with his dissection in a more leisurely manner." They concluded that a "tranquilly pliant," controlled, unfeeling patient allowed the surgeon to proceed with "all convenient deliberation," and a degree of mechanical throroughness previously unattainable.[30]

Anesthesia found advocates in internal medicine, as well as in surgery and obstetrics. Following their usual procedure of prescribing drugs for their general effects on the system rather than for specific diseases, nineteenth-century physicians used anesthetics to treat all forms of pain, convulsions, and many other so-called diseases of the nerves. The ailments listed included tetanus, epilepsy, puerperal convulsions, delirium tremens, chorea, asthma, hysteria, hiccup, whooping cough, colic, cholera, menstrual cramps and neuralgia.[31] Anesthetics were also prescribed as sleeping aids for insomnia and tranquilizers for the insane.[32]

The Utility of Power

The advantages claimed for anesthesia did not end with the suspension of pain. The ability to control sensation and consciousness, to produce a "tranquilly pliant" patient, conferred a great deal of power, a power that many physicians welcomed despite fears that it might be misused. In fact, some supporters heralded as beneficial the very same uses of anesthesia that critics had denounced as abuses.

Many eminent physicians found the absolute control over their patients conferred by anesthesia to be one of its key advantages. As one major surgery text put it, "Its benefits are not confined to the abolition of pain; . . . it circumvents the opposition of the timid and unruly." Dr. Samuel D. Gross, in his widely used *A System of Surgery* agreed. "Anaesthetics . . . by placing the patient in a passive condition give the surgeon a control over him which he could not possibly obtain in any other manner." An article in the *American Journal of the Medical Sciences* listed among the main advantages of obstetric anesthesia, "To quiet particularly noisy patients." Anesthetics were also frequently advocated to control the violence of manic asylum patients, and as a truth serum to detect malingerers feigning illness. The ability to subdue noisy, disruptive, and uncooperative patients was an increasingly important advantage as hospitals and asylums grew larger and more efficiency minded.[33]

Doctors commonly lauded anesthesia for fostering medical paternalism and relieving patients from the painful knowledge of what was in fact being done to them. "It is, indeed, not an unheard-of thing that a surgeon's presence of mind should fail him in a difficult operation, even at the present day; but at least the patient, unconscious through the blessing of anaesthesia, does not know it . . . to the great comfort of all concerned," one physician recalled in 1897.[34]

While many doctors thus hoped the profession could use anesthetics to increase their power over patients, others welcomed the new painkillers as a means of decreasing medical power and allowing greater patient autonomy, especially in obstetric cases. Dr. Simpson rejoiced that the ease of administering anesthetics gave patients the option to choose their own treatment.[35] Dr. J. F. B. Flagg of Philadelphia advised the husbands of expectant women, "If her doctor is disposed to act the alarmist [regarding anesthesia], you had better put him in the next room with the rest of the children, and allow of no one to be present who cannot be useful."[36] Nor was this medical support for patient autonomy limited to obstetrics. Proponents of anesthesia welcomed patient demand as a counterweight to what they saw as excessive professional timidity. Dr. Jackson quoted with approval the observation of Velpeau in 1850, that "with the knowledge the public has already acquired, the surgeons will hardly be partisans, but the patients know enough already to force them to make use of this method."[37]

Even the use of anesthetics to intoxicate could be an advantage, as well as an abuse, of its powers. Surgeons, dentists, and patients alike saw virtue in a drug that would make operations not merely painless but fun. Even that paragon of sobriety John Collins Warren marveled, "Who could imagine that drawing the knife over the delicate skin of the face might produce a sensation of unmixed delight!" Dr. Bigelow reported that one of Morton's first patients declared the extraction of two teeth " ' was the best fun he ever saw,' avowed his intention to come there again, and insisted upon having another tooth extracted upon the spot." "Staid demure, elderly gentlemen, in the most abandoned gayety, insisted on the operator forthwith joining them in a joyous Polka," chuckled a young medical student.[38]

Bigelow confirmed from his own experience that pure ether was as "pleasant" and "exhilarating" as "the Egyptian haschish."[39] He claimed there was "scarcely a school or community in our country where the boys and girls have not inhaled ether, to produce gayety," with no recorded ill effects. Dr. Jackson alleged that "college and school boys often amused themselves by breathing it." Several doctors advocated ether intoxication as a safer substitute for alcohol.[40]

J. F. B. Flagg reported that students in the 1840s used ether for "the purposes of amusement, and 'the development of character,' "—an explanation remarkably like the defense of "consciousness-expanding" psychoactive substances in the 1960s.[41] Among those to praise the mystic experience of anesthetization were William James and Tennyson.[42] Claims that every school was full of ether-sniffers may well have been gross exaggerations by physicians eager to prove the safety of the new drugs. But the fact remained that for a variety of reasons, many people condoned and openly encouraged ether intoxication.

Even the forcible use of anesthetics by laymen could be defended as beneficial, at least on the level of popular humor. In fact, the popular cartoons and jokes that circulated throughout the nineteenth century, about laughing gas and other anesthetics, provide an explicit insight into the tension-filled Victorian association between anesthesia and power—sexual dominance in particular. British artist Robert Seymour pioneered the genre in 1830 when he portrayed the forcible use of laughing gas as a remedy for nagging wives (plate 5).[43] Years before the introduction of surgical anesthesia, Seymour's image won immense popularity on both sides of the Atlantic (if plagiarism be taken as the highest form of flattery—see plate 2 for an American example). Following the discovery of anesthesia, the use of laughing gas, ether, and chloroform in the taming of the shrew became a staple of the Victorian humor magazines. In February 1847, less than four months after Morton's demonstration, a *Punch* cartoon extolled the "WONDERFUL EFFECTS OF ETHER IN A CASE OF SCOLDING WIFE."[44] By the end of the year, the theme had even been set to music.

> Scolding wife and squalling infant—petulance
> and fretfullness,
> Lulling with its magic power, *instantèr,* in
> forgetfullness;
> Peace in private families securing, and in
> populous
> Nurseries, whene'er their little inmates prove
> "obstropolous."[45]

Under the thin veil of humor, Victorians could express the anxious association of anesthesia with sexual power, in an era when sexual conflict could not be discussed openly.

Thus, the promoters of anesthesia, like its critics, divided sharply over the use of its immense powers. What one group denounced as dangerous abuses another group praised as advantages. And neither defenders nor detractors agreed on who should control these powers, nor on what effect anesthetics actually would have on

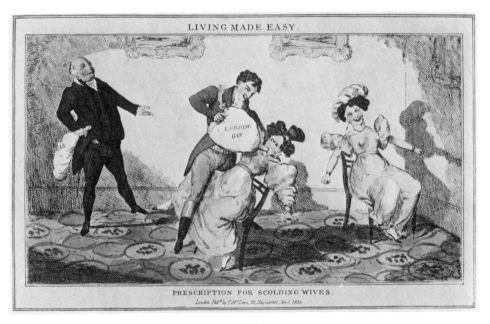

PLATE V

"Living Made Easy: Prescription for Scolding Wives"
National Library of Medicine

the balance of medical authority. In short, anesthesia was both attacked and defended, both for weakening and for strengthening physician control over patients.

Power and Potency: The Advantages of Danger and Quackery

The list of anesthesia's reported risks was massive. But most nineteenth-century physicians evaluated each alleged danger separately. Any given doctor accepted some of the charges and rejected others. While virtually all agreed anesthesia had some harmful consequences, only a handful of charges were accepted by a consensus of medical opinion.[46] The many other alleged side effects were debated on a case-by-case basis, with a large number of physicians prepared to refute or minimize the importance of any particular charge.[47]

However, instead of attempting to disprove the alleged dangers of anesthetics, a few physicians interpreted these risks as benefits in disguise. Advocates of professional monopoly sometimes used the hazard as an argument for limiting anesthesia to trained experts. Danger could be turned to an advantage, because it could justify increased professional control. Warning that chloroform can be "a prompt and certain poison," the AMA Committee on Medical Science concluded that "chloroform should be used with great caution, and only by professional men." Since ether too could "cause the complete destruction of life," the *Western Lancet* advised "that its use should be restricted to those who are competent." "In view of the fact that death has been known to occur," medical texts warned dentists that "administration of the ether should be confided to a well-trained physician." Most medical authors recommended that anesthesia be made the sole responsibility of a designated expert at each operation.[48] Critics charged that British physicians preferred chloroform over ether because the greater danger of the former agent ensured it would remain under professional control.[49]

There is no direct evidence that American physicians deliberately exaggerated the dangers of anesthesia. However, in other areas of nineteenth-century medicine, the adoption of dangerous practices as a means of demonstrating the superior skill, training, and daring of the profession and of frightening off competitors was not unheard of. In an unusually frank example, the *American Journal of the Medical Sciences* advocated adoption of a particularly mutilating new type of forceps on the grounds that it would prove too dangerous for any but trained obstetricians to employ. The *Journal* even tried to apply the same strategy against hydropathy, solemnly warning patients that bathing could be lethal unless prescribed by a regularly trained doctor![50]

Some defenders of anesthesia also tried to cast the unsavory activities of its discoverers in a more favorable light.[51] Even ether's association with previous disreputable attempts to prevent pain was in some ways an advantage. Some opponents of patent medicines and of mesmerism saw the similarity as a benefit, in that anesthesia would drive such "quackery" off the market. "Rejoice! Mesmerism, and its professors, have met with a heavy blow," the English surgeon Liston wrote following his first anesthetic operation. "Unlike the farce and trickery of mesmerism, this is based on scientific principles and is solely in the hands of gentlemen of high professional attainment," agreed the *Boston Medical and Surgical Journal*.[52] Still others, who had gone out on the limb of mesmerism, saw this new discovery as a chance to claim vindication of their visions and return to the professional fold.[53]

Benefits and Drawbacks: A Summary Scorecard

Most nineteenth-century Americans, regardless of their medical or social opinions, found at least a few things to like and a few things to oppose in the new painkillers. The debate over anesthesia thus crosscut many ideological and organizational lines. However, different groups did differ in the particular mix of specific benefits and drawbacks they anticipated.[54]

Of all medical sects, the hydropaths, vegetarians, Grahamites, and similar natural healers offered perhaps the most developed and intense antianesthetic critique. They attacked anesthesia because it was "unnatural": it encouraged operative surgery, and employed poisonous, intoxicating chemicals, instead of relying on nature's healing powers; it cheated nature by depriving unhealthy living habits of their deservedly painful consequences. But these same sects also exceeded all others in portraying pain as an evil that could and should be totally eliminated. They applauded the goal of the new painkillers, even though they abhorred the means.

Midcentury homeopaths, too, usually attacked anesthesia as unwise interference with both nature's healing and nature's punishments.[55] However, most homeopaths were less doctrinaire than the hydropaths. They were willing to use some drugs and even surgery to help natural recovery, and most assumed that some pains either should not or could not be eliminated by any means. They shared both the hydropaths' hopes and their fears concerning anesthesia, but to a lesser degree.[56]

Members of the Eclectic sect also worried that anesthesia would promote the use of the knife instead of their drugs. And they too attacked anesthesia as an "unnatural" state. But, unlike either homeopaths or hydropaths, they based this latter conclusion on a vitalist view that pain was essential to the life force.[57] Also unlike these other sects, Eclectics saw pain as a valuable counterirritant to fight disease and sometimes advocated very painful remedies as substitutes for anesthetics.[58] Eclectics further tended to see spiritual, as well as medical, compensations in suffering.[59] And more than other sects, they reported long lists of specific side effects and contraindications.[60] Eclectics did cite advantages to anesthesia, however, especially in the prevention of such pain-induced diseases as shock and in the improved control of patients.[61]

The botanic, physio-medical and other neo-Thomsonian sects shared most of the Eclectic position on the pros and cons of anesthesia; a reflection of their common roots in the teachings of Samuel Thomson. However these latter-day Thomsonians criticized the Eclectics for abandoning Thomson's exclusive reliance on "natural," i.e., vegetable, remedies for pain.[62]

Different groups of orthodox physicians also differed in their enumeration of the specific pros and cons of anesthesia. Those who still accepted Benjamin Rush's theory of counterirritation worried that anesthesia led to increased wound infection because anesthetics prevented the pain necessary to drive out the disease. However, these same advocates of counterirritation also often considered pain itself a serious disease, more than capable of counteracting any poisonous effect of the painkiller.[63] Likewise, vitalist physicians split between those who believed that pain enhanced the life force and those who warned that pain depleted it.

By midcentury most orthodox physicians tempered their therapeutic heroism with a new appreciation of natural healing. To the extent that they adopted environmental therapies and relied on nature's healing powers, these orthodox doctors shared the concern of the hydropaths and homeopaths that anesthesia was an unwise chemical circumvention of nature's beneficent punishments. However, only the most radically perfectionist physicians believed that nature could cure all pains; most orthodox physicians who advocated natural healing accepted anesthesia as a useful, though artificial, adjunct to nature, especially in such unnatural situations as surgery.

Leaders of several medical associations feared anesthesia would further divide and discredit the profession. Those who clung to the eighteenth-century vision of professional gentility also spurned anesthesia as fatally tainted by commercialism; many shunned the whole field of pain relief as rife with quackery. Yet anesthesia also offered organizational advantages, especially increased public gratitude and patronage. Those who viewed professionalism as requiring paternalistic authority over patients rejoiced in the new powers anesthesia provided; yet they also despaired of maintaining a medical monopoly on its use. Others whose vision of professional-client relations exalted patient autonomy conversely welcomed the lay demand for anesthesia but sometimes bemoaned the anesthetized patients' inability to participate during the procedure.[64] Dentists saw in anesthesia both the elimination of the greatest public complaint against their craft and a serious challenge to their professional aspirations.

Though lay opinion on medical issues is often fragmentary and hard to locate, the available evidence indicates that, like physicians, Americans from a broad range of ideological perspectives saw both advantages and dangers in the new pain remedies. Antebellum social reformers often claimed anesthesia as part and parcel of the benevolent spirit of the age. Yet many of the more radical reformers shared the perfectionist view of nature that led the hydropaths to oppose anesthetics as ''unnatural.''

Advocates of specific social causes often had specific concerns about the new painkillers as well. Temperance leaders denounced anesthetic drunkenness. Feminists feared both the moral and the political consequences if a woman surrendered her consciousness to a male anesthetist. Many nineteenth-century women also protrayed their sex as closer to "nature" than men were; attacks on anesthesia as "unnatural" held a special appeal for them. And others valued the spiritual power of female suffering as the most potent force for feminism possible within the confines of Victorian society. Yet feminists also saw certain advantages in anesthetics. Anesthesia gave medical legitimacy to the treatment of obstetric pain and could be used to increase, as well as decrease, the power of women patients.

Physicians often blamed Calvinist theology for creating antianesthetic sentiment, and such denominations as the Old School Presbyterians certainly did regard suffering as the predestined fate of man (and woman). Yet only one or two explicitly predestinarian attacks on anesthetics can be documented, while many biblical literalists publicly thanked God for conferring the gift of anesthesia. The major theological challenge to anesthesia came not from predestinarians but from radical perfectionists, who saw painlessness as possible but regarded anesthesia as an unacceptable shortcut.[65]

CHAPTER FIVE

THE PROFESSIONAL CALCULUS: ANESTHESIA AND THE ORIGINS OF UTILITARIAN PROFESSIONALISM

The Lesser of Two Evils

FitzWilliam Sargent, surgeon to Wills Eye Hospital in Philadelphia, spoke for most of the profession in 1852 when he declared that, with anesthesia, as with any other drug, "the blessing is not unalloyed."[1] Almost all midcentury practitioners concluded that anesthesia offered at least some potential advantages and some likely disadvantages. Even New York's Valentine Mott, a most outspoken proponent of painlessness, conceded that anesthetics had some inherent dangers. And virtually all admitted that anesthesia had at least some real benefits. John B. Porter, for example, denounced anesthesia as an emotional and physiological "evil" that "never" failed to produce harm; yet even he accepted that the new painkillers could be of real benefit in preventing lethal shock.[2]

Thus the evaluation of anesthesia did not stop with a simple listing of its pros and cons. Most practitioners felt obliged not only to decide the absolute merits of each individual charge and countercharge but, in addition, to decide the *relative* importance of those advantages and disadvantages that they considered pertinent. "Of two evils we must choose the least, and this is the case in all surgery," explained the *American Journal of the Medical Sciences*. The general problem was best expressed by the AMA Committee on Surgery. "The great question, which still divides medical opinion, is: . . . do the risks and evils attendant upon the use of these agents in surgery, counterbalance the advantages afforded by exemption from pain, and to what extent and under what circumstances is it proper to use them?"[3]

The issue was not the objective magnitude of the danger but the values by which any degree of danger might be legitimated. The debate went beyond a disagreement over the facts of anesthesia's benefits or drawbacks to a controversy over the value system by which physicians should choose between the advantages and disadvantages. This dispute was not over the scientific merits of the arguments about anesthesia but instead reflected a fundamental ideological conflict within nineteenth-century medicine over priorities among professional obligations and the ethics of professional decisionmaking.

How did physicians attempt to weigh such benefits as the relief of suffering and the prevention of shock against the danger of harm from anesthesia? The analysis below shows that each of the three major definitions of professional duty in midcentury America provided a different judgment on the medical ethics of anesthesia. The ideology of natural healing rejected the use of harmful artificial drugs either for the prevention of suffering or for averting the physical effects of pain. The heroic version of medical duty also opposed the use of anesthetics to avoid suffering. However, heroic concepts of medical ethics did sanction the use of anesthesia to combat the physical effects of pain.[4]

Only conservative professionalism permitted the cautious use of anesthetics, both to relieve emotional suffering and to prevent physical damage. This new utilitarian approach to professional duty sanctioned the use of anesthesia whenever the probability of mental or physical harm to the patient was demonstrably greater without anesthetics than with them. The extent to which a practitioner shared the naturalistic, heroic, or conservative view of medical duty thus profoundly influenced his or her reception of the new painkillers.

The Calculus of Safety: Choosing Between
Natural and Artificial Dangers

Anesthetics, many nineteenth-century physicians claimed, could lessen or avert the physical damage done by pain—damage that allegedly included shock, infection, chronic disease, and death. Avoiding these *physical* effects of pain constituted an important benefit of anesthesia, separate from such other benefits as the relief of suffering.[5]

But, granted that anesthetics might prevent physical harm, a practitioner still had to decide whether that advantage was worth the costs. Which was the "lesser evil"—the harm likely to be caused by pain or the harm that might be caused by the painkiller?

Deciding on the relative safety of anesthesia thus raised an ancient problem common to all forms of therapy: how to determine whether the "cure" is worse than the "disease." It may be hard for modern readers to see that there could be room for debate in such a decision. Today, we expect most physicians simply to measure the probability and extent of possible damage from the cure and from the disease and to adopt the least harmful course.[6] But many nineteenth-century Americans vehemently denied that the "natural" effects of untreated disease (or untreated pain) could be equated with the "artificial" effects of active therapy. Early-nineteenth-century practitioners of heroic medicine had argued that human intervention was almost always necessary for successful therapy, whereas midcentury natural healers believed unaided natural recuperation to be inherently the most effective.

Furthermore, this seemingly technical debate subsumed a more fundamental ethical dispute over the physician's proper professional role. For many nineteenth-century physicians, weighing the respective dangers posed by disease and by treatment meant not simply measuring which risk was larger but evaluating which type of risk was morally worse. This choice thus reflected the ancient moral distinction between acts of commission and acts of omission. Heroic practitioners regarded active intervention as the physician's primary ethical obligation; natural healers preferred to passively "do no harm" rather than risk causing harm directly. The heroic professional tradition encouraged risk-taking whenever a life might be saved; the ethics of natural healing sanctioned only safe and supportive therapies.[7] In short, heroic medicine and natural healing offered two opposing value systems by which physicians could judge whether the physical benefits of anesthesia were worth the risks.

Though early nineteenth-century heroic medicine is (correctly) remembered as extremely harsh and painful, heroic therapy did provide an important precedent for legitimating the use of anesthetics. Benjamin Rush and such disciples as William Potts Dewees taught that pain "must be regarded as [a] disease." If pain was a disease, then the doctrine of counterirritation demanded the use of strong active remedies to drive it from the body.[8]

Physicians like Rush and Dewees urged that such dangerous pains be fought by the infliction of damaging remedies, like blistering, cupping, and above all, copious bloodletting.[9] Rush and Dewees were among the first modern physicians to attempt to treat the pain of ordinary childbirth. They insisted that the pangs of parturition were not beneficial but a cause and a symptom of several dangerous illnesses. As such, they urged venesection, to the point of unconsciousness, to cure the throes of labor.[10] To be sure, in the specific medical system taught by Rush, a "tonic" drug like ether would not have been used often. Only "depleting" remedies were considered harsh enough to be used to fight such dangerous pains. But the theory of heroic counterirritation could be separated from Rush's depletive therapies; it retained its appeal long after Rush's system as such had been discarded.

As late as the 1860s, physicians used such heroic doctrines to justify the use of anesthetics. The theory of counterirritation was often cited as proving that the dangerous effects of pain neutralized the dangers of using anesthesia. "Pain and loss of blood may both be considered as counter-agents, which neutralize [ether's harmful] effects, and render them more safe," declared one physician. "I believe pain to be a preventive to the fatal effect of chloroform, because the sensory portion of the great nervous center will resist its influence with more tenacity and force than if there be no pain present," proclaimed a report of the Illinois State Medical Society in 1859. Practitioners attributed the effectiveness of anesthetics directly to their physically irritating or harmful properties, while others combined anesthesia with bloodletting to make it safer![11] "To say that any particular remedy is without danger—is entirely safe, is almost equivalent to saying it is of but little value," declared William M. Boling, professor of obstetrics at Transylvania University. "Every" drug "capable of producing a . . . curative influence, is more or less dangerous." Thus, he concluded, anesthetics had to be dangerous to work.[12]

Such arguments were especially common in obstetrics, because in childbirth, anesthetics were usually given only after the onset of pain. In labor, the anesthetic danger was neutralized by an already present pain, while in surgery, the anesthetic poison preceded the pain.[13]

Heroic therapies extended beyond the confines of the regular profession. Thus, the heroic defense of anesthesia was not limited to orthodox physicians. The Eclectic sect of healers also lauded the counterirritant benefits of ether and recommended violent counterirritation as an accompaniment or substitute for anesthetics.[14]

In addition to such technical theories, heroic medicine offered a more general precedent for anesthesia as well. The professional legitimacy accorded so many other potentially injurious medicines in the heroic era made it possible to justify the risks of anesthesia by ethical analogy. If the danger of inflammation justified calomel, purging, blistering, and bleeding, then surely the danger of pain ought to warrant the use of anesthetics. Thus, a report of the Medical Society of Virginia warned that the effects of anesthesia resembled "fatal disease or injury of the brain," and asked rhetorically, "Is it not rash presumption to lead a human being so close to the portals of death?" But, the 1851 report continued, bloodletting to unconsciousness was "even a more alarming condition" than etherization; yet "we do not hesitate to induce this state, not only in the treatment of those diseases whose fatal course requires them to be promptly and boldly arrested, but even when a dislocated limb is to be replaced, or an inflamed eye is to be relieved."[15] Concern over the risks of anesthetics, declared another physician, "if tenable at all would exclude by a parity of reasoning our most valuable articles from the materia medica."[16] Heroic medicine thus provided both a technical rationale and an ethical precedent for the use of dangerous anesthetics, to cure the dangerous "disease" of pain.

At the opposite pole of nineteenth-century medicine, the tenets of natural healing barred the use of anesthetics even when pain threatened life itself. Such prohibitions drew upon the scientific theory that natural pains were healthful and that human intervention was detrimental. But they owed their force to the underlying ethical theory, that no amount of benefit could justify a physician's actively inflicting harm. Dr. Samuel Gridley Howe, an orthodox physician turned hydropath, proclaimed the fundamental ethical doctrine of natural healing: "we have no right to do evil that good may come out of it." "The hydropath will never do harm even when he can do no good," declared the founders of the Elmira, N.Y., Water-Cure.[17] Natural healing linked the Hippocratic injunction to "do no harm" to the biblical commandment "thou shalt not kill," to prohibit the use of dangerous drugs, regardless of benefits.

Philadelphia obstetrician Charles Meigs cited both the technical objection to relieving natural pain and the ethical imperative to avoid harm, in a widely reprinted 1848 letter to James Simpson.

But should I exhibit the remedy for pain to a thousand patients in labor, merely to prevent the physiological pain . . . and if I should in consequence destroy only one of them, I should feel disposed to clothe me in sack-cloth, and cast ashes on my head for the remainder of my days. What sufficient motive have I to risk the life or death of even one in a thousand?[18]

John Upton Riggs, a University of Michigan medical student, captured the essence of this ethical doctrine in an 1868 attack on chloroform. "If a patient is killed while under its influence, does the fact that ten thousand others who have taken the same amount and escape unharmed, restore him to life, console his friends, or afford maintenance to his family."[19]

Rigid adherence to such values would have banned not only anesthesia but all surgery as well. Yet, by the 1860s, only a few extreme hydropaths practiced such pristine medical nihilism. Most of those who claimed to follow natural healing gave *priority* to passive measures without totally banning active remedies. They believed nature morally and medically preferable to art but still allowed some use of dangerous therapies sometimes including surgery and anesthesia. Such physicians would incur a very slight risk of doing harm, provided that the benefits were vastly greater than the dangers.[20] Still, the more closely a practitioner adhered to the doctrines of strictly natural healing, the less medically and morally acceptable anesthesia became.

Conservative medicine offered mid-nineteenth-century

physicians an alternative to both heroic and natural healing. What distinguished conservative decisionmaking was the assumption that a balance could be struck between natural and inflicted dangers, a middle course in which the distinction between acts of commission and acts of omission would no longer influence professional decisions. New York physician Austin Flint's second law of conservative medicine stated it well: "Not to do harm is no less an object of treatment than to do good."[21] "There is a vantage ground between the two extremes," another conservative spokesman claimed, "neither verging towards meddlesome interference on the one hand, nor imbecile neglect on the other."[22]

Applied to anesthesia, medical conservatism demanded a "middle course"[23] between the dangers of pain and the dangers of painkillers. As the Philadelphia *Medical Examiner* explained, "We deprecate alike the excessive enthusiasm which insists that under no possible circumstances, ether can be, or ever has been prejudicial, and the unreasonable timidity which prevents the employment of a useful agent, because, in a few cases, injurious effects have been apparently occasioned by it."[24]

This conservative search for a "middle course" between Art and Nature was closely tied to nineteenth-century advances in medical statistics, particularly the revolutionary applications of mathematics to assessments of drug safety and efficacy developed in Paris by Pierre Louis. These techniques, combining recent advances in calculus and probability theory with the utilitarian ethics of Bentham, allowed physicians to measure the risks and benefits of a drug, without invoking such ethical absolutes as the traditional injunction to "do no harm." Louis and his followers taught that neither the inflicted harm done by therapeutic side effects nor the natural damage of untreated pathology was inherently preferable to the other. Rather, the physicians's task was to compare directly the objective statistical magnitude of each harm regardless of its source and act so as to maximize the overall benefit to the patient. The British scientist Sir John Herschell captured the newness and wonder of this therapeutic calculus in 1850.

Men began to hear with surprise, not unmixed with some vague hope of ultimate benefit that not only births, deaths, and marriages, but . . . the comparative value of medical remedies, and different modes of treatment of disease . . . might come to be surveyed with the lynx-eyed scrutiny of a dispassionate analysis.[25]

This new calculus of safety formed a central tenet of American conservative professionalism. Worthington Hooker, for example, insisted on the "accurate adjustment of remedial means to the ends to be accomplished." When deciding on the use of a dangerous drug, "the truly judicious physician is neither bewildered nor precipitate" but carefully chooses his course by measuring the benefits and risks—"this nice balancing of probabilities." Hooker's one specific illustration of this crucial process involved the decision to prescribe opium for severe pain.[26]

Hooker's insistence on careful measurement and direct comparison between means and ends in therapy was reflected in the advice of many conservative American physicians concerning the relative dangers of pain and of anesthetics. "If the injurious effect of the means used be less than that of the pain prevented, we are justified in employing them" proclaimed Valentine Mott's handbook on anesthetics.[27] Anesthetics "should be administered in all cases where the danger would be greater without than with them," a University of Pennsylvania medical student explained. The *New York Journal of Medicine* ruled "that etherization may be expedient where the danger from the shock of an operation is greater than from inhaling the poison." A University of Michigan medical student summed up the conservative view, in 1871: "If a remedy is dangerous we are morally bound not to use it, unless withholding it involves a greater danger still."[28]

Only statistical measurement could determine which danger was greatest. The editor of the *Western Lancet* explained, "The question then for solution, is, whether the immediate effects and the secondary consequences of the inhalation of ether may not be more prejudicial, than the effects of pain during a surgical operation." He concluded that "the only method by which this can be accomplished is *statistical observations*."[29] A medical student of 1853 put it this way: "Men of science have differed in opinion" concerning how to weigh "that most terrible of obstacles, *pain,* and the nervous shock produced thereby," against "the injurious effects following the use of these valuable agents." "Statistics can afford the only unfailing criterion and are indispensable to the formation of a judgment—they should be allowed to speak for themselves."[30] The problem thus became entirely technical. The risks and benefits of pain-relievers could be measured and the decision made according to a "rational" calculus. The physician's duty was to minimize total harm—not to make value distinctions between one type of harm and another.

By the 1850s, this mathematical approach to medical ethics enjoyed considerable professional acceptance in the United States.[31] Thus, in the decade following Morton's ether demonstration, medical journals repeatedly attempted to quantify the relative value of anesthetics. Though many of these studies suffered from a very primitive understanding of statistics, they clearly reflected the importance of mathematics in the conservatives' attempt to choose between conflicting versions of professional duty.[32]

But, as Austin Flint repeatedly pointed out, medical conservatism did not simply follow from medical statistics. Such explanations of conservatism, Flint declared, "will go only a little way. The change is one of sentiment." The desire to find a moderate course between conflicting approaches in medicine preceded acceptance of Louis' methods. Medical statistics did not create medical conservatism; rather it was because conservatives were already seeking a way to synthesize the divisive ethical and therapeutic conflicts of nineteenth-century medicine that they turned to statistical techniques. Conservative medicine was more than simply the result of quantitative measurement; it was an *a priori* ideological commitment to moderation, reunification, and synthesis in a badly divided profession. The key to understanding medical conservatism, according to Dr. Henry I. Bowditch, was the deep conviction that, in all areas of medicine, "evil is good run mad."[33]

Faced with the need to choose between the dangers of pain and the dangers of anesthesia, nineteenth-century physicians could turn to three different professional ideologies for both scientific and ethical guidance. Heroic medicine sanctioned aggressive risk-taking to combat the disease of pain, while natural healing rejected all dangerous drugs, regardless of the alleged benefits. Only the new doctrines of conservative medicine attempted to combine the competing claims of Art and Nature, to equate acts of omission and commission. In an explicit attempt to synthesize the scientific and ethical conflicts racking the profession, conservative medicine sought to reduce morality to mathematics, to measure objectively whether the "cure" or the "disease" constituted the "lesser evil."

MEDICINE AS METAPHOR: NATURE VS. ART

At least on the level of metaphor, mid-nineteenth-century Americans saw parallels between the conflicts rending medicine and those in many other areas of life. Like physicians, American social reformers divided sharply over the choice between active and passive means.[34] Some preached a passive strategy of "moral suasion" and "nonresistance." Others advocated a violent confrontation with the forces of evil. Each side drew upon medical images to justify themselves or attack their opposition. In education and penology, for example, opponents of active means denounced forceful and physical punishments as "the calomel of culture,"[35] while opponents of passive techniques labeled moral suasion as moral "homeopathy."[36]

The climax of this conflict was, of course, the apocalypse of Civil War. Not surprisingly, activist supporters of war justified themselves by reference to heroic medicine; just as heroic practitioners had previously portrayed themselves as warriors against disease. "The American People are under treatment, they need to be cured" explained the *New York Tribune* in 1862. "The disease is chronic and deep-seated; but the treatment is heroic, and must ultimately prevail. Have faith, be patient, and on with the War for the Union!" For activist reformers, there could be no cure except to purge the land with blood.[37] Conversely, nonresistant Garrisonians of the 1840s had used the same analogy between force and heroic medicine to denounce both.[38]

Moderate reformers, who sought some limited means of action short of all-out heroic battle, often portrayed themselves as conservative physicians. Free-Soilers, for example, spoke of themselves as limiting the disease of slavery to the affected areas, while allowing nature to cure the seat of the illness.[39] For Walt Whitman, the conservative physician's careful straddling between Art and Nature offered virtually the only guiding principle for moderates in the immoderate days of war.[40]

But as the Civil War dragged on it became apparent that society and medicine were changing in opposite directions. While physicians were abandoning heroic medical remedies, the nation was subjected to increasingly heroic social remedies. By war's end even the staunchest opponents of heroic medicine came to use heroic therapy as a metaphor to justify the vast national bloodletting.[41]

The Calculus of Suffering: Choosing Between Suffering and Death

Anesthesia not only lessened the physical impact of pain; its main benefit was the prevention of suffering. Thus, the most crucial choice physicians faced in using anesthetics was to decide the relative priority of suffering and safety. If the prevention of suffering could be achieved only by risking the side effects of anesthetic drugs, were the benefits worth the cost? How much suffering had to be averted; how safe did anesthesia have to be, to justify taking the risk?

The discovery of anesthesia thus raised one of the most basic dilemmas in defining a doctor's professional duties. "I most conscientiously believe that the proud mission of the physician is distinctly twofold—namely, to alleviate human suffering, as well as preserve human life," wrote Dr. James Y. Simpson, the Edinburgh pioneer of chloroform anesthesia. Doctors in Western cultures are expected to restore health and preserve life; they are also expected to combat suffering. But what is the proper professional behavior when these obligations conflict? What should a physician do when pain relief requires giving a dangerous drug—or conversely, when curing a dangerous disease requires the use of painful remedies? Should life be preserved absolutely, no matter what the cost in anguish? Should all suffering be relieved regardless of the risk to life? No sane person would want to inflict more suffering or more risk than necessary; but what constitutes "necessity," and for what ends? Should an agonized cancer patient be given a potentially deadly dose of painkillers? Should painful therapies be used to gain a brief prolongation of life in a terminal illness? Most physicians today would agree there is *some* point at which the duty to relieve suffering overrides the duty to prolong life. But what is that point? Clearly, no one standard can provide a universal response to such conflicts. Some people risk death itself to avoid even minor pain; others suffer intense agonies to avert slight dangers. This problem of choosing between relieving suffering and preserving life is as old as medicine itself. The prehistoric healer who first discovered the blessing and the curse of the opium poppy faced an identical dilemma.[42]

One way physicians have sought to resolve such conflicts has been to develop a common set of professional values—formal or informal ideals, which serve to guide practitioners when weighing a choice between such basic duties.[43] The ideology of professionalism, whether expressed in formal ethics codes or imparted through informal traditions, can provide an agreed-upon set of general values that may guide doctors in reaching a specific course of action in such situations. Thus, in deciding on the use of anesthetics, midcentury surgeons had available a long tradition of preexisting professional values, ideals, and standards of behavior created over centuries of medical practice to deal with many other more or less similar choices.

But the values that constitute professionalism are not static. They are constantly subject to change, both as a result of new medical techniques and of new social conditions. In conflicts between relieving and curing, for example, the medical profession has decided very differently at different times.

The mid-nineteenth century was one period of great change and conflict over such basic questions of professional values. A new social awareness of, and sensitivity to, suffering helped shape such disparate movements as antislavery and antivivisection. Looking back on this era, philosopher Charles Peirce reportedly proposed that the nineteenth century be remembered as the ''Age of Pain.''[44] Accompanying this change in social values, midcentury physicians experienced a technical revolution in the treatment of pain: the isolation of morphine, cocaine, and heroin; the invention of the hypodermic syringe, and, most dramatically, the discovery of inhalation anesthesia. These changes, both in social attitudes and medical techniques, combined to alter profoundly the professional values of nineteenth-century doctors; the new professional outlook in turn shaped medical use of the new painkillers.

At the start of the nineteenth century, the majority tradition in Western medical ethics was hostile to any efforts at relieving suffering if they involved a risk to life. But in the mid-1800s, a growing number of practitioners turned toward the more utilitarian standards of conservative medicine. The conservative model of professionalism allowed, even required, a degree of risk-taking proportional to the degree of pain relieved. This revolution in professional attitudes drew upon the sentimental romanticism of literature and the arts, the benevolent humanitarianism of social reformers, the calculating mentality of the new medical statisticians, and the sharp competition from rival medical sects. But, most fundamentally, the new medical approach to suffering was rooted in American physicians' search for a moderate consensus ideology, to reunite their seriously divided profession.

"SHARP COMPASSION": THE SUPREMACY OF LIFE

> The wounded surgeon plies the steel
> That questions the distempered part;
> Beneath the bleeding hands we feel
> The sharp compassion of the healer's art
> —T.S. Eliot[45]

It is hard for us today to re-create the impact of pre-anesthetic practice on the feelings of the surgeon. The emotional ability to inflict vast suffering was perhaps the most basic of all professional prerequisites. A nineteenth-century anesthesia promoter recalled the once commonly required procedure to repair a dislocated hip.

Big drops of perspiration, started by the excess of agony, bestrew the patient's forehead, sharp screams burst from him in peal after peal—all his struggles to free himself and escape the horrid torture, are valueless, for he is in the powerful hands of men then as inexorable as death. . . . At last the agony becomes too great for human endurance, and with a wild, despairing yell, the sufferer relapses into unconsciousness.[46]

Under such conditions, the professional values adopted by surgeons for most of Western history emphasized that the saving of life held absolute priority over the avoidance of suffering. The Hippocratic tradition even forbade physicians from providing pain relievers to patients judged incurable. The intent of such prohibitions may have been to prevent euthanasia, to protect the physician's reputation, and/or to save the patient's money. But the implication was clearly that cure, not pain relief, was the overriding medical duty.[47]

Surgical practice was no license to torture. "On no account should one cause needless pain," Hippocrates cautioned surgeons. But no suffering which might save lives was defined to be "needless."[48] "Now a surgeon should be . . . filled with pity, so that he wishes to cure his patient, yet is not moved by his cries, to go too fast, or cut less than is necessary; but he does everything just as if the cries of pain cause him no emotion," insisted the first century A.D. physician Celsus. His injunction helped define surgical professional duty for centuries thereafter. Like Hippocrates, Celsus sanctioned neither callousness nor indifference. He required the surgeon to feel "pity" for the patient. But feelings of pity ought neither to affect the surgeon's actions nor to interfere with the infliction of the vast suffering necessary to fight death. Thus Celsus also opposed the use of dangerous painkillers and narcotics.[49] Surgeons were required to inflict tremendous suffering whenever "necessary" to save life yet without losing their humanity in the process.

For many early-nineteenth-century surgical students, learning to inflict pain according to these dicta of Celsus constituted the single hardest part of their professional training. Benjamin Rush's student Philip Syng Physick, the first American to gain prominence as a full-time surgeon, became so sick at his initial amputation that he had to be carried from the room in midoperation.[50] A British doctor recalled one of his earliest surgical experiences.

As the operation, which was necessarily a lengthy and slow one, proceeded, her cries became more and more terrible; first one and then another student fainted, and ultimately all but a determined few had left the theatre unable to stand the distressing scene.

Another reminisced in 1887 that "the pupils of the present day do not faint as *we* used to do before . . . anaesthetics."[51] Those who could not learn to believe the suffering was worth it had to leave the profession. Samuel Cooper's early-nineteenth-century textbook cautioned prospective young surgeons to heed the example of the Swiss physiologist Haller. According to Cooper, Haller studied diligently to become a surgeon but he failed in practice, due to his "fear of giving too much pain." Young Charles Darwin likewise witnessed two operations at Edinburgh but was so upset by the pain that he fled from the hospital and abandoned all plans for a medical career. Cooper told aspiring young surgeons to learn well the "excellent" precept of Celsus: "this undisturbed coolness, which is still more rare than skill, is the most valuable quality in the practice of surgery."[52]

The emotional outlook required to practice such painful cures was an acquired skill gained through professional training and experience. Asa Fitch of New York, a student at Rutgers in the winter of 1828, kept a journal of the process by which the emotions of a young man were transformed into the emotions of a professional surgeon. At the beginning, the sight of a leg amputation left him devastated.

> But, oh, how my feelings recoiled at the sight! To behold the keen shining knife drawn around the leg severing the integuments, while the unhappy subject of the operation uttered the most heart rending screams in his agony and torment, . . . to hear the saw working its way through the bone, produced an impression I can never forget.

But after only a few weeks of witnessing such pain and copying the impassivity of his professional mentors, Fitch could boast about "a most tedious and painful operation" on a young child, "I had none of the tenderness which I have always before felt on such occasions."[53]

Not surprisingly, those who managed to overcome their revulsion and master the professional ability to inflict suffering took a certain pride in their accomplishment. British surgeon John Hunter claimed that there was a certain "*éclat* generally attending painful operations, often only because they are so." And, also not surprisingly, the practice of surgery did sometimes produce callousness, despite Celsus's careful injunction.[54] (Henri de Mondeville, the thirteenth-century surgeon to Philip the Fair, believed the two professional prerequisites for a surgeon were a strong stomach and the ability to "cut like an executioner.")[55]

While the traditions and training of pre-anesthetic surgeons thus sanctioned the infliction of agonizing remedies whenever necessary to save life, practitioners varied widely in their concept of "necessity." For most, operations generally remained the surgeon's last resort, employed only when every other hope of cure was gone. Such surgical reticence derived mainly from the appalling mortality rates, the product of uncontrollable infections, hemorrhage, and shock. In major limb amputations, 30 to 50 percent death rates were not uncommon.[56] As a result, both surgeons and patients avoided operations as long as possible (thus perhaps further inflating the surgical mortality). But, at least some surgeons cited suffering, not simply mortality, as their reason for avoiding the knife. An eighteenth-century British surgical text declared, "Painful methods are always the last remedies in the hands of a man that is truly able in his profession; and they are the first, or rather they are the only resources of him whose knowledge is confined to the art of operating."[57]

Within this general pre-anesthetic tradition, early-nineteenth-century American physicians and surgeons gained a reputation for the particularly unrestrained infliction of excruciating remedies. Central to the notoriety of American practice as uniquely harsh and cruel was the medical system of Benjamin Rush. Rush employed heroic doses of painful remedies, based on the belief that pain could cure illness. Rush held that a body could have only one disease at a time. Since he considered pain itself to be a disease, inflicting great pain on a patient could drive the disease from his body. For example, Rush speculated, "whipping" and "hot iron" would cure a case of poisoning.[58] In short, Rush recommended "that bold humanity which dictates the use of powerful but painful remedies in violent diseases."[59]

A skilled propagandist, Rush promoted his therapies in part by convincing practitioners and patients alike that they were "heroic," "bold," courageous, manly, and patriotic. Americans were tougher than Europeans; American diseases were correspondingly tougher than mild European diseases; to cure Americans would require uniquely painful doses administered by heroic American physicians.[60]

Whether or not American physicians really inflicted more pain than Europeans, Rush's rhetoric led observers on both sides of the Atlantic to assume they did. In the West especially, "mildness of medical treatment is real cruelty," wrote a popular Cincinnati medical author. What was needed, he declared, was a "vigorous mode of practice; the diseases of our own country especially require it."[61]

The heroic reliance on extreme measures regardless of pain was hardly limited to orthodox practitioners. Thomsonians, botanics, and Eclectics also burned, bled, or blistered their patients to drive out life-threatening diseases.[62]

In surgery as in medicine, Americans portrayed their

practice as uniquely painful. "Frontier" surgeons like Ephraim McDowell, Nathan Smith, and J. Marion Sims developed new operations that, they bragged, Europeans had been too sensitive and timid to perform. Nationalistic Americans pointed with vast pride to the agonizing accomplishments of their surgeons as examples of the virile new culture of the young Republic. American surgeons attributed their successes in part to a frontier stoicism lacking in effete Old World practitioners; European critics denounced American practice as an example of frontier barbarism and cruelty.[63] William Gibson's popular textbook summed up the spirit of American surgical practice in the first decades of the nineteenth century. Gibson advised that even the most "severe pain should never be an obstacle" to the performance of life-preserving operations.[64]

Thus, in the half-century before the discovery of anesthesia, American physicians and surgeons generally defined professional duty as demanding the unhesitating infliction of extreme suffering in order to save lives. Reared in this tradition, many midcentury practitioners found it understandably difficult to sanction the use of drugs that had the power to relieve suffering at the risk of life. This response can be seen most starkly in the reaction of some American practitioners to the discovery of anesthesia. Not surprisingly, more than a few insisted that the duty to preserve life absolutely outweighed the duty to relieve what one doctor revealingly termed "mere anguish."[65] Writing in the prestigious *American Journal of the Medical Sciences* in 1852, David F. Condie declared flatly, "It may be our duty to inflict pain to *save life*, but [we] can scarcely be warranted in *risking life* merely to avoid pain."[66] An opponent of chloroform based his position on "the absolute and supreme respect for human life which gives grandeur and dignity to our art." An 1857 editorial by Jonathan Dawson in the *Ohio Medical and Surgical Journal* stated, "Better suffer a little pain, than not be perfectly . . . *safe.*" The *New York Journal of Medicine* ruled that "immunity of pain merely, should never be purchased at the risk of life."[67]

For these practitioners, the duty to preserve life was absolute; the duty to prevent suffering was recognized, but only when there was virtually no degree of physical danger involved. Thus, a Philadelphia medical student admitted, "The mission of the physician is undoubtedly two-fold—to relieve human pain as well as to preserve human life." Yet one had clear priority over the other. "En-

dangering the life of our patient, merely for the purpose of relieving
. . . from pain,'' he found totally ''unjustifiable.'' These physicians,
it must be emphasized, did not claim suffering was necessarily good
nor that doctors should not try to prevent it; only that no risk to life
should be taken for that purpose. Their position did not rule out the
use of anesthetics, if they could be shown to have other advantages,
such as saving life or preventing disease, or if the dangers could be
totally eliminated. The AMA Committee on Obstetrics ruled anesthesia an acceptable cure for uterine spasms, declaring, ''Here, the
question being not to relieve pain or obtain other minor advantage,
but to cure a disease always dangerous and often fatal, the argument
against the use of etherization, that we endanger life for inadequate
reasons, does not apply.'' Although ''immunity of pain, merely'' never
justified ''the risk of life,'' the *New York Journal of Medicine* agreed
''that etherization may be expedient'' where there was ''danger from
the shock of an operation.'' Even Samuel Gregory conceded that, in
''surgical operations, where, in addition to the pain, the shock to the
system might be perilous to life, the use of ether would be advisa-
ble.''[68] The question here was not whether anesthesia had any legitimate uses but whether the relief of *suffering* ever justified the risk to
life anesthetics were believed to pose. On that narrower issue, many
midcentury physicians answered, ''never.''

A MEASURE OF RELIEF

However, a growing number of other physicians angrily
disagreed with such an absolute standard. They urged the use of anesthesia, based on what they claimed was a professional duty to prevent
suffering, even when that meant taking some risks with life. ''Pain is
only evil . . . . We are not required to possess an innocuous agent''
to fight it, declared New York surgeon Valentine Mott. John Erichsen's
influential textbook, *The Science and Art of Surgery,* urged students
to accept the fact that ''we cannot purchase immunity from suffering
without incurring a certain degree of danger.'' In an 1851 textbook,
one New York surgeon told students that the relief of suffering was
worth the cost, even though ''I know that, in urging upon the profession the *duty,* . . . . of using anaesthetics, I may be instrumental in
the destruction of human life.''[69]

The most extreme form of pain relief at the expense of
life is, of course, euthanasia. While no mid-nineteenth-century Amer-

ican physician openly advocated using anesthesia for "mercy killing," several came close. In 1860, Samuel Dickson defended the use
of chloroform, even though it proved "fatal to a considerable number" of patients, by arguing that

> in the great majority of these death was already impending, and there was
> only the substitution of a prompt and painless termination of life for a
> succession of cruel and protracted tortures. There was probably great gain
> in the exchange.[70]

Others went so far as to urge its use for the painless execution of
condemned criminals.[71] And, as early as 1848, the surgeon in Morton's initial demonstration, Boston's eminent John Collins Warren,
published the case histories of patients for whom he had used ether
to provide "euthanasia"—a painless (but not more rapid) death—in
terminal cancer.[72]

The new willingness to take risks purely for the relief of
suffering can be seen not only in the use of anesthetics but in other
areas of medicine as well. The prescription of alcohol and opiates to
relieve suffering (not simply to treat disease or prevent shock) appears to have increased by the mid-nineteenth century, particularly in
surgery.[73] An even clearer indication of the new attitude was the gradual
introduction of surgical operations whose only anticipated benefit was
the mitigation of suffering. Thus in 1848 J. Mason Warren urged the
AMA to sanction operations "as a palliative" for painful incurable
breast cancers. Philadelphia surgeon Henry H. Smith taught his students in 1855 to operate on such cases "not with any view of curing
the patient but simply for purposes of making Life pleasant and death
easier."[74] During the Civil War, Silas Weir Mitchell began experiments with neurosurgery for the relief of chronic pain in nonterminal
injuries.[75] In each of these cases, patients were subjected to the dangers and mutilations of an operation, with little if any hope of curing
an organic disease, but purely for relief. The growing legitimacy of
risk-taking for the relief of suffering may also be seen in the accel-
erating number of experiments using mesmerism, freezing, compres-
sion, and other unproven or hazardous techniques to reduce the agony
of surgical operations. In this experimental series, Morton's ether
demonstration was neither the first nor the last.[76]

What led to this new level of medical concern for suffering? The decision to risk life for the sake of relieving suffering did have some roots in ancient professional traditions, although few nineteenth-century physicians besides James Simpson sought out such precedents. One of the earliest proponents of this position was Aretaeus of Cappodoccia, who in the first century opposed the Hippocratic ban on giving pain relievers to the terminally ill.[77] In the following century, Galen also advocated the cautious use of some potentially dangerous anodynes.[78] At various times, other ancient and medieval practitioners employed potentially harmful substances to relieve the sufferings of disease and as surgical anodynes. The best known efforts involved opium, alcohol, and mandragora. In his diligent scholarly attempt to find precedents for the professional use of anesthetics, Dr. Simpson unearthed several similar experiments with potentially dangerous painkillers. But such practices appear to have declined in number and respectability long before the nineteenth century. In seventeenth-century France, for example, a barber-surgeon who attempted to develop an herbal anodyne was prosecuted by the medical establishment and fined heavily for endangering the lives of his patients.[79]

The modern revival of emphasis on the duty of doctors to relieve suffering began with Sir Francis Bacon. "I esteem it the office of a physician not only to restore health, but to mitigate pain and dolors; and not only when such mitigation may conduce to recovery, but when it may serve to make a fair and easy passage," he declared in attacking Hippocratic professionalism in 1605.[80] A century and three quarters later, the Scottish medical essayist John Gregory still had an uphill fight to legitimate the relief of suffering for the dying, against the influence of Hippocratic tradtion.

Let me exhort you against the custom of some physicians, who leave their patients when their life is despaired of, and when it is no longer decent to put them to farther expense. It is as much the business of a physician to alleviate pain, and to smooth the avenues of death, when unavoidable, as to cure diseases.[81]

The most influential statement of this position came in Thomas Percival's *Medical Ethics*. Percival defined the physician's role as uniting "tenderness with steadiness" and urged that pain relievers be provided the terminally ill. His views were closely echoed by such American conservatives as Worthington Hooker and in the AMA code of ethics.[82]

Sectarian attacks on the painfulness of heroic treatment also played a role in raising the priority of pain relief among orthodox physicians. Those sects that advocated natural healing, groups like the homeopaths and hydropaths, routinely denounced the suffering inflicted by heroic practice. Patients, too, repeatedly cited painlessness as their major reason for choosing homeopathy over heroic practice. "Gladly would we see banished from the sick chamber the nauseous drugs, the offensive draughts, the pill, the powder, the potion, and all the painful and debilitating expedients of our present system, in favor of the mild and gentle measures of Homeopathy," declared the Boston *Christian Examiner*.[83] Just as the heroic physician's attitude toward pain was portrayed as particularly manly, homeopaths claimed that their own mildness attracted children and their mothers.[84] In fact, homeopathic founder Samuel Hahnemann denied that disease existed at all, apart from such symptoms as suffering. "There is nothing to cure but the sufferings of the patient," he declared.[85] A Philadelphia homeopathic student took this doctrine to mean that "the relief of suffering" was "the sole object" of the homeopathic profession.[86]

The rise of natural healing sects thus called attention to the importance of relieving suffering and offered patients an alternative to the agonies of heroic therapy. But, contrary to the claims of its practitioners, natural healing was not always less painful than heroic treatment. The active infliction of suffering was certainly a small part of these sects' practice. But when followed strictly, natural healing banned clinically effective use of opium, morphine, alcohol, ether, chloroform, nitrous oxide, and most other painkillers. The natural healing sects did not require the doctor to inflict much suffering but they offered little active relief. As Dr. Oliver Wendell Holmes pointed out, the only "natural anaesthetics" were "sleep, fainting, death."[87]

Natural healing taught sympathy with suffering but would not sanction active, artificial, or risky measures to relieve it. As late as 1892, a New York practitioner held to the stern commandments of pure homeopathic medical ethics.

To stand at the bedside of a sufferer whose groans and moans bespeak his agony and excite the sympathies of his sorrowing family; to listen to their entreaties to the doctor to "do something" for the relief of the patient; and surrounded thus . . . calmly to watch the development of the case, . . . truly, this is a great test of moral character.[88]

Jacob Beakley likewise denounced the use of anesthesia, in the 1865 *Transactions of the Homoeopathic Medical Society of New York:* "the conscientious surgeon can never cease to reflect that the great object of his art is the preservation of human life, and that the lessening of human suffering is only the second."[89]

On most issues, heroic and natural healing represented opposite poles of nineteenth-century medicine. Yet for opposite reasons, both heroic and natural healers equally condemned the use of drugs to relieve suffering, if the painkillers posed a risk to life. Both doctrines banned anesthetics as too dangerous to use purely for suffering. Sectarian competition may have helped mitigate the painfulness of heroic therapy, but natural healing itself provided no sanction for the use of active painkillers.

Nineteenth-century criticism of medical callousness was hardly limited to sectarian natural healers, however. Popular sentimentalist authors across the nation produced a torrent of demands for more sensitivity to feelings in the practice of the professions. This romantic outpouring clearly played a role in heightening medical concern over suffering, though its effect in legitimating dangerous pain relievers was subtle and indirect.

Public pressure for physicians to feel more emotional involvement with their patients grew increasingly insistent over the antebellum years.

Assuredly it is not a pulseless, tideless being that is desired to officiate at the couch of sickness. Rather is the man most acceptable as a physician who most approximates the feminine type; who is kind, and gentle, and cautious, and sympathetic, and truthful, and delicately modest,

according to a typical expression of such sentiments in the *Philadelphia Bulletin.*[90] One of the most caustic attacks on unfeeling surgery was Herman Melville's 1850 portrait of Dr. Cadwallader Cuticle in *White-Jacket.* Cuticle is hard, callous, and unfeeling.

Nothing could exceed his coolness when actually employed in his imminent vocation. Surrounded by moans and shrieks, by features distorted with an-

guish inflicted by himself, he yet maintained a countenance almost super-
naturally calm. . . . Yet you could not say that Cuticle was essentially a
cruel-hearted man. His apparent heartlessness must have been of a purely
scientific origin. It is not to be imagined even that Cuticle would have harmed
a fly, unless he could procure a microscope powerful enough to assist him
in experimenting on the minute vitals of the creature.[91]

But Cuticle's cold, mechanical science is an external shell, designed
to cover his real feelings—not the pangs of compassion, but perverse
and sadistic pleasure.

Cuticle, on some occasions, would affect a certain disrelish of his profession, and declaim against the necessity that forced a man of his humanity to
perform a surgical operation. Especially was it apt to be thus with him, when
the case was one of more than ordinary interest. In discussing it, previous
to setting about it, he would veil his eagerness under an aspect of great cir-
cumspection; curiously marred, however, by continual sallies of unsuppress-
able impatience.[92]

Conservative physicians generally endorsed such criticisms of the unfeeling practice of medicine. In 1849, Henry J. Bigelow urged curriculum reform at the Harvard Medical School in order "to re-establish a facility in the manifestation of that kindly feeling
which is generally upon the surface in early youth, but which sometimes in the process of education gets embedded beneath a stratum of
indifference and insensibility." Conservative spokesmen like Worthington Hooker insisted that "humane sympathies" actually exceeded technical "skill" in medical importance. In 1848, the New
York surgeon Alexander H. Stevens told the AMA, "Our profession,
gentlemen, is the link that unites Science and Philanthropy."[93]

As expressed by such physicians, the demand for senti-
ment and feeling contained more than a little elitist bias. The callousness of heroic medicine was blamed on the general decline of those
genteel graces that supposedly had elevated the tone of the eighteenth-century professional. Elitist physicians equated the lack of sensitivity in treatment with a lack of sensibility in manner. They dismissed the average nineteenth-century practitioner as "uncouth in his
manners, vulgar and indelicate in his language, slovenly in his dress,
and harsh and unfeeling in his treatment."[94] While followers of Rush
had expounded the need for harshness in democratic and especially

Western medicine, critics scorned the resulting insensitivity as a form of rustic barbarism increasingly limited to "country physicians." [95]

Midcentury romanticism, with its denunciation of scientific callousness and its appeal for more attention to feelings in medicine, clearly played an important role in legitimating a new medical sensitivity toward suffering. To a young medical student like John Wesley Thompson, the surgeon's duty seemed to derive entirely from sentimentalism.

Who can realize what is meant by intense pain and not feel himself called upon to relieve its victim? Surely no one who has a spark of sympathy within his breast. There are some who think a Surgeon, or Physician should not feel, or heed such things; but as well bid the ocean be still, or the mother forget her first-born, as to enforce such a sentiment. It is treason against humanity. [96]

But despite such purple prose, medical willingness to take active risks for the relief of human agonies did not derive directly from romantic sentimentalism. As Worthington Hooker emphasized, *sympathizing* with pain did not necessarily lead to *relieving* it. Hooker insisted upon distinguishing between attacks on medical callousness that sprang from a mawkish wallowing in misery, and true medical benevolence, which came from "active" risktaking to relieve suffering.

The single most important source of support for the profession's new willingness to risk life in the relief of suffering was the ideology of conservative medicine. Natural healing sanctioned sentimental concern for suffering but prohibited dangerous drugs; heroic medicine legitimated risk-taking but not for the relief of suffering. In their effort to mediate between these two rival doctrines, conservatives combined the heroic tolerance for danger with the sensitivity of natural healing. Their synthesis of art and nature thus led to a new concept of medical duty, a hybrid that Hooker termed "active sympathy." While neither heroic nor natural healing sanctioned active remedies for suffering, the new conservative synthesis did. Hooker summarized the new approach.

It has sometimes been said, that the physician, from his familiarity with scenes of distress, becomes unfeeling, and incapable of sympathizing with others.

. . . True, he will not have that mawkish sensibility which vents itself in tears, and sighs, and expressions of pity, but stops short of action . . . . If he ever had any of such romantic and unpractical sensibility, he has cast it off in his actual service in the field of benevolence, into which his profession has necessarily led him. He has learned over and over, the lesson of *active* sympathy. . . . He may seem to be devoid of sympathy, as he goes to work midst scenes of suffering, without a tear, or even a sigh, performing his duties with an unblanched face, a cool and collected air, and a steady hand, while all around are full of fear, and trembling, and pity. Yet there *is* sympathy in his bosom, but it is *active*. It vents itself in the right way—in doing.[97]

Likewise Jacob Bigelow declared the alleviation of suffering to be a basic professional duty. This goal could be accomplished by passive, active, or "cautious" means, though the more active the painkiller, the greater the danger. Thus, in deciding which course to follow, the rational conservative physician needed to balance the total "good" against the total "harm" and act to maximize overall benefit. Bigelow clearly expected this calculus to favor the moderate "cautious" use of potentially harmful painkillers.[98]

MEDICINE AS METAPHOR: BETWEEN BENEVOLENCE AND BRUTALITY

The nineteenth-century cult of the sentiments originated outside of medicine. It pervaded Victorian literature, art, religion, and reform; its most popular mass exponents were the women's magazines. In this world, suffering constituted a peak of emotional sublimity. The Christlike suffering and death of innocent mothers and infants for the redemption of a heartless masculine world constituted the stock theme of such immensely popular periodical writers as Lydia H. Sigourney. Sentimentalists denounced the infliction of pain not only for damaging the victim but also for dehumanizing and brutalizing the perpetrator. "Thou wilt give them hardness of heart, thy curse unto them," summarized the text upon which Sigourney warned husbands, employers, slave owners, and animal drivers to refrain from cruelty.[99]

But, as Hooker pointed out in a medical context, the relation between such sentimental rhetoric and the active relief of human suffering was quite ambiguous. To sentimentalists, pain was degrading, but suffering could be ennobling. Sentimentalism thus called attention to suffering in a new and vivid way but provided two conflicting behavioral responses. In the case of *Uncle Tom's Cabin,* sentimentalism lent a dramatic new urgency to the attack on human misery. In the writings of Lydia Sigourney, it provided only bathos and catharsis. Sentimentalism remained an ambiguous force in nineteenth-century America, equally capable of inspiring a crusade against pain or a self-indulgent wallow in perpetual suffering.[100]

And although sentimentalism deeply influenced some segments of American thought, it left other parts of society unmoved. In contrast to the emotional outpourings over suffering that dominated liberal theology, belles lettres, humanitarian reform, and the popular periodicals, midcentury America also witnessed the growth of a masculine cult of toughness and callousness. This anti-sentimental glorification of insensitivity took two very different forms: one, a reaffirmation of the traditional manly ability to endure pain; the other, a newer, more mechanical form of indifference to suffering.

The traditional cult of manly endurance especially filled the mythology (and perhaps the reality) of the violent frontier. Americans who adopted the scarred and bullet-riddled figure of Andrew Jackson as the "symbol for an age," were responding to Old Hickory's ability to take it and dish it out. And Jackson's Democratic Party had no monopoly on such virility, as the monotonous succession of military presidents testified. America remained largely immune to such sophisticated, aristocratic European devotees of pain as de Sade or Swinburne, but the antipathy was based on class and anti-intellectual prejudices rather than on repugnance toward the enjoyment of suffering itself. Thus, the Republic spawned its own virile, populist, backwoods de Sades, like George Washington Harris. Harris, a prototypically obscure folk humorist from Tennessee, created in Sut Lovingood a character for whom violence and sadism were the epitome of good clean American fun.[101]

But the machine age brought a new form of masculine insensitivity, more in tune with an era of commerce and technology. American commercial boosters bragged that our new indifference to the price of progress—steamboat explosions, railroad accidents, factory mutilations—was what enabled us to surpass the effete and decadently sensitive Europeans. In the more traditional world of Andrew Jackson, the pains of war had offered the rewards of manly glory. But following the mechanical butchery of the Civil War, combat was reduced to a meaningless hell. Hardened insensitivity, not heroic endurance, now seemed the only appropriate response.[102]

To resolve the paradoxical nature of nineteenth-century social attitudes toward pain, *both* the romantic preoccupation with suffering and the antiromantic cults of hardness and unfeeling must be seen as interrelated aspects of the midcentury penchant for dichotomizing all facets of human life. Victorian social iconography divided the world into two separate and distinct spheres—Head vs. Heart, Reason vs. Sentiment, World vs. Home, Art vs. Nature—all seen as reflections of the great division between Masculine and Feminine.[103] But although these were two antithetical worlds, the existence of each depended on the existence of its opposite. To regard either the sentimental benevolence of Dorothea Dix or the mechanical, ruthless efficiency of William Tecumseh Sherman as uniquely characteristic of midcentury America would be to overlook the process of polarization by which each helped produce and define the other. Between romanticism and antiromanticism existed a profound dialectic of pain.[104]

While most nineteenth-century Americans dichotomized intellect and feelings (and, like Melville, thought of the surgeon as the archtypical unfeeling male), one American writer self-consciously set out to reverse the growing polarization of sensitivity and hardness, of male and female. And in so doing, he seized on the new conservative medical profession as the perfect metaphor to embody the balanced combination of contraries he glorified. That poet was Walt Whitman.

While sentimentalist writers regarded pain as the brutal, physical antithesis of the spiritual and sublime, Whitman rejected all such distinctions. Physical sensations were identical with the sublime. "Seeing, hearing, feeling, are miracles."[105] Perfectionists tended to view pain as merely useful, an evil necessary for punishing violators of God's natural laws. Whitman upheld the natural goodness of all bodily senses in and for themselves.

> All this I swallow, it tastes good, I like it
> well, it becomes mine,
> I am the man, I suffer'd, I was there.[106]

To live is to feel, and if living is good, then all feelings are good. Pain is a part of life; "Agonies are one of my changes of garments." [107] Even the pangs of death are a part of life and therefore partake of joyousness. [108]

In poetry and in life, Whitman found a powerful metaphor for this synthesis in the language and outlook of the new conservative medical ethic. The key to understanding Whitman's use of medical images is to realize that, like "Walt," nineteenth-century American doctors were striving to synthesize what others saw as contraries. Whitman's poetry presumed the validity of the conservative physician's claim to be "the link that unites Science and Philanthropy." Whitman once told some friends, "Were I looking about for a profession, I should choose that of a doctor. Yes; widely opposite as science and the emotional elements are, they might be joined in the medical profession." [109] For Whitman, the doctor, the surgeon, the accoucheur, the wound dresser, become the personae through whose being and language the union of benevolence and science, passive sympathy and active hardness, find expression.

> To his work without flinching the accoucheur comes. [110]

> I am firm with each, the pangs are sharp yet unavoidable, . . .
> These and more I dress with impassive hand
>   (yet deep in my breast, a fire, a burning flame.) [111]

Medicine, like sex, unites male hardness with female benevolence: "I do not hurt you any more than is necessary for you." [112]

Competition and Consensus

The revolution in nineteenth-century therapeutics is often portrayed as a struggle between the advocates of painful and brutal heroic medicine and the sectarian followers of gentle, painless natural healing. [113] Like all caricatures, this image captures one aspect of reality, but the full picture is more complex. Heroic physicians did inflict great suffering to preserve life, but they also would take risks to cure the "disease" of pain. While heroic professionalism would not sanction anesthesia to relieve suffering, it did justify anesthetics to prevent the damage done by pain. On the other hand, the doctrines of natural healing banned all dangerous drugs, regardless of benefits. While natural healers preached sympathy for suffering and inflicted no pain, they rejected anesthesia, and all other potent painkillers.

In fact, while sectarian pressure did help push orthodox physicians into moderating their painfully heroic therapies, it was probably competition with orthodox medicine that eventually forced many natural healers to adopt at least occasional use of active pain remedies.

By the 1870s, some use of anesthetics had been accepted by all but the most extreme natural healers. A survey of student theses at Philadelphia's Homoeopathic Medical College of Pennsylvania shows anesthesia in use by 1857, but only as a life-saving measure in surgery.[114] As late as 1869 students continued to denounce as unnatural the employment of anesthetics simply to relieve suffering or in even surgical obstetrics.[115] The Philadelphia *Hahnemannian Monthly* claimed in 1869 that "Homeopaths are far less inclined to the use of anaesthetics than allopaths."[116]

But by then, at least one of the college's students had adopted the conservative view in its entirety. John M. Criley's thesis of that year declared that "it is the Physicians duty to prescribe so long as the good resulting from his practice exceeds the evil. And why should not Ether or Chloroform be judged by the same rule as other medicine."[117] Similar developments took place at the University of Michigan's homeopathic department, where a cautious approval of anesthesia was the only view taught in J. G. Gilchrist's 1877 lectures on surgery.[118] By 1882 one Hahnemann Medical College student contemptuously dismissed both the "moral" and the "physiological" objections in reporting a series of 2,100 anesthetic deliveries.[119] Some even claimed ether as a homeopathic discovery.[120]

A minority of twentieth-century practitioners, those who still followed "good old fashioned simon-pure homeopathy," continued to denounce a homeopathic user of active painkillers as "a medical bastard."[121] But by 1915 homeopaths actually pioneered the dangerous but popular "twilight sleep" method of obstetric anesthesia.[122]

A similar schism between pure natural healing and a more conservative approach developed among hydropaths. By the 1870s, anesthetic surgery was performed at water-cure spas, from Elmira, New

York, to Battle Creek, Michigan, though the founders of the movement still denounced such unnatural acts.[123]

The new doctrines of conservative medicine thus served
to legitimate the use of anesthetics, for both suffering and pain, by
both orthodox and sectarian healers. In this new version of professional duty, a doctor's choice between the pros and cons of anesthesia depended, not on the distinction between Art and Nature, but
on a synthetic, utilitarian measurement of the ''lesser evil''—a calculus of suffering.[124]

The Calculus of Suffering and the Ethics of Professional Decisionmaking

In today's world, where cost-benefit analysis is a profession in itself, routinely used to decide questions from drug safety to
war and peace, it may be hard to recapture how radically the calculus
of suffering revolutionized the techniques of professional decisionmaking in medicine. It reflected a utilitarian philosophy, a social
moderation, a numerical frame of mind, and a quest for consensus,
none of which were prominent in American medicine before the
1830s.[125] The novelty of this calculus can be seen in the understated
incredulity of one 1859 British anesthesia textbook writer. ''Of late
it is even found necessary to give what is called a 'quantificative' value
. . . and it is said a patient . . . incurs a certain appreciable or definite decimal of danger from chloroform.''[126] It is perhaps even more
difficult for us to see any validity in alternative approaches, views
like those of Charles Meigs, that ''any surgical operation founded . . .
on some cold and calculating computation of benefits possible, I regard as of doubtful propriety.''[127] Yet a careful consideration of such
criticism reveals some major difficulties unsolved by the ''rational''
conservative calculus.

One problem faced by conservative physicians grew out
of the fact that most of the nineteenth-century *materia medica* flunked
the statistical test. To the surprise and discomfort of many conservatives, giving equal moral weight to natural and inflicted dangers did
not result in sanctioning an equal mixture of active and passive rem-

edies. Conservative medicine had seemed to offer a middle ground between heroic dosing and natural healing, a justification for the limited retention of such increasingly unpopular remedies as bleeding and purging.[128] But the statistical calculus that was supposed to be an alternative to therapeutic nihilism wound up more often than not simply confirming the natural healer's position that all drugs were unsafe. Such findings may have been good science, but they did not solve the problem of the doctor who saw conservatism as a moderate synthesis between action and inaction, the clinician who still felt some duty to *do something* for sick patients.[129]

For these conservatives, moderation and synthesis were the guiding principles; statistics and a utilitarian calculus were useful because they were expected to confirm the preconceived balance between Art and Nature. But if the calculus produced an answer that seemed too extreme, the scales could still be tilted to conform to moderate values. Most conservatives thus continued to employ some bloodletting, long after Louis' statistics had discredited the practice.[130] Conversely, a few conservatives tended to discount anesthesia statistics that leaned too far in the direction of art. A leading conservative surgical text of 1860 concluded its analysis of the pros and cons of anesthesia: "If pain is bearable, and not injurious, let it be borne."[131]

A second problem raised by opponents of the calculus concerned the distribution of costs and benefits. Using a commonplace example, let us say the shock of unanesthetized surgery were discovered to kill a larger percentage of patients than would be poisoned by anesthesia. By the calculus of conservative medicine, the physician should proceed with anesthetization. But that course would still require the poisoning of some patients. At what point does the saving of other people's lives justify the taking of even one?

"It is said one death in ten thousand cases is sufficient to condemn chloroform on moral grounds," a British textbook warned in 1859, recalling Charles Meigs' pledge to don sackcloth and ashes for life to atone for such a murder.[132] Few critics went this far in rejecting utilitarianism, but many remained unsure *how much* benefit it would take to justify one fatality. Death rates between one per thousand and one per ten thousand were frequently cited as sufficient to restrict anesthesia to capital surgery,[133] while the *American Journal of the Medical Sciences* held in 1867 that a (nonfatal) complication rate of about one percent would be bad enough to ban anesthesia completely.[134]

Another problem raised by critics of the calculus of suffering concerned the fundamental utilitarian assumption that all pains and injuries can be objectively compared in magnitude, that some common unit of measurement can be found for such things as suffering or disability. But do such units exist? For example, anesthetics can occasionally cause circulatory collapse leading to permanent brain damage. Is the idiocy that might thus result from anesthesia a bigger or smaller evil than the suffering that might result from unanesthetized major surgery? In a modern example, the potent antibiotic necessary to cure certain drug-resistant eye infections can result in hearing loss as a side effect. How can we measure whether blindness causes more suffering than deafness? And, as another nineteenth-century critic asked, how can we compare the magnitude of a present pain with the suffering from a future side effect?[135]

A final problem that deeply concerned nineteenth-century physicians was at what level of generality the calculus should be applied. Should the sum of the risks from all possible uses of anesthesia be weighed against the cumulative total of benefits, to produce a simple universal rule that pain relievers should (or should not) be used? Or did the doctor also have to weigh and measure the pros and cons for each individual patient? This problem of selecting the appropriate level of individualization seriously divided mid-nineteenth-century conservative physicians in their application of the new calculus.[136]

CHAPTER SIX

FROM THE UNIVERSAL
TO THE PARTICULAR:
PROFESSIONALISM, ANESTHESIA,
AND HUMAN INDIVIDUALITY

> I adapt myself to each case and to temperaments.
> —Walt Whitman [1]

Most mid-nineteenth-century physicians had to decide between what they saw as the benefits and drawbacks of using anesthetics. But at what level of generality was the choice to be made? Could the decision be embodied in a universal law—"the advantages of using anesthesia do (or do not) justify the risks"—or did the doctor have to make a separate decision for each individual patient? To what extent do the benefits and drawbacks of anesthetics differ from case to case, and what influence, if any, should such variations have on the physician's choice? Might a safe, effective dose for one person kill another and leave a third unaffected? Do some people suffer more from pain than do others? Do some patients require the control afforded by anesthesia more than do others? And if so, how and how much should the doctor take such variations into account?

Tension between the universal and the particular in medicine long predated the discovery of anesthesia.[2] In reconciling such conflicts, surgeons once again drew upon centuries of professional precedent. But here too, midcentury practitioners found professional traditions in turmoil and change. Whereas heroic professionalism had emphasized a relatively uniform therapeutics, midcentury conservative professional doctrines demanded a much greater degree of individualization. The conflict over individualizing anesthetic prescriptions thus reflected important changes in medical professionalism. Furthermore, the degree to which the profession particularized its prescriptions in turn reflected fundamental social changes, created by the increasingly uncertain role of the individual in a socially diverse industrializing democracy.

Anesthesia and Human Individuality

Mid-nineteenth-century physicians repeatedly stressed the overwhelming importance of a wide range of individual variations in modifying their use of anesthetics, with ether, and especially with chloroform.[3] Because the effect of anesthesia "in one set of cases is so diametrically opposite to that met with in others," prescriptions must vary accordingly, warned an editorially endorsed article in the 1851 *American Journal of the Medical Sciences*.[4] "Every circumstance connected with the health of the patient should be taken into consideration before exhibiting chloroform as these circumstances may influence its effect," declared another physician in 1860.[5] "Many enjoy the chloroform as they would a good dinner," wrote a Female Medical College of Pennsylvania graduate in 1866, but "others live a life time of agony," during the inhalation.[6] Henry Lyman's 1881 textbook of anesthesia listed three pages of "conditions, which may be considered accidental or peculiar to the individual," which were "capable of modifying the effects of anaesthesia."[7] "Although the general effects produced by the inhalation of ether are similar, yet peculiarity of temperament, and particular states of the system, have an important influence in modifying the phenomena which manifest

themselves," reported the AMA Committee on Surgery.[8] Dr. David
Meredith Reese blamed "lack of discrimination [among] the subjects" for causing most of the reported mishaps with ether.[9]
     The most important individual variations involved differ-
ences in reactions to drugs and differences in sensitivity to pain, according to FitzWilliam Sargent. The proper balance between "too intense pain" and "too powerful" anesthetics varied widely from person
to person, his 1856 text explained, because "different individuals are
susceptible of pain and of the influence of narcotics in very different
degrees."[10]
     Alexander Hosack summed up this common opinion of
many midcentury medical writers. If anesthetics can act *"differently
on different constitutions,"* he concluded, *"we have to enter into a
calculation of the good to be derived"* in each individual case.[11] Young
John Wesley Thompson of the University of Pennsylvania agreed that
every aspect of an individual's makeup could influence that calculation. "As long as there is a difference in the moral or physical character of individuals, a difference in temperament and in nerve force,
so long will treatment have to vary."[12]
     While they emphasized the variability of anesthesia, these
physicians also insisted that anesthetics were neither more nor less
uncertain than any other useful drugs.[13] "The peculiarities of condition or constitution" which affect anesthesia, are probably the same
as those which govern "the use of all the more potent articles of the
materia medica," declared the AMA Committee on Obstetrics. "In
this respect these agents present a striking analogy to anodynes and
stimulants generally," the Committee on Surgery agreed.[14]
     These practitioners did not rest their case for individual-
ization simply on the observed specific properties of anesthetics. Instead they repeatedly claimed that their opposition to indiscriminate
anesthetization depended on a much larger issue of professional principle. They considered individual differences important in anesthesia,
not simply because of the unique individual aspects of pain or of these
particular drugs, but because they felt there was something inherently
unprofessional about any universally applicable panaceas—any automatic cookbook systems of therapy that could cure all pains in all
people.
     Administration of anesthesia in a *"wholesale* manner,"
without regard for the necessity of "confining its use to its legitimate

limits," constituted the trademark of the "totally unqualified" practitioner, J. F. B. Flagg warned. "The fact that this powerful agent
was in the hands of irresponsible men; used by them *indiscriminately*,
. . . has been enough of itself to create disgust." [15] Another physi-
cian-dentist denounced "the hazardous chances from the indiscriminate uses of these subtle fluids or gases," as an "outrageous" violation of professional standards, [16] characteristic of *"mechanical"*
practitioners, "who play with people's constitutions whilst they are
entirely ignorant of the . . . elementary principles of medicine and
surgery and the physiology of the system." [17] A student at the University of Pennsylvania College of Medicine in 1857 warned that
"reckless and indiscriminate employment" of anesthetics would un-
doubedly "bring discredit upon the practitioner." [18]

The *St. Louis Medical and Surgical Journal* satirized the
indiscriminate use of anesthesia as a panacea.

> So pleasant, and at the same time so powerful are the exhiler-
> ating *[sic]* and anodyne effects of chloroform, that the day is probably not
> distant when it will not only be used by every physician, but be "hung on
> some rusty nail" . . . in every log cabin in the land . . . . If a little child
> has a belly ache or an old woman a face ache, a few pleasant whiffs from
> the green bottle will dissipate it all—and when the pipe or the quid fail to
> drive away devils or bring angels to minister to the hypochondriac or the
> hysterics, a few inhalations from a fashionable pocket inhaler will accom-
> plish both—make ugliness beauty, and transport from hell to heaven without
> a change of heart. [19]

John Wesley Thompson provided a full and clear summary of how anesthetic individualization derived from fundamental
issues of professional ideology.

> It is the part of the empiric to say, that for certain afflictions there must be
> administered a specific article in specific doses; but the educated and judi-
> cious practitioner examines well his case, . . . ascertains not only the na-
> ture of the ailment, but of his patient also, and then graduates his treatment
> accordingly. . . .
> The ignorant world having seen [anesthesia's] action, and heard
> its fame in skillful hands, must have it used, or use it themselves in every
> trivial occasion. They view it merely as a "pain-killer," and so to speak,
> more in the light of a mechanical, than of a powerful physiological, agent;

and if . . . the slightest unpleasant sensation or pain [was] to be felt, an anaesthetic must be administered; if by a proper person, well; if not, still it must be given.[20]

To physicians like Thompson, "specifics"—chemical magic bullets which worked in every single case of a given medical condition— were the mark of ignorance or quackery. "Few if any have been the specifics discovered, and no doubt such will ever continue to be the case."[21]

In a recent widely discussed study, Ivan Illich has charged that nineteenth-century medical professionalizers exaggerated the utility of anesthesia in order to encourage popular belief in medical omnipotence. However, this criticism clearly does not apply to the brand of professionalism espoused by physicians like Thompson.[22] It was the peddlers of Perry Davis' patent "Pain Killer," not professionals like Thompson, who fed the public's demand for instant relief and panaceas for pain; it was "Pond's Extract," not anesthesia, that was advertised as the *"Universal* Pain Extractor."[23]

Mid-nineteenth-century physicians regarded the ability to make careful individual therapeutic distinctions among patients as the mark of a true professional. Conversely, they used the alleged need for such fine discrimination as a powerful argument for attempting to erect a professional monopoly on the use of anesthetics. Thus, the *Western Lancet* cited the variation of anesthetic effects according to individual "idioseneracy" *[sic]* as one reason why "its use should be restricted to those who are competent."[24] The AMA claimed the varying reactions that occurred upon administering chloroform "to some constitutions" required that it be used "only by professional men."[25] The Medical Society of Virginia warned that practitioners "who were not physicians, . . . were less competent than physicians to discriminate between those who were and those who were not suitable subjects for the administration of anaesthetic agents."[26]

Carried to its logical conclusion, this argument implied that, because of the complexity of individual variations, even the average general surgeon should not attempt to use anesthesia. For precisely this reason, by the 1860s, many experts urged some form of specialization in administering anesthetics. An 1863 text, for example, declared that "the peculiarities of individuals" made it necessary to have a designated surgical assistant administer the anesthetic and "nothing else."[27] The extreme variability of chloroform, it was argued, created a need for full-time specialists. The use of ether also supposedly required the attention of a specially designated trained individual, though such persons were not expected to devote their professional careers exclusively to anesthesia.[28] Thus, on the basis of their concept of medical professionalism, many conservative physicians concluded that it was their duty to discriminate very carefully among individual patients before using anesthetics.

There were a few physicians, however, who insisted that such individual differences among patients were of little significance in anesthetization. Perhaps the most radical such proponent of indiscriminate anesthesia use was James Y. Simpson. As early as May 1847, even before his discovery of chloroform, Simpson wrote, "I am etherizing all my Obstetric cases. The ladies *all* demand it here—Nothing but good results." Dentist Mayo G. Smith of Boston published a long list of individual variations reported by others, yet he denied the importance of such differences and urged the use of ether for all types of patients. At the Poor House Hospital in Westchester County, New York, anesthetics reportedly were "used almost indiscriminately" (although a number of qualifications were stated). A Confederate manual of military surgery urged that anesthetics be "used as liberally in allaying the pain of surgical affections as cold water is now used for keeping down inflammation. *We do not hesitate to say, that it should be given to every patient requiring a serious or painful operation.*"[29]

These advocates of more or less universal anesthetization, no less than their opponents, based their position on broad professional principles, with implications that far transcended the specific properties of anesthesia. In his 1854 M.D thesis, John Harvey Jr. claimed that individual variations could be ignored in anesthesia because heroic professionalism had always ignored such differences in the choice of a remedy.

As a general rule, the same agents will produce similar effects upon all men; and those, upon whom, owing to some peculiar idiosyncracy, a different effect is produced, are few and far between. I have known four common Cathartic pills to salivate a person; but on that account, would any one fear to administer Calomel.[30]

One of Simpson's colleagues declared that, except for a few specified individual circumstances,

The surgeons of Edinburgh have used chloroform in all their operations . . . ; and that no one amongst them would deem himself justified, morally or professionally, in now cutting and operating upon a patient in a waking and sensitive state. Every professional principle, nay, the common principles of humanity, forbade it.[31]

Simpson also opposed the individualization of anesthesia because he felt it gave physicians too much control over their patients. When Ramsbotham doubted that even physicians could *"always* calculate the exact dose,'' for each individual obstetrical patient, Simpson replied with equanimity, "The ladies themselves will keep medical men right about the proper quantity."[32] Giving physicians the power to judge such individual variations gave them the power to decide which patients must suffer and which would be relieved, an authority Simpson (and most feminists) felt that doctors should not have.[33]

However, even Simpson limited his advocacy of obstetric anesthetization to all *patients*—not to all pregnant *women*. In a published letter to Meigs, Simpson emphatically denied that he believed all parturient women should receive anesthesia; rather he was referring only to "the class of patients in civilized life upon whom you and I attend, . . . patients in the higher ranks of life." Simpson felt comfortable in not making distinctions among his patients, not because he adhered to principles of biological or social equality, but because he limited his practice to a highly homogeneous patient population. Simpson always described his own clients as "ladies"; he reserved the term "females" for other classes of women. "Females in the lower and hardier grades of civilized society"—not to mention "the parturient female" of the "uncivilized tribes"—were not very likely to be attended by Sir James Y. Simpson, "M.D., F.R.S.E., Professor of Midwifery in the University of Edinburgh, Physician-Accoucheur to the Queen in Scotland, Etc. Etc. Etc."[34]

In summary, mid-nineteenth-century medical writers were split between a majority who felt that professionalism required wide individual variations in the use of anesthesia and a minority who more or less denied the relevance of such particularization. To understand the origins and importance of this conflict, it is necessary to examine in some detail the momentous revolution underway in nineteenth-century attitudes toward human individuality in medicine, in other professions, and throughout society.

Professionalism and the Individual in American Society

GALEN AND INDIVIDUALITY

Ancient medicine took cognizance of human variation through the doctrine of the "four humors." According to Galen, individuals possessed these four bodily elements in an infinite variety of combinations. Human individuality was thus infinite, yet limited to these four variables;[35] each person's "constitution" was a unique individual variation on just four basic types.[36]

Disease resulted when a person's mixture of humors became too unbalanced. The task of the physician was to restore an equilibrium among these elements. Thus the Galenic medical system generalized all of medicine into only eight basic therapies—the augmentation or depletion of each humor—but it required that these procedures be carefully proportioned to the individual patient's constitution. For example, a patient suffering from an excess of blood required depletion of that humor, but only to the precise extent of that patient's specific individual surfeit.[37] In modern terms, Galenic therapy was infinitely individualized in "dosage" but limited to a handful of basic "procedures." Galen's specific theories had been long discarded by the nineteenth century, yet both his terminology and his approach to human individuality still deeply influenced discussions of professional duty.

RUSH AND ENLIGHTENMENT UNIVERSALITY

The professional ideology developed by Benjamin Rush restricted the selection of therapies even more than had Galen's humoralism, while retaining some of the classical emphasis on individual variations in dosage. The majority of diseases, Rush taught, were merely different forms of inflammation, caused by excess vascular tension or "excitability." Thus, most diseases could be cured by "depletion" of the blood.[38] This almost universal therapy of depletion could be accomplished by any of several different purgative drugs, such as calomel, jalap, and ipecac, as well as by bloodletting. But Rush declared, "a fourth part of the medicine now in use, would be sufficient" under his system.[39]

The extreme universality of Rush's system is only somewhat exaggerated in the following anecdote relayed by his student Charles Caldwell. At the height of the 1793 yellow fever epidemic, a large crowd had gathered to seek the doctor's aid. Finding himself unable to visit them all, he addressed the throng from his carriage, advising them that the disease could be cured "by bloodletting, and copious purging."

"What," said a voice from the crowd, "bleed and purge every one?"

"Yes," said the doctor, "bleed and purge all Kensington!—Drive on, Ben."[40]

Rush based the uniformity of his therapy on his explicit Enlightenment faith in the simplicity, predictability, and rationality of the universe[41] and on his Jeffersonian conviction that, in real and important ways, all men had been created equal. Universally applicable medical therapies accorded with human equality in three different ways. First, they were simple enough to be practiced by anyone. They did not require long, expensive, or exclusive training. "All that is necessary might be taught to a boy or girl twelve years old in a few hours." Second, the unrestricted supply of potential practitioners made such therapy cheap enough for all to afford. Third, the same basic form of therapy worked for all, rich and poor, black and white, men and women.[42]

These egalitarian implications of Rush's therapy were not carried to the point of abolishing either academic training or professional distinctions. Rather, they formed an important part of Rush's attempt to replace eighteenth-century genteel values with a new Republican American professional ideology. Rush cautioned, "let it not be supposed that I wish to see the exercise of medicine abolished as a regular profession."[43] Instead, he hoped that the diffusion of a demystified, simple, and universal medical science would lead the public to appreciate the medical profession and to abandon quackery.[44]

Thus, Rush advocated universally applicable therapies to further both Republicanism and Enlightenment in medical professionalism.[45]

But while Rush radically restricted individual variations in therapeutic modality, his system did require the practitioner to adjust the dosage to the variety of individual patient constitutions and circumstances. Everyone might be cured by bleeding and purging, but the amount of depletion necessary varied from patient to patient, depending on how much excess stimulation was present. "Our prescriptions," Rush explained, "are to be regulated chiefly by the force of morbid excitement," and since "this force be varied in acute diseases by a hundred different circumstances, even by a cloud, . . . lessening for a few minutes, the light and heat of the sun, it follows that the utmost watchfulness and skill will be necessary to accommodate our remedies to the changing state of the system."[46]

In addition to weather and climate, Rush took careful note of "the different habits and constitutions of his patients, and varied his prescriptions with their strength, age and sex," according to his eulogist, Dr. James Thatcher.[47] Nationality, geographic origin, and economic class likewise modified the extent of depletion necessary: Americans needed to be bled more than Englishmen, the middle classes more than the rich or the poor.[48]

This recognition of individuality in dosage circumscribed both the universality and the egalitarianism of Rush's system. The conflict is particularly apparent in Rush's explicit comparison between the whipping of criminals and the practice of heroic medicine. Like bleeding or purging, corporal infliction had to be modified in dosage to account for individual differences in sensitivity. "In order to render these punishments effectual, they should be accommodated to the constitutions and tempers of the criminals."[49] But in both medicine and penology Rush realized that such individualization seriously limited the equality of treatment provided by a uniform, universal therapy. In the case of punishment Rush admitted, "I am aware of the prejudices of freemen, against entrusting power to a discretionary court." In medicine too the egalitarianism of a system that could be learned by all and practiced on all alike was clearly circumscribed by requiring that the doses be differentiated by race, class, nationality, and sex, especially if these variations required years of experience and study to master. For Rush, the basic goal was to produce a uniform level of depletion (or pain), but to do so required individualizing the dosage of bleeding (or whipping). The therapy had to fit the disease (or crime), but the extent had to fit the individual patient (or criminal).[50]

Thus, under Rush's system, dosage was individualized to fit the patient, although the variations almost always stayed within the "copious" to "heroic" range. The therapeutic modality itself was almost uniformly depletion, effected through a very limited choice of drugs and procedures. Rush encouraged some sensitivity to the individuality of patients, but only within the confines of an extremely uniform therapeutic system. On balance, Benjamin Rush's heroic professional ideology favored the universal over the particular. Though the amount of blood drawn might vary, "all Kensington" would be bled.

More universalist than even Rush's therapy was the botanical system of Samuel Thomson. Thomson's original practice reduced the entire *materia medica* to the use of lobelia and steam (prescribed according to a mail-order cookbook). For Thomson, as for Rush, medical uniformity was justified by both political and professional concerns. But Thomson was far more radical than Rush was. While Rush saw his circumscribed version of universality as a means of Republicanizing and Americanizing professionalism, Thomson expected his truly universal formulary to do away with doctors and professionalism entirely.[51]

MEDICAL CONSERVATISM AND THE INDIVIDUAL

Compared to Thomson or Rush, midcentury physicians practiced much more highly individualized therapeutics. Among the sectarians, hydropaths did use a universal drug, water, but in individualized applications, from steam baths to enemas to ice packs. In homeopathy, the doses were relatively uniform—minuscule—but the choice of drugs was more varied and individualized than in heroic practice.[52]

However, by 1846, the leading critics of therapeutic uniformity were not sectarians but conservative regular physicians. In fact, Rush's insistence upon universal depletion never enjoyed complete acceptance among orthodox physicians, even in early-nineteenth-century America.[53] His early opponents believed physicians should be able to choose between depletion and "stimulation" (with tonics, wine, beef, and opium), depending on the state of the individual patient.[54]

Physicians like Josiah Goodhue of the Berkshire Medical Institution in Massachusetts argued that the poor and malnourished needed a completely different form of therapy than the rich did. Such "debilitated" patients required active stimulation with food and tonics, not simply smaller amounts of bloodletting. These early critics had little influence in their own day, but their argument that different people required different kinds of treatment, as well as simply different doses, formed the basis of the ideas that, by 1846, led conservative American physicians to reject as unprofessional the uniformity of Rush's system.[55]

Midcentury conservative textbooks declared it a basic professional principle that the therapy itself, not just the dose, had to be carefully matched to the individual patient. Hooker's *Physician and Patient* declared that both "the *quantities* and *forms* in which remedies are administered . . . must, of course, be varied to suit each individual case. Sometimes a very nice adaptation is necessary."[56] Even once the therapy was selected, the dosage had to vary much more widely than the "heroic" system had allowed. "The variations, in these respects, required by different cases, have a wide range— some demanding large doses to produce the needed effect, and others being strongly affected by small ones." Significantly, Hooker chose as his sole example of this need for variation the case of severe pain.[57] Austin Flint listed among the "maxims" of "Conservative Medicine": "*first,* that we are not so much to treat diseases, as patients affected with disease."[58]

Thus, conservative spokesmen rejected, not the use of Rush's remedies, but their purported universality. "We know and feel the value of these great and powerful agents; but it is because of their value and power, in suitable cases . . . , that we fear their indiscriminate use," explained one enormously popular midcentury textbook.[59] It was the "injudicious and indiscriminate" use of depletives as a universal panacea, not the remedies themselves, which Austin Flint repudiated.[60] "It is the *abuse,* and not the judicious use, of the lancet to which we object," wrote Dr. Stephen W. Williams; "the doctrine that every pain the patient felt was an inflammation, and that consequently the lancet or leeching must be resorted to."[61] Even heroic doses might still be employed, so long as they were not used indiscriminately.[62]

This conservative view of therapeutic individuality was

best summarized in 1850 by Paul Eve, a leading Southern surgeon and an important founder of the AMA.

No two human constitutions are precisely alike. A London medical periodical has just affirmed that what cured cholera in one street, would not cure it in another. None of us can predict the full effect of even a single dose of medicine. We cannot, therefore, adopt any routine practice, any invariable system of treating diseases; this is the blind and reckless course of empiricism; but we must, in order to apply our agents intelligently and effectually, vary them, according to the peculiar and ever changing circumstances attending each case.[63]

This new medical emphasis on individuality was not without supporting scientific evidence. Conservatives carefully amassed considerable data to show that people did vary widely in their reactions both to disease and to drugs. Furthermore, most drugs available in nineteenth-century America themselves varied widely in potency from batch to batch, owing both to primitive pharmacological technique and to sophisticated forms of adulteration.[64] But, as Flint repeatedly emphasized, the differences between conservative and heroic practice were not simply questions of fact but of value. The conflict was not simply over what therapies worked but over what behavior was professionally acceptable. For Rush, varying the mode of treatment to fit the individual case was empiricism—not just a mistake but a form of quackery. Likewise, to conservatives, Rush's universalism was not merely a factual error but an unprofessional search for panaceas. In both cases the ideological decision about what a legitimate professional form of therapy should look like preceded and helped shape the specific types of therapy each group adopted.[65]

Conservative medicine's emphasis on individuality served a wide variety of professional purposes. First, it explained to an uneasy public why medicine failed to provide the specific, certain panaceas they demanded. Likewise, it prohibited practitioners from inflating public expectations about the possibility of ever finding such remedies. Conservative physicians declared the search for specifics to be "as vain as that of the ancient alchemists for the philosopher's stone . . . . It is a *humbug* resorted to alone by designing charlatans who would batten on the ignorance and credulity of the people."[66]

Second, the need for complex individualized variations in

therapy limited the practice of medicine to those trained in these intricate skills. Conservative insistence on the need to hand-tailor therapy to fit each individual patient thus led to the reemergence of mystery in professionalism. This repudiation of Rush's universalism constituted a conservative attempt to preserve a professional monopoly over medical knowledge, in the face of mounting Jacksonian antimonopoly agitation and opposition to licensing legislation. In this sense, "conservative" medicine was socially and politically "conservative" as well. Rush's hopes for an open, egalitarian profession based on simple uniform treatments were anathema to practitioners who had to struggle for their livelihood in the wide-open midcentury medical marketplace.[67]

Third, conservatives hoped that by restricting and individualizing the use of depletion and heroic doses, they might salvage some legitimacy for the continued use of these increasingly unpopular techniques.[68] Thus, while conservatives approved attempts to limit and individualize the use of calomel, they did not generally rally behind efforts to have mercurials banned entirely from the medicine chest.[69] Fourth, cookbook medicine, what conservatives denounced as "routine practice," was boring to practice. It lacked challenge to the physician and thus gave medicine an air of intellectual stagnation.[70]

Conservatives also expected their decreased uniformity would encourage practitioners to exercise greater sensitivity toward the unique needs and individual worth of each patient. Such was the clear intent of Flint's first law.[71] In the same spirit, the *Boston Medical and Surgical Journal,* in an 1883 editorial attacking "Routine Practice," denounced physicians who "slight their work, and . . . treat the cases merely with reference to a diagnosis (itself more or less imperfectly formed) rather that with reference to the individual needs." The dependent poor, the *Journal* noted, would suffer the most from such depersonalized, inhumane, "routine" medicine.[72] In contrast, conservative medicine offered careful attention to the differing needs of every individual. In this manner, conservative professionalism shared something of the romantic individualism of Emerson and Thoreau.

But there was a dark facet to such individualization. The conservative attack on therapeutic uniformity also made it possible for blatantly discriminatory treatment to gain professional sanction. Thus, an article on bloodletting reprinted in the 1853 *American Journal of the Medical Sciences* declared, "The error consists in a vain effort to discover a uniform rule of treatment . . . adapted to all cases." Bleeding, for example, was indicated only for certain patients, such as cases of nymphomania, insanity caused by repressed menstruation, and "where the patient has been in the habit of living *above par.*"[73] Not surprisingly, conservative physicians began to discover that the rich needed more (and more expensive) medicine than did the poor.[74]

By rejecting universal therapies as unprofessional, conservative medicine transformed every aspect of a patient's person, background, and habits—and thus every bias, dislike, and prejudice of the physician—into a potentially legitimate factor in selecting the appropriate course of treatment. Applied to anesthesia, this discretion to decide who shall suffer and who shall be relieved constituted an enormous source of power for the physician, in maintaining authority and control over the patient. The *North American Medico-Chirurgical Review* published an 1857 case in which the frustrated physician decided against the use of anesthetics on a disruptive young child with a dislocated thigh. "I determined to let him suffer a while, in order to impress upon his mind more forcibly the necessity of keeping quiet."[75] Carried to its logical conclusion, the conservative attack on uniform therapies sanctioned the doctrines of physicians like Samuel Cartwright, Josiah Nott, and others, who insisted that Negroes and whites required fundamentally distinct medical treatment. Though few conservative physicians endorsed Nott's monomaniacal preoccupation with race, lesser degrees of racial discrimination in therapy were perfectly consistent with their professional ideology.[76]

The conservative rejection of therapeutic uniformity in medicine paralleled similar trends in other nineteenth-century professions as well. Teachers, for example, insisted that the methods of pedagogy, not just the content, be adapted to the personality and capacity of each individual child. The professional organ of the New York State Teachers' Association urged teachers to emulate physicians and reject "the folly of the same treatment" for different patients. "Our wisdom will be to accommodate ourselves to the peculiar temperament and habits of all, treating each according to his particular character and peculiar development."[77]

The evangelical clergy were among the earliest professional advocates of such individualization. "The minister must address his hearers," explained the Reverend Charles G. Finney. "He will never do them any good, farther than he succeeds in convincing each individual that he means him.''

     I have been in many places in times of revival, and I have never been able to employ precisely the same course of preaching in one as in another. . . . In one place, one set of truths, in another, another set.[78]

    In fact, the growing particularism of conservative medicine reflected an increased awareness of human individuality and variation manifest throughout mid-nineteenth-century American society. Political factionalism, religious sectarianism, economic liberalism, immigration, and ethnic conflict drastically altered the assumption of social harmony on which Benjamin Rush's version of medical universalism had depended. The rapid cultural fragmentation of nineteenth-century America created a growing awareness of and concern over human diversity. The attempt to combine Romantic sensitivity to the uniqueness of each individual with Enlightenment concepts of law, rationality, and fairness—to protect social cohesion in a period of expanding individualism and cultural diversity—constituted perhaps the most vexing problem of social ideology facing the nation.[79]

    This attempt to contain the contradictions between individuality and unity in American life produced the greatness of Walt Whitman. To embrace the distinctiveness of human individuality, the poet significantly chose the language of conservative medicine: ''I adapt myself to each case and to temperaments.''[80] In poems like ''Salut au Monde!'' he catalogued page after page of human diversity—biological, moral, and intellectual. But love transcended particularism. In spite of diversity, even because of it, Man was everywhere Man, and therefore equally worthy of love. *E Pluribus Unum.*

    Have you ever loved the body of a woman?
    Have you ever loved the body of a man?
    Do you not see that these are exactly the same to all
      in all nations and times all over the earth?[81]

    In summary, the debate over individual variation in the use of anesthesia can be seen as part of a larger social and professional conflict over the role of individuality in American life. Conservative professionalism required discrimination and individualization in the use, as well as dosage, of every remedy, from bleeding to bathing,[82] including, of course, anesthesia. The many denunciations of indiscriminate anesthetization as quackery reflected this growing particularism of both professional and social ideology. Conservative professionalism required physicians to vary the use of anesthesia according to each patient's individual circumstances. This adaptation to individual needs at its best reaffirmed that each patient was a unique and valuable individual; at its worst it legitimated discriminatory treatment and the monopolization of knowledge.

Rules and Regulations for Individualizing Anesthesia

Conservative physicians insisted that the use of anesthesia be adapted to individual patient differences, but most also believed such variations were neither random nor unpredictable. Differences in people's reactions to pain and to anesthesia, they assumed, could be studied, classified, and codified into detailed rules that would govern the use of such drugs in each particular situation. The AMA Committee on Surgery confidently looked forward ''to rules which shall regulate their employment, and shall indicate the class of cases to which they are inapplicable.''[83] The Committee on Obstetrics agreed.

There is every reason to believe that farther experience and closer observation will enable us to adopt rules for their use as precise and as definite as have been laid down with respect to ergot.[84]

The result would be a detailed and particularized codification of rules governing the types of individual situations in which anesthesia was either indicated or contraindicated.

Such particularized rules, indeed, were not long in forthcoming. Throughout the 1850s, a battery of journal articles and surgical textbooks laid down a barrage of proposed indications and regulations to govern the use and dose of anesthetics in every conceivable individual situation.[85] By the 1860s, the rules had become numerous enough to warrant textbooks of anesthesia. The promulgation of such regulations proceeded most rapidly in the areas of medicine most affected by the demands of large organizations. One of the earliest texts devoted exclusively to anesthesia was Valentine Mott's, published by the United States Sanitary Commission for the use of the Union Army medics.[86] Hospital managers too began urging that staff physicians record and regularize their use of anesthetics.[87] In places where the more unpredictable chloroform was preferred to ether, the growth of such specialized procedures and rules occurred faster than elsewhere, but even with ether the trend was clear.[88]

Not all physicians approved of such formal rationalized rules, especially when it came to precise numerical measures of dosage. "Such precision sounds very fairly," but it was both useless and impractical, the *British Medical Journal* warned. One practitioner in 1870 scoffed that the attempt to classify individual differences would create such an elaborate technical "array of rules and procedures" that anesthesia would become a narrow, illiberal, unprofessional specialty. Already "almost a little science has grown out of the nominal and mostly fruitless precautions, which are brought out in showy opposition to possible . . . effects of chloroform,"[89] he noted. His remarks in fact constituted a fairly accurate appraisal of efforts by chloroform anesthetists in England to create a full-fledged specialty of anesthesiology.[90] But such criticisms remained largely confined to opponents of medical conservatism, until the 1870s.

Rules, Bureaucracy, and Professional Discretion

In rejecting universal therapies most medical conservatives sought, not unlimited individualization, but a moderate balance between the universal and the individual, between Science and Art. Once again, midcentury conservatives adopted as their guide the principles of moderation counseled by Bacon in 1625:

Physicians are some of them so pleasing, and conformable to the humor of the patient, as they press not the true cure of the disease; and some other are so regular in proceeding . . . for the disease, as they respect not sufficiently the condition of the patient. Take one of a middle temper.[91]

The majority of conservative medical writers stopped short of saying that no two patients could be treated identically. Instead, they sought to define and classify human differences—making sure that the resulting generalizations remained detailed enough to cover all the important particulars. Thus, from the late 1830s on, a growing number of medical journals and textbooks began to formulate a variety of rules to govern the particular "types" of patients for whom a particular remedy was or was not indicated. Instructions concerning the appropriate therapies for different classes of cases grew increasingly detailed and particularized, compared to the generalities of early pharmacopoeias and texts (though quantitative measures of dosage were still rare throughout the nineteenth century). These classifications often included the patient's age, sex, race, economic class, and nationality, as well as overall health, and the precise nature of the symptoms. Thus, for the first time, physicians began to consider the special medical needs of women and of children distinctive and important enough to warrant creation of such specialties as gynecology and pediatrics.[92]

The formulation of such therapeutic regulations drew heavily on the development of medical statistics by Pierre Louis and the early-nineteenth-century Paris clinicians. To Louis and his American disciple Henry I. Bowditch, people and diseases might vary widely but the variations were always measurable and categorizable at some level of generality greater than the individual.[93]

The emergence of large, incipiently bureaucratic medical institutions, a development closely linked to medical statistics, also helped foster the growth of detailed therapeutic rules. As early as the 1830s the handful of urban public hospitals in America began to follow highly particularized but clearly regularized indications in the use of remedies from bloodletting to beef soup.[94] The growth of such regulations accelerated dramatically with the efforts of the United States Sanitary Commission during the Civil War. The bulletins, circulars, and pamphlets of the Commission disseminated across the Union standardized therapeutic rules and regulations, part of the Commission's overall effort to turn a random assortment of volunteer doctors into a systematic medical corps.[95] With several hundred patients a day per doctor, with millions of dollars in supplies to order and route, Civil War therapy had to be reduced to standardized rules. The codification of therapeutics also constituted an attempt to retain some semblance of order and rationality in dealing with the increasingly diverse patient populations of the cities. Codification offered conservative physicians a middle course between the universalism of Rush's system and the possible anarchy of unrestrained individualization.

However, not all physicians welcomed this temporizing.

A few mid-nineteenth-century practitioners insisted that no effort to provide rules for therapy could ever be individualized enough, no matter how particular such regulations were. Initially, such criticism came from those with only slight commitment to conservative professional principles. For example, Charles D. Meigs wrote in 1848 of the physician's essential qualifications, "He should be able to make nice discriminations; quickly perceiving the slightest shades of difference." "Method in medicine is beneath contempt; because, owing to the infinite variety and differences existing . . . there never were, nor can be, two absolutely similar cases."[96] Another critic in 1863 ridiculed the attempt to derive statistical rules of therapy "accurately graduated to the square of the [patient's] constitution."[97] Any system of therapeutic rules, no matter how narrowly particularized, still destroyed the "noble" uniqueness of each human being; it still reduced a patient to a list of symptoms, conditions, and diseases.[98]

By 1883, even the conservative *Boston Medical and Surgical Journal* had reached the same conclusion, and for the same reasons. The *Journal* termed medicine

> that profession where the work is never alike in any two cases[.] No two patients have the same constitution or mental proclivities. No two instances of typhoid fever, or of any other disease, are precisely alike. The intelligent and efficient care of any case of illness demands a consideration of all the circumstances which are peculiar to itself and of the traits of body and mind which are peculiar to the patient. No "rule of thumb," no recourse to a formula-book, will avail for the proper treatment even of the typical diseases.[99]

A cookbook was still a cookbook, no matter how many and how detailed the recipes.

And, unlike Meigs, by 1883 the *Journal* was able to give a name to the specific culprit that was fostering medical codification—hospital bureaucracy. "Hospital service is, . . . often debased to the merest routine. . . . This is especially true of dispensary [charity outpatient] practice. . . . [W]ith the large number of cases, many of them uninteresting personally and professionally, . . . the tendency would be very strong toward superficial, unconsidered, and routine practice," rather than to attend to the "individual needs."[100]

By the 1860s, conservatives had discovered other problems with such regulations as well. For example, the detail required to develop particularized rules for all of medical practice would prevent any one general practitioner from mastering all of medicine. Thus, such formularies would foster illiberal, merely technical specialization and would eliminate the integrative, personal function performed by a doctor who could treat the whole patient.[101] Even more ominously, if medicine could be reduced to a mechanical formula, no matter how complex, it implied that people too might be no more than complex machines.[102]

Not all the arguments against therapeutic regulations, however, were so altruistic or so philosophic. Meigs scorned the codification of therapeutic rules as an unbearable infringement upon his paternalistic discretionary authority over his patients.[103] And while a complex enough code might suffice to keep the untrained and unskilled from practicing and to hold down economic competition, even the most difficult and complex rules might still be mastered by the wrong people. If medicine were reduced to a technical formula, no matter how complicated, "there is nothing to prevent a Jew peddler . . . from passing himself off as a distinguished professor."[104]

The development of specific therapeutic rules was designed to rationalize the process of fitting the cure to the individual patient. At their best, such rules of practice could combine the efficiency, regularity, and objectivity of Rush's system with the romantic's sensitivity to human diversity. But at their worst, such formulae produced a maze of petty mechanical rules, devoid of any true individual concern. Likewise, such regulations could elevate into formal, objective-sounding laws the most blatant inequities. While it was the individualism of conservative medicine that lent legitimacy to Josiah Nott's personal medical racism, it was the codification of such views that elevated his personal biases into the proposed medical specialty he called "niggerology."[105]

In antebellum America, however, this incipient conflict among conservatives over the legitimacy of therapeutic rules remained for the most part unarticulated and muted. Most conservatives seemed only dimly aware of the contradiction between romantic individualism and particularistic regulations. Worthington Hooker was one of those who tried to straddle the difficulty. Hooker, as we have seen, insisted that therapy be individualized. Yet he did not claim that every case was unique, nor that medicine had no rules, but simply that these rules could not be completely codified or taught. They had to be *felt.*

> Experience gives to the shrewd and judicious physician a sort of tact in detecting these contingencies, and in so modifying his practice as to meet with some good degree of fitness the various indications which they present. This tact is to be acquired at the bed-side of the sick, by patient watching of the workings of disease, and of the influence of remedies upon it; and though the experience of others is a valuable auxilliary in acquiring it, it is only an auxilliary and cannot communicate it alone.[106]

Before the Civil War, the conflict in medical therapeutics was not between universalism and discretion but between universalism and particularism; not between rules and no rules but between big rules and little rules. Advocates of therapeutic rationalization, such as Henry I. Bowditch, and advocates of individualistic discretion, such as the *Boston Medical and Surgical Journal,* could both unite in opposition to universalistic systems of therapy like those of Rush or Thomson. Only when the demands of medical bureaucracy during and after the Civil War forced the issue did most conservatives have to confront the difference between particularized rules and individual discretion. Whitman could speak of adapting himself "to each case and to temperaments,"[107] without quite realizing that classifying and stereotyping people by "temperaments" infringed upon the unique individuality of "each case."

Conservative physicians were not alone in their slowness to perceive such distinctions. Antebellum school teachers too, preoccupied with opposition to the undifferentiated teaching of the one-room school house, failed to grasp the inherent contradiction between the demands of a particularized bureaucracy and true individualism. In the same breath, teachers' journals praised the instructor whose classroom ran "like clock-work," but denounced the notion that the educator should be a "teaching machine" or "teaching-jenny."[108] The same journal that called "the centralizing or unit-izing of authority, and systematizing of schools" the "corner stone of progress" went on to label the imposition of standardized classroom methods "Prussian" and "despotic."[109] From a twentieth-century viewpoint, the nineteenth-century creation of large, age-graded, ability-tracked, factory-style school systems seems the height of impersonal bureaucracy. But to antebellum educators, preoccupied with replacing the undifferentiated one-room school, the particularization possible in a finely graded bureaucracy seemed to be a move toward *greater* recognition of pupil individuality.[110] Teachers, like doctors, confused the recognition of diversity with the recognition of individuality. Herein lies the explanation for what Michael Katz called the "irony of early school reform"—the paradox of a massive mechanical bureaucracy erected by educators in the name of individualization.[111] Virtually the same irony characterized antebellum conservative medical therapeutics.[112]

In summary, most antebellum physicians, preoccupied with dismantling the universal therapy of an earlier era, created a maze of new particularized indications and contraindications for different patient "types" without realizing until the 1860s that such rules still might conflict with the recognition of patient individuality and with practitioner discretion. The attempt to draw up specific detailed regulations for the use of anesthesia was thus one small part of a critically important change underway in many midcentury professions and throughout society.

CHAPTER SEVEN

"THEY DON'T FEEL IT LIKE WE DO": SOCIAL POLITICS AND THE PERCEPTION OF PAIN

Most nineteenth-century Americans and Europeans who paused to reflect on the subject believed that human beings differed widely in their sensitivity to and endurance of both natural and inflicted physical pain.[1] "The causes which modify the external or internal sensations are innumerable: age, sex, temperament, the seasons, climate, habit, individual disposition," noted the renowned neurophysiologist François Magendie.[2] Such an all-inclusive list of factors made cultural stereotypes and prejudices an integral part of professional judgments concerning which kinds of people were most susceptible to pain. Conversely, differences in pain sensitivity attributed to different individuals and groups provided scientific legitimacy for discriminatory treatment, both by the profession and by society at large. The belief that people varied widely in their ability to feel pain influenced almost every aspect of nineteenth-century social and professional life, including, of course, the use of anesthesia.

A Great Chain of Feeling

From the earliest history of empirical science to the present day, biomedical researchers have attempted to specify which types of people feel the most pain.[3] Among the earliest efforts to generalize about variations in human sensitivity was Galen's doctrine of the four humors. Of the four types of "temperaments," fat, sluggish, "phlegmatic" people usually were assumed to feel the least pain; thin, excitable, "choleric" people the most.[4]

But with the growing cultural and professional importance nineteenth-century Americans placed on accurately differentiating and categorizing detailed individual human differences, such broad rules of thumb no longer sufficed.[5] A vast number of additional specific biological, social, and moral distinctions began to assume significance as predictors of human sensitivity to pain.

GENDER

Sex seemed to be one factor that clearly influenced the perception of pain. Several ancient societies possessed the notion that women felt pain much more severely than did men.[6] In mid-nineteenth-century America, such traditional beliefs gained added significance as a result of the Victorian penchant for polarizing and dichotomizing sex roles in society.

"The nerves themselves are smaller, and of a more delicate structure" in women. "They are endowed with greater sensibility," explained one male physician. According to a standard midcentury American physiology textbook, all female "senses, as a general rule, are more acute." A leading American gynecology text declared woman to be "more delicate" in "her whole economy." Dr. Oliver Wendell Holmes marveled, "She is so much more fertile in capacities of suffering than a man. She has so many varieties of headache." "In consequence of her greater sensitiveness to external impressions," declared Dr. Morrill Wyman of Cambridge, Massachusetts, "a blow of equal force produces a more serious effect" on a woman than on a man.[7] Medical opinion that women possessed a low perceptual threshold for pain both drew upon and reinforced common Victorian cultural values. Romantic writers, from Edgar Allan Poe to Lydia H. Sigourney, saw feminine sensitivity to pain as a reflection of women's overall physical frailty and heightened spiritual "sensibility."[8]

Conversely, traditional concepts of virility presumed a truly masculine man to be almost impervious to physical pain. Thomas Trotter, surgeon to the British fleet, warned physicians not to "confound the complaint of the slim soft-fibred man-milliner, with that of the firm and brawny ploughman." When a real man feels pain, it is serious. As the paragons of virility, soldiers and sailors exhibited masculine insensitivity to the fullest. Heroic manly fortitude, heightened by the "excitement" of battle, rendered soldiers insensitive to the pain of "almost any operation." At least such was the opinion of British military surgeon Rutherford Alcock, as quoted approvingly by American army surgeon John B. Porter.[9] Even humanitarian reformers like Horace Mann agreed that "sensitiveness to bodily pain . . . impairs manliness," especially among soldiers.[10]

AGE

Age, like sex, exerted a powerful influence on the perception of pain, according to most nineteenth-century theorists. Old age, it was generally agreed, diminished all perceptual acuity, including the ability to feel pain.[11] But there the agreement ended. The degree of sensitivity in children proved an especially controversial issue. Dr. Abel Pierson of Massachusetts declared that infants could sleep insensibly even while undergoing surgery.[12] Pierson, Henry J. Bigelow, and others who believed in infant insensibility, assumed that the ability to experience pain was related to intelligence, memory, and rationality; like the lower animals, the very young lacked the mental capacity to suffer.[13] In contrast, others who felt children to be especially sensitive emphasized the feminine rather than the animal aspects of child nature. "The constitutions of children, in point of debility and irritability, approach to the female"; therefore, a child's "nervous power is . . . easily affected by stimuli," noted Dr. Trotter. As the idea that "women and children" comprised a single biosocial category gained popularity in Romantic Era America, the view that young children were extremely vulnerable to pain gradually came to predominate.[14]

SOCIAL CONDITION

In addition to age and sex, social and economic class played a major role in determining which people were believed most sensitive to suffering. As explained by Tocqueville, the European pauper had become inured to perpetual misery and was hardly even aware of it. But, he declared, in the egalitarian United States, there were no such permanently degraded people (except for slaves). Everyone shared equally the extreme hypersensitivity of the middle classes. America's constantly fluctuating fortunes prevented anyone from becoming accustomed to the physical pains of poverty, while exposing everyone to the risk of having to undergo them.[15]

Although Tocqueville could locate no hardened poor in white Jacksonian America, the wealthy Connecticut novelist John W. De Forest found them easily by 1863. "We waste unnecessary sympathy on poor people," he asserted. "A man is not necessarily wretched because he is cold & hungry and unsheltered; provided those circumstances usually attend him, he gets along very well with them; they are annoyances, but not torments."[16]

Alcohol further hardened the poor to their lot, at least for the time they were actually drunk. But the chronic alcoholic, though insensible when intoxicated, became agonizingly hyperaesthetic when sober. "Mania a potu" resulted in a morbid sensibility of the nerves, whose painfulness rapidly drove the sufferer back to the bottle. Criminals too seemed highly insensitive to both physical and moral pain, according to one late-nineteenth-century physical anthropologist. Immigrants, especially Germans and Irish, were also deemed less sensitive than were native Americans. Hydropath Thomas Low Nichols contrasted "our Teutonic friend's harder strung nerves, blunter sensation," with "the nicer sensibilities and consequent greater capacity of suffering of finer grained humanity."[17]

And if poverty and degradation produced numbness, the combination of wealth, status, and femininity could breed a truly exquisite sensitivity. According to the Brothers Grimm, a genuine princess could invariably be distinguished from the ordinary herd by her royal hypersensitivity—even a pea hidden under many mattresses would produce pain.[18] Such precious creatures were almost too sensitive to carry out normal bodily functions. Menstruation caused "almost all women in the better classes" to suffer pathological levels of pain, according to a midcentury obstetrics text. But "the nervous system of the poorer classes [of women] in our cities, fortified by constant exercise in the open air, and strengthened by frugal habits," was not subject to such "morbid action," in the opinion of the noted gynecologist Dr. Gunning S. Bedford. "Pain is in various proportions among women who are equally well formed," Dr. William Potts Dewees declared; "we generally find the women of the country more obnoxious to it, than those of cities." [19]

Education and cultural refinement, factors closely correlated with class, comprised another influence long believed to alter human perception of pain. "For in much wisdom is much grief," warned Koheleth, the Preacher of Ecclesiastes; "and he that increaseth knowledge increaseth sorrow." From the story of Eve to the myth of Pandora the ancient teachings agreed—sensitivity to pain is the result of knowledge. [20] Many nineteenth-century Americans took such concepts to heart. The leaders of the common school movement in particular stressed the importance of avoiding overcultivation of the intellect, lest public schooling produce a generation of overly sensitive children. Unlike Koheleth, Horace Mann did not conclude that all knowledge increased human suffering; yet he demanded that mental development proceed in step with physical education, to prevent excessive nervous sensitivity. [21] Since women were already very sensitive, intellectual education for girls had to be especially circumscribed and carefully counteracted by physical exercise. [22]

It was not just education, but culture and civilization itself that produced excessive sensibility. Nineteenth-century writers repeatedly contrasted the pain-free "natural" life of the savage with the hypersensitive nervous disorders of "artificial" civilized existence. The difference could be explained either theologically or naturalistically. Religious romantics called the savages' freedom from suffering a result of the primitives' almost prelapsarian innocence. Since pain was punishment for eating the fruit that gave knowledge of good and evil, those tribes still living in almost Edenic ignorance of moral responsibility were of course less subject to suffering. More naturalistic observers, like Dr. Dewees, rejected the notion that physical pain was punishment for original sin and that innocence could be any protection against the pain of violating natural laws. Dewees viewed the savage life as conferring freedom from pain simply because it was "natural"—because savages lived the way nature intended. [23]

In *A View of the Nervous Temperament,* Thomas Trotter

developed and expounded the idea that the spread of civilization "never fail[s] to induce a delicacy of feeling, that disposes alike to more accute pain, as to more exquisite pleasure." Writing in 1806, he introduced a concept that remained a source of concern throughout the nineteenth century when he warned that the growing "general effeminacy" of modern sensibility was leading to the self-destruction of civilization.[24] American public health activists like Dr. John H. Griscom of New York agreed, blaming excessive "irritability of the nervous system" and the consequent "Degeneracy of the Human Race" on the poor ventilation and polluted air characteristic of civilized urban life. The morbid sensitivity produced by city life would lead to the self-induced fall of civilization. To avoid such a catastrophe, however, it was not necessary to abandon civilized living entirely, so long as city dwellers and sophisticates could be lured back to the pure air, hard work, natural habits of life, and simple virtues of the yeoman farmer.[25]

The effect of civilized living conditions on female sensitivity constituted a special threat to human survival, by making the function of reproduction unbearably painful. Dr. Dewees of Philadelphia, perhaps the foremost American obstetrician of the early nineteenth century, blamed "civilized life" for the fact that childbirth was "usually observed" to be "exceedingly painful . . . especially in the upper walks of life." Even domesticated animals suffered more exquisitely than did their wild sisters. The same sentiments were echoed at the other end of the century by Dr. Henry M. Lyman, professor at Chicago's Rush and Woman's Medical Colleges. "Really normal labor is not a painful process. . . . But in civilized society the majority of mankind are living under quite abnormal conditions. . . . Hence, in civilized society, it is the rule, rather than the exception, to find parturition attended with a high degree of suffering." Such opinions were not limited to male physicians. Even a homeopathically inclined feminist like Elizabeth Cady Stanton agreed that "refined, genteel, civilized" women suffered inordinate pain in childbearing.[26]

While civilized women suffered excessively from pregnancy and childbirth, their savage sisters supposedly felt no pain at all. "Woman in a savage state . . . enjoys a kind of natural anaesthesia during labor," noted Dr. James Y. Simpson, the Scottish pioneer of artificial obstetric anesthesia. "Am I not almost a savage?" Stanton exulted, following her own painless delivery.[27]

Concern over the implications of pain for the future of civilization heightened following the spread of Darwinian theory. The excessive sensibility produced by refined, artificial living clearly gave the uncivilized both an economic and reproductive advantage in the struggle for survival.[28] But while evolutionary theory increased the frequency with which such fears were voiced, the basic idea, that civilization produced a self-destructive level of sensitivity to pain, remained unchanged throughout the entire nineteenth century. "There can be no question as to whether the nervous systems of highly cultivated and refined individuals among civilized peoples are more complex and refined in structure and delicate in susceptibility and action . . . than the nervous system of savages," declared a leading American neurologist in 1881. The distinguished founder of American neurology, Dr. Silas Weir Mitchell, agreed. "In our process of being civilized we have won, I suspect, intensified capacity to suffer. *The savage does not feel pain as we do.*"[29]

RACE

Nineteenth-century white Americans viewed savagery and race as highly interrelated concepts. Both as a correlate of savagery and as an influence in its own right, race was believed to be crucially important in influencing human perception of pain. The archetype of savagery, the Indian, was believed almost incapable of feeling. "Every skin has its own natur'," the Pathfinder proclaimed to the sailor Master Cap. "Until you can find me a Chinaman, or a Christian man . . . who could sing . . . with [his] flesh torn with splinters and cut with knives . . . you cannot find a man with redskin natur'." Benjamin Rush asserted that Indian men could often "inure themselves to burning part of their bodies with fire, or cutting them with sharp instruments."[30] Enlightenment America's foremost race theorist, the Reverend Mr. Samuel Stanhope Smith of Princeton, believed that no women suffered less from childbirth than American aborigines did. "We know that among Indians the squaws do not suffer in childbirth," Stanton lectured. "Among your red Indian and other uncivilized tribes," agreed Dr. Simpson, "the parturient female does not suffer the same amount of pain during labour, as the female of the white race."[31]

The Negro constituted the Indian's closest rival for insensibility, according to a wide variety of observers on both sides of the

Atlantic and all sides of the slavery issue. Early European voyagers to Africa noted black imperviousness to suffering. One medical explorer reported that blacks felt no pain even under the most radical surgery. "I have amputated the legs of many negroes who have held the upper part of the limb themselves," he asserted. The eighteenth-century English physician and expert on race, Dr. Charles White, cited such accounts as evidence for his contention that Negro immunity to pain resulted from the excessive thickness of black skin. Owing to their primitive "sensibilities," blacks could undergo, "with few expressions of pain, the accidents of nature which agonize white people," according to a West Indian plantation handbook.[32]

But the most elaborate account of black insensibility came from an American—the controversial midcentury New Orleans physician Samuel A. Cartwright. Dr. Cartwright was the discoverer of "dysaesthesia Aethiopis," an hereditary disease of blacks, which caused such "obtuse sensibility of body" that its victims "seem to be insensible to pain when subjected to punishment."[33] While few, even among slaveholders, adopted Cartwright's peculiar terminology, or his unscriptural conclusion that the Negro was a separate subhuman species, the basic "fact" of black insensibility won almost unquestioned Southern white acceptance. Dr. A. P. Merrill declared,

Nervous action in the negro is comparatively sluggish, but his senses of seeing, hearing, and smelling, are apt to be acute and active; those of touch and taste, obtuse. He requires less sleep than the white man; has greater insensibility to pain . . . .
They submit to and bear the infliction of the rod with a surprizing degree of resignation, and even cheerfulness. . . . They differ from their white masters in no one particular more than in this.[34]

"What might be grievous misery to the white man, . . . is none to the differently tempered black," declared Virginia essayist George Frederick Holmes; "identity of sensibilities between the races of the free and the negroes" was preposterous.[35]

Several Southern physicians performed excruciating experiments on black patients, in the clear belief that their victims lacked the ability to feel pain. America's most eminent gynecological surgeon, Dr. J. Marion Sims, explained that he carried out his lengthy and agonizing experimental operations on slave women, not because he could force slaves to submit to them, but because white women were too sensitive to pain. A Virginia physician experimented with a cure for pneumonia that involved pouring water "near the boiling point" over the bare back of the Negro subject; the treatment "seemed to arouse his sensibilities somewhat." A Georgia doctor trying the same experiment expressed genuine astonishment when the patient "leaped up instantly and appeared to be in great agony."[36]

Even many opponents of slavery propagated the belief that blacks did not feel as much pain as did whites. Dr. Rush, one of the earliest American abolitionists, blamed the Negroes' morbid insensitivity on congenital leprosy (an explanation that also accounted for the blacks' supposedly distinctive odor). The cheerful demeanor of slaves, even "where the lash of the master" was at its cruelest, proved to Abraham Lincoln that black insensibility was evidence of God's compassion. Abolitionist Lydia Maria Child likewise praised the "merciful arrangement of Divine Providence, by which the acuteness of sensibility is lessened when it becomes merely a source of suffering." Tocqueville earlier had drawn the same conclusion, though he clearly recognized its moral ambiguity. "Am I to call it a proof of God's mercy, or a visitation of his wrath, that man, in certain states, appears to be insensible . . . ? The Negro, plunged in this abyss of evils, scarcely feels his own calamitous situation." Fugitive slaves and freedmen like Henry Watson and Jermain Loguen agreed that bondsmen eventually became incapable of feeling.[37]

Black women, like their Indian sisters, supposedly enjoyed racial immunity from the extreme sensitivity that characterized white womanhood. Negro mothers "were not subject to the . . . pain which attended women of the better classes in giving birth . . . ," according to the Southerners interviewed by Frederick Law Olmstead. Like black men, black women supposedly experienced little suffering, even from major surgery. "Negresses . . . will bear cutting with nearly, if not quite, as much impunity as dogs and rabbits," reported the *London Medical and Chirurgical Review* in 1817.[38]

But while the "full-blooded" Negro was depicted as nearly without feeling, the "mulatto" was stereotyped as exceedingly sensitive. From the scientific-racist tracts of Alabama's Dr. Josiah C. Nott, to the most sentimental antislavery novels, nineteenth-century Americans unanimously declared the offspring of racial "amalgamation" to be almost as hypersensitive as white women. In *White-Jacket*,

Melville's vignette, describing a "Head-bumping" contest between "a full-blooded 'bull-negro' " and a mulatto named "Rose-Water," assumes that the reader understands the two characters to be at virtually opposite poles of human sensibility. Melville, like the sentimentalist opponents of slavery, used the mulatto's almost feminine sensitivity to dramatize the injustice of a system that treated all nonwhites alike. Dr. Nott and the Southern apologists saw in the same phenomenon nothing but nature's ordained punishment for race-mixing.[39]

Thus all living things might be arranged in a hierarchy of sensitivity, a great chain of feeling. Brute animals, savages, purebred nonwhites, the poor and oppressed, the inebriated, and the old, constituted the lower orders. The most sensitive included women; the rich, civilized, educated, and sophisticated; sober drunkards; and mulattoes. Children were usually considered feminine in sensitivity, though infants were sometimes believed not to feel. Occupying the virtuous middle ground were the sturdy yeoman farmers.[40]

The Causes and Curability of Perceptual Differences

Although most Americans agreed that race, sex, age, and social condition were all good indicators of sensitivity to pain, they divided sharply over whether these factors themselves were the real *causes* of such perceptual differences. Granted, for example, that blacks and Indians felt less pain than whites did, two issues remained: first, was the difference a normal and a proper result of "racial nature," or was it an abnormal, "unnatural" condition caused by other factors such as disease, ignorance, poverty, or oppression; and second, could the difference in sensibility be changed or was it permanent?[41]

For the Pathfinder the answers were clear-cut—"redskin natur' " itself produced an unalterable level of insensibility. Living an Indian's life would never enable a white to fully duplicate the natives' natural insensitivity; living the life of a white man would never completely erase it from an Indian. In like manner, Southern defenders of a rigid status quo took great comfort in the knowledge that blacks by their very nature were unalterably adapted to the rigors of slavery.[42]

But reformers of all shades vehemently denied that blacks or Indians were insensible by nature. From committed abolitionists to Southerners seeking to strengthen slavery by making it more humane, advocates of racial meliorism chose to interpret differences in human sensibility as "unnatural"—as the result of something other than permanent racial nature.[43]

The most obvious alternative explanation was brutality. Reformers like Horace Mann, Lemuel Shattuck, and Dr. Morrill Wyman reminded middle-class whites that they too would grow insensitive to pain if they were subjected to repeated floggings, degradations, and privations. Lydia Maria Child, Tocqueville, and Lincoln saw black insensibility as a form of numbness—a result of the conditions of slavery rather than an inherent racial characteristic. These reformers did not deny that blacks felt less pain than whites did, but they interpreted the difference as a remediable, abnormal effect of slavery rather than as a natural justification of it. By treating slaves with kindness or by freeing them, it might well be possible to restore their normal sensibility.[44]

Some slaves agreed. One runaway, subject to repeated brutality, reportedly "began to grow less feeling . . . and even indifferent to my own punishment."[45] Such testimony bears remarkable similarity to that of modern-day victims of prolonged brutality. "I arrived at that state of numbness where I was no longer sensitive to either club or whip," wrote a survivor of Auschwitz.[46]

Oppression was not the only nonracial cause invoked to account for racial variations in the perception of pain. As noted before, the "uncivilized" conditions and habits of the darker races and the influence of hard work in the open air also seemed to play a role. Trotter and Dewees, early in the century, denied any differences between nonwhites and such white "savages" as Calabrians or Scandinavians.[47] In the case of the Indians, Benjamin Rush pointed out that their childrearing practices were carefully and deliberately constructed to produce insensibility.[48] Those who sought to meliorate the treatment of slaves and of Indians suggested a wide range of plausible alternatives to race itself as being the actual cause of racial perceptual differences.

However, blaming insensitivity on brutality or other environmental factors did not guarantee that sensibility could be restored simply by improving conditions. Imposing civilization on the

Indians, for example, revived their sensitivity so rapidly that they died in great numbers.[49]

Furthermore, most nineteenth-century Americans believed that acquired characteristics could become hereditary, that brutalization repeated over many generations might eventually lead to hereditary numbness, and that within the span of one lifetime the hardening produced by long mistreatment would thus be difficult or impossible to erase. Southern slaveholders and frontier army officers who lived in daily contact with supposedly hardened savages might agree with reformers that environment, not race, had originally inured nonwhites to pain; yet they rejected the reformers' claims that it would be easy or safe to reverse the process through kindness or better conditions. Dr. Merrill regarded the insensitivity of blacks as due more to "their condition and habits of life . . . than . . . any inherent and distinctive liability of the colored race." Yet he doubted whether any such characteristics could or should be changed after centuries of ingraining. "Admitting that all his peculiarities of deterioration are the result of forty or more centuries of constant decline . . . however much may be done by mankind, toward the promotion of the civilization [of the blacks] . . . , many thousand years must necessarily elapse, before he can be brought up to the present position of the white man."[50] In addition to undermining hopes for restoring sensitivity to blacks and Indians, belief in the heritability of acquired traits also cast great doubt on the chances for curing sensory brutalization among the oppressed, violent, drunken Irish or among American poor whites.[51] Because acquired insensibility might become hereditary, environmentalist explanations did not necessarily guarantee the efficacy of change.

But if blaming the environment did not guarantee the efficacy of reform, blaming heredity did not completely rule out change either, so long as the inherited insensibility was still seen as "unnatural." Belief in the malleability of heredity cut both ways. Thus, even when racial differences in sensitivity were blamed on inherited biological abnormalities, such as thick black skin or other hereditary diseases, antislavery optimists like Dr. Rush still did not have to conclude that the differences were permanent. By the proper sensitivity-inducing environmental therapy, even thick, malodorous, and leprous black skins could eventually be restored to white levels of perceptual acuity. Enlightenment rationalists like Rush implied that all human differences in pain sensitivity were unnatural, pathological, and thus potentially curable.[52]

Like racial differences, the influence of sex on pain perception raised questions of underlying causes and of permanence. Many male physicians who wrote on the subject considered female sensitivity to be the normal result of natural physiological differences inherent in gender. Because sensitivity was a fundamental aspect of feminine nature, such arguments concluded, women could never compete successfully in the brutal masculine world and would always require the protection of men.[53]

Victorian women themselves sometimes seemed to believe that their gender rendered them naturally hypersensitive to pain. Those who completely internalized the hegemonic stereotype found that their extreme sensitivity gave them a degree of usable manipulative power—within the confines of "woman's sphere." "Domestic feminists" like Sarah Josepha Hale, and sentimentalist reformers like Dorothea Dix, declared that female sensitivity conferred not simply physical vulnerability but spiritual strength. Suffering made women morally superior to men, and therefore justified for them a vital role in the reformation of the home and society.[54]

However some nineteenth-century Americans rejected the idea that women were naturally prone to suffering. Dr. Mary Putnam Jacobi denounced "women who expect to go to bed at every menstrual period . . . . Constantly considering their nerves, urged to consider them by well-intentioned but short-sighted advisors, they pretty soon become nothing but bundles of nerves."[55] Radical feminists like Elizabeth Cady Stanton admitted that most women in fact were exquisitely sensitive to pain, but she blamed Victorian culture, including the male medical profession, for creating this unnatural, pathological state of affairs.[56]

The question of whether female sensitivity sprang from nature or nurture particularly confounded the issue of the origins of labor pain. Early obstetricians like Dewees and midcentury practitioners such as Augustus K. Gardner agreed that most birth pain was unnatural, pathological, environmental—the curable result of violating natural laws. However, many biblical literalists like obstetricians Charles D. Meigs, Hugh Hodge, and Francis Ramsbotham believed painful birth to be a normal, inescapable facet of feminine nature.[57]

Likewise, Victorian Americans disagreed over whether manly toughness was natural or environmental in origin, whether the insensitivity of seamen and soldiers was born or made. Diverse, often conflicting efforts by such humanitarians as wartime nurse-organizers Florence Nightingale, Dorothea Dix, and Clara Barton; nurse-authors Louisa May Alcott and Walt Whitman; and sailor-authors Herman Melville and Richard Henry Dana all contributed to a growing suspicion that military insensitivity was the result of training and conditions rather than innate heroism. And while Alcott, Whitman, Melville, and the Sanitary Commission agreed that some insensitivity was a virtue in a fighting man, they warned that American troops could have too much of a good thing; hardening must not proceed to the point of brutalization.[58]

Furthermore, the explanations for such sexual differences were not always internally consistent. Some Americans viewed sex differences in sensitivity as a normal condition of biology while simultaneously portraying womanly tenderness and manly insensitivity as forms of virtue that required careful training. Dr. Meigs came under sharp attack for repeatedly contradicting himself on whether female sensibility was natural or learned. Horace Mann consciously sought to appeal to both sides, implying that sexual variations in sensitivity were inherent in the nature of gender, but only as ideal types; woman's natural tenderness and man's natural hardness still required careful artificial cultivation lest they be nipped in the bud. Because "sensitiveness to bodily pain . . . impairs manliness," the educator declared, boys need to be "trained to a disregard, and even a contempt of bodily pain, so that they may not be unnerved and unmanned." The eminent British-American physiologist Robley Dunglison was somewhat calmer but no more committal. Women are generally more sensitive then men, he wrote, "whether from original delicacy of organization, or from habit, is not certain; probably both."[59]

Sensitivity and Endurance

Nineteenth-century commentators carefully distinguished between "insensitivity"—the inability to feel pain, and "endurance"—the ability to bear it. They insisted that the differences discussed so far were real differences in the way pain was perceived, not simply differences in the capacity to withstand it.

But the difference between insensitivity and endurance is

easier to define than to apply. Suppose a slave is vigorously whipped, yet shows none of the reactions we have learned to associate with pain. Who is to say for sure whether his behavior is the result of insensitivity or endurance? All the observer has to go on is the slave's behavior (including his verbal accounts), but what certainty can that provide about what the slave was "really feeling?"

The problem of knowing another person's actual feelings has intrigued philosophers for centuries. Well-educated midcentury Americans could not have avoided some exposure to the issue, while those who had completed a liberal college course might have been expected to reflect an awareness of the ways in which Descartes, Hume, the Scottish realists, Kant, and Bentham had attempted to resolve it.[60] Yet American and European writers who claimed to detect real differences in human sensitivity often showed no concern over the philosophical difficulties; from Alexis de Tocqueville to Dr. Silas Weir Mitchell, nineteenth-century commentators seemed convinced that they could readily distinguish between endurance and insensitivity.[61] Very few of these observers felt troubled enough to add even such mild qualifiers as "*seem* to be insensible to pain" or "with few *expressions* of pain" to their accounts quoted above.[62]

How could these commentators have been so sure of their practical ability to resolve a thorny philosophical issue? In what sense can endurance and insensibility be so different as to be distinguished at a glance?[63] Perhaps the answer is simply that "endurance" is a word with many positive connotations in Western cultures, while "insensitivity" may often be used to imply some very negative judgments. Endurance requires heroic effort; insensitivity can come from brutish stolidity. Endurance involves strength and character; insensitivity can result from a moral or physiological defect. Thus, if someone who is admired undergoes a normally painful ordeal without flinching it is likely to be called "endurance;" if a hated or contemptable person performs exactly the same feat it is likely to be called "insensitivity."[64]

Nineteenth-century commentators explicitly recognized this moral distinction between insensibility and endurance. Dr. Trotter noted that moral judgments "depend in great measure" upon the individual's "capacity for feeling." "One man is condemned for sinking under adversity, as proof of deficient virtue and spirit; while another is extolled for his courage, as a token that he possesses nobleness of mind. Yet . . . . [t]he first may be a weak nerved being, and a good man; and the other, under apparent resolution of soul, may possess nothing beyond want of feeling.'' Since Trotter believed the ability to diagnose true insensibility constituted a fundamental medical skill, he concluded that only a doctor could ''best decide with impartiality on their respective merits.'' Thus Trotter deduced that moral judgments should be based on a medical evaluation of sensitivity; it did not occur to him that, conversely, his boasted ability to diagnose true sensibility might actually depend on moralistic prejudice.[65]

Nineteenth-century writers clearly reserved the term ''endurance'' for people of whom they approved. For example, while most whites (and a few blacks) spoke of the slaves' ''insensibility,'' most blacks attributed their seeming lack of feelings to heroic endurance instead. The twentieth-century black poet Langston Hughes wrote,

> Because my mouth
> Is wide with laughter
> And my throat
> Is deep with song,
> You do not think
> I suffer after
> I have held my pain
> So long.
>
> Because my mouth
> Is wide with laughter,
> You do not hear
> My inner cry,
> Because my feet
> Are gay with dancing,
> You do not know
> I die.[66]

His predecessors simply sang, ''Nobody knows the trouble I seen / Nobody knows but Jesus.'' ''Oh God! I can feel the torture now— the terrible, excruciating agony of those moments. I did not scream; I was too proud to let my tormentor know what I was suffering,'' remembered one former slave.[67] To hide one's pain from the oppressor became an act of defiance. To have private feelings, unknown and unknowable by the master, provided a sense of autonomous personhood, a realization that there was something no master could own.

Like these blacks, white antislavery sentimentalists Alexander Kinmont of Cincinnati, William Ellery Channing, and Harriet Beecher Stowe also attributed the Negroes' seeming insensitivity to praiseworthy qualities of endurance. However, these sympathetic whites wanted to believe that black endurance constituted a submissive Christian turning of the other cheek, rather than a desperate and defiant form of resistance.[68] White abolitionist Thomas Wentworth Higginson, who commanded black troops in the Civil War, was amazed to discover that their supposed Christlike resignation had more aggressive aspects.[69]

White admirers defended the Indian in identical terms with the black.[70] Samuel Stanhope Smith denounced those who "imputed to the aboriginal natives of America . . . *insensibility* because they suffer torture with a *patience* not to be paralleled in any other country." Jefferson's *Notes on Virginia* likewise boasted that the noble native American "*endures* tortures with a firmness unknown . . . with us," yet "his *sensibility* is keen, . . . though in general they endeavor to appear superior to human events."[71]

The Jeffersonian praise of Indian endurance contained more than a little nationalistic pride—a response to Buffon's assertion that American fauna were puny and degenerate.[72] In similar chauvinistic fashion most nineteenth-century Americans considered themselves better able to endure pain than were effete Europeans. Westerners supposedly had an especially high tolerance for suffering because of the almost savagely natural existence they led. From Walt Whitman to the leaders of the AMA, nineteenth-century Americans accepted the idea that the frontier environment produced actual physiological changes that made all Americans, and especially Westerners, a tougher breed of human beings.[73]

The distinction between sensitivity and endurance is vital to unraveling the tangled Victorian romantic conception of femininity. While women supposedly felt pains that men would not even notice, female spirituality enabled women patiently to submit to pains that no man could endure.[74] Women were exalted as excellent sufferers, true Christian martyrs, whose role was "to suffer and to be silent."[75] The Massachusetts General Hospital praised one such woman, "She was to the last a great sufferer."[76] Feminine endurance derived, not from physical strength, but from its opposite, the moral power of innocent suffering. Victorian physicians recorded with sacred awe the case histories of frail, hypersensitive women, to whom every headache and heartache was excruciating, yet whose spiritual powers of endurance enabled them to bear agonizing surgical and medical torments without complaint. "What angelic serenity!" gushed Dr. Gardner over his female patients afflicted with "lingering suffering." "What beautific gentleness and love! What a mild radiance pervading the whole being of one of those afflicted!"[77] According to Victorian sentimentalist ideology, this combination of hypersensitivity and submissive endurance placed medical men under a double obligation to protect women from pain—both because women could be hurt so easily and because their silent submission could evoke such intense male guilt. Thus, despite his adoration of women in pain, Gardner was among the first to use anesthetics in childbirth.[78]

If women had both high sensitivity and high endurance levels, the urban poor, and especially the Irish, had neither. Habituation to personal violence, generations of poverty, oppression, and ignorance combined to render the poor almost hereditarily insensible.[79] Yet the same factors that destroyed their capacity to feel simultaneously undermined their powers of endurance and resistance, as even a cursory glance at the urban mortality bills demonstrated.[80]

The very old also scored relatively low on both sensitivity and endurance. But unlike the poor, the elderly could not really be blamed for causing their own frailty and thus might still be entitled to gentle treatment. As with children, innocent helplessness entitled the old to a patronizing solicitude for their sufferings.[81]

Pain, Equality, and Human Rights

Though they argued bitterly over the causes and implications, almost all nineteenth-century American commentators agreed that human beings differed widely in their sensitivity to and/or endurance of pain. Yet earlier observers had sometimes denied such differences. Alexander Hewat, a South Carolina Presbyterian minister, declared in 1779 that Negroes, in their natural African habitats, "are by nature . . . , equally susceptible of pain and pleasure, equally averse from bondage and misery, as Europeans themselves." Nineteenth-century antislavery writers interpreted such data to prove that the observed insensitivity of *American* blacks must be an "unnatural" result of bondage. But Hewat instead implied that the belief in unequal sensitivity itself was mistaken.[82]

In 1605, William Shakespeare had written that

> The poor beetle, that we tread upon,
> In corporal sufferance finds a pang as great
> As when a giant dies.

But mid-nineteenth-century medical journals quoted Shakespeare only to reject his literary conceit.[83]

Nineteenth-century authors occasionally did remind their readers that all sentient creatures shared the experience of pain to some degree, and thus all merited sentimental concern. But only a handful went on to affirm *equality* of sensitivity among different people. Dr. Eliza L. S. Thomas proclaimed that "man's corporeal nature is averse to pain. The stoutest heart will quail under its afflictions. Even the *stern indian* of the forest, whose haughty nature has been so much the theme of poets; will unbend *his* kingly dignity and briny tears will flow afresh at even a simple tooth-ache." In the words of New York's eminent surgeon Valentine Mott,

> Pain reduces all ranks to a level—it makes all men cowards. Some constitutionally and physically suffer very little from surgical operations; while others, from moral courage or religious culture, are enabled to endure great bodily torture. These, however, form but a very small item in the great mass of the family of mankind, and therefore deserve to be named only as exceptions to the great and general rule.[84]

For these few egalitarians, no less than for their opponents, the issue of sensitivity to pain went beyond theoretical neurology. All assumed that their conclusions ought to have some important implications for the actual treatment of human beings. From Southern extremists who justified the harshest slavery on grounds that blacks could not really feel it, to Reverend Hewat, who opposed slavery because blacks did indeed feel it, virtually everyone assumed that people who really did feel pain differently somehow ought to be treated differently.

Nineteenth-century observers still accepted almost by reflex the idea that everything in nature was created for a Purpose; that man's ethical obligation was to discover and obey nature's Design. If differences in sensitivity existed, it meant they had been created for a reason that human beings were obliged to respect. Only if mankind had been created literally equal would it be right to treat all men equally.[85] Thus, Jeremy Bentham carefully designed his utilitarian calculus to correct the supposedly obvious injustice of treating equally those with unequal sensitivity to pain. Implicit in Horace Mann's dedication to common schooling was the effort to create a common level of sensibility among the electorate; without an equality of sensitivity, political equality was assuredly temporary.[86]

But a few nineteenth-century Americans did resist the alluring fallacy of ethical naturalism. They alone insisted that, even if someone could be proved totally insensible to pain, such biological facts could not determine how that person ought to be treated by others. As the *New York Tribune* explained following the Emancipation Proclamation, *"Human Rights do not depend on the equality of Man or Races,* but are wholly independent of them."[87]

PART THREE: Who Received Anesthetics: Theory and Practice

CHAPTER EIGHT

INDICATIONS AND CONTRAINDICATIONS: RULES FOR USING ANESTHETICS

Different people differed widely in their sensitivity to pain, susceptibility to drug effects, and resistance to medical authority. And
different operations involved differing amounts of pain and risk. Thus
conservative physicians expected that the benefits and drawbacks of
anesthesia would vary significantly from patient to patient. To aid in
assessing all the pros and cons for each individual patient, mid-nineteenth-century medical journals, textbooks, and medical school lec-
turers attempted to provide detailed particularized rules and guide-
lines by which the practitioner could determine which types of patients
most needed anesthesia. While few conservative physicians believed
all of these suggested rules and regulations were applicable, almost
all believed in at least some.

THE YOUNG AND THE OLD

Children were one group whose susceptibility to pain made them especially likely candidates for anesthesia. One of John Collins Warren's correspondents, for example, cited the common nineteenth-century operation of lithotomy (removal of bladder stones) as too minor to require anesthesia in adults. But in young children, he rejoiced, it "is a great relief both to patient and to surgeon."[1] The editor of the *American Journal of the Medical Sciences* strongly endorsed an article that specifically cited lithotomy in children as one of the few instances for which anesthesia was always indicated.[2] In 1851, Samuel D. Gross' definitive American textbook on bladder surgery agreed.[3]

A more sentimental endorsement of the need to anesthetize children came from Dr. Eliza L. S. Thomas. Of all the effects of anesthesia, Dr. Thomas found "none more peculiarly beautiful than in its administration to children who are the subjects of Surgical interference. Operations agonizing to the Surgeon particularly if he be a father, can be performed with ease. . . . [E]verything repulsive to the impressive spirit of childhood is out of sight." Children also should receive preferential anesthetization because, unlike adults, the young were "innocents unconscious of the motive" for the surgery, and their pains did not result from willful, responsible violations of natural law.[4]

With very young children, however, there were two schools of opinion, based on two different viewpoints regarding infants' sensitivity to pain. While Thomas held that babies had a hypersensitive and "impressive spirit" that demanded anesthesia, Henry J. Bigelow adopted a less romantic, more Lockean view of pain sensitivity in the "young infant." "The fact that it has neither the anticipation nor remembrance of suffering, however severe, seems to render this stage of narcotism [full anesthesia] unnecessary," he wrote in a special report published by the AMA.[5]

Considerations of patient management and control reinforced the verdict of benevolence in prescribing the particular use of anesthetics on the young. For children too little to be restrained by reason, yet too big to be restrained easily by force, anesthesia was especially valuable. Lyman's anesthesiology text of 1881, for example, considered anesthetics unwarranted in dental surgery in adults. "But if the patient be a child," ether was indicated, to render the patient "more easily manageable." Dr. Gross agreed that children required anesthesia more than did adults, not only because of the child's tender sensibilities but because, with the squirming young patient "being rendered perfectly quiet and tractable, the surgeon may deliberately proceed."[6] Many other printed reports agreed that, even in the most minor surgery, anesthetics were permissible to control children, especially those of a "wayward disposition."[7] With the newborn, however, "the facility of controlling a child of this age" contributed to making full anesthetization "unnecessary," according to Dr. Bigelow.[8]

Children were believed particularly susceptible to the effects of the anesthetic itself. Whether this susceptibility was an advantage or a danger, however, was a subject of some dispute. Most physicians concluded that the dangers of anesthesia were less for children than for adults. University of Pennsylvania medical students in 1860 were taught, "It is very important that the age should be taken into consideration for in the very young it acts very favourably."[9] A number of midcentury surgical textbooks and journals supported this position, and as late as 1881, Lyman's anesthesiology text declared, "Children support anaesthesia with remarkable tolerance. They yield promptly to the anaesthetic influence, and their sleep is peaceful and profound. A fatal result is among these little patients exceedingly rare."[10]

Some surgeons, however, interpreted the ease of anesthetizing children as a danger that required greater caution and/or smaller doses, especially with chloroform. Morton (who certainly had an axe to grind) wrote, "In females and children, in whom there is generally a greater susceptibility of the nervous system, the action of chloroform is quicker, more complete, and therefore more dangerous," though this danger supposedly did not exist with his ether.[11] For the vast majority of authorities, however, the combination of high sensitivity to pain, difficulty in managing the patient, and ease of anesthetization made children from about two years old to adolescence unexcelled subjects for the use of anesthetics.[12]

Interestingly, old age was rarely considered as an independent factor in anesthetization; rather the "old and infirm" formed a single medical category. Those texts that commented specifically on the elderly believed that old people felt less pain, were more liable to shock, and were more susceptible to the effects of anesthesia, than were other patients.[13] The Medical Society of Virginia declared, "Old and infirm persons yielded more readily than the middle-aged and the robust'' to the influence of anesthesia. While some texts considered this susceptibility a sign that ''after the age of sixty-five years, it was devoid of danger,''[14] Lyman and most others denied that anesthesia was safe for the elderly and recommended ''great deliberation'' before ''the administration of an anaesthetic to an elderly person.''[15] In general, however, anesthetization of the elderly was assumed to follow the general rules governing debilitated patients, discussed below.

WOMEN AND MEN

Even before the discovery of anesthesia, physicians and other professionals advocated the use of less painful procedures on sensitive women than on hardy men. ''She is more sensitive to internal emotions and external sensations; and I assert, without fear of contradiction, that no physician can be safely trusted . . . who disregards even in the child the distinction of sex,'' wrote Dr. Morrill Wyman. ''In medical colleges, in medical books, in medical practice, woman is recognized as having a peculiar organization, requiring the most careful and gentle treatment,'' according to Reverend John Todd of Pittsfield, Massachusetts. Applying these widely shared views, Dr. Edward Warren concluded that anesthesia was especially vital in the treatment of women patients. ''In many individuals of the softer sex there is so great a degree of physical as well as mental sensibility, that they cannot bear a great amount or long continuance of pain. The patient either sinks at once under her sufferings, or a lingering disease is induced,'' Dr. Warren declared. ''In many of these cases, life might have been saved . . . by the use of anaesthetic agents.''[16]

The anesthetization of women was also especially indicated, not only to soothe their delicate physical sensibilities, but to overcome their moral sensibilities and subdue their resistance to medical authority. Women were generally believed to be particularly troublesome patients because of their shame at exposing themselves to male doctors, their supposedly child-like lack of reasoning power, their resentment of male authority, and their seeming proclivity for natural, noninterventionist modes of medical practice.[17] A leading surgery text of 1860 recommended that anesthesia be used to do ''away with the scruples of the over-modest woman, to whom the shame of exposure is worse than the pain of the knife.''[18] Dr. Edward Horner recommended anesthesia for operative obstetrics "in cases where manual or instrumental assistance is imperatively demanded, and is strenuously resisted by the patient."[19] An article in the *American Journal of the Medical Sciences* declared it "occasionally admissible, particularly in children," to involuntarily anesthetize troublesome patients—the "child" in this case being a "young lady, of highly cultivated mind, aged about 25 years."[20]

Like children too, women were believed especially susceptible to the effects of anesthetics.[21] Generally, this susceptibility was seen as a sign of greater safety. As explained by Lyman,

> The influence of sex is quite apparent among the phenomena of anaesthesia. Women pass more readily than men into the stage of insensibility, and the anaesthetic sleep is more profound. As a consequence of this fact, syncope is less frequently observed among them than among men. They resemble children in this particular. The mortality of the male sex is accordingly greater than that of the female.[22]

But this greater female susceptibility also indicated greater caution and smaller doses when anesthetizing women. "Females, and especially those of a nervous temperament, require a much smaller quantity than males," declared one surgical text of 1863. The same author specified a dose of ether for women only one-eighth that prescribed for strong or alcoholic men.[23] Anesthesia was thus no exception to Robley Dunglison's general rule that, compared to men, women should be given a "much smaller dose" of all medicines.[24]

In addition, a variety of other factors had to be taken into account with women. According to Lyman, "The menstrual period would seem to expose the female to greater risks of nervous disturbance . . . ; so that, unless absolutely necessary, the employment of anesthesia should be deferred till the monthly interval is established."[25] Women were also supposedly prone to suffer from hysteria. "Hysterical females, and lively excitable animals are much more susceptible" to the effects of anesthesia, according to a British surgeon whose views appeared in the *American Journal of the Medical Sciences* in 1851.[26] However, in the opinion of a University of Pennsylvania medical student, "An hysterical diathesis does not form any objection to the use of chloroform as the pain would bring on an attack" if the anesthetic were omitted.[27] In summary, as in the case of children, the combination of greater advantages and lesser dangers made women particularly likely candidates for anesthesia; though in both cases the dose administered might be smaller than that for an adult man.

So far as anesthesia was concerned, medical texts discussed the active healthy male patient mostly for purposes of contrast with women and children. Thus the average man, supposedly less sensitive, more reasonable and cooperative, and less susceptible to drugs, required anesthesia in fewer cases but in larger doses than women and children did. Midcentury American medical writers agreed almost unanimously that strong, vigorous men were resistant to the effects of anesthesia; the more manly the more resistant. "A strong, full-blooded man is pretty sure to resist the approaches of anaesthesia under any circumstances," declared the Boston Society for Medical Improvement in 1861.[28]

SOCIAL CONDITION

"In considering the selection of cases for anaesthetic agency," the *American Journal of the Medical Sciences* insisted, "habits of previous life should be inquired into."[29] This advice held true for all patients, though it was especially true for women. Simpson declared class, race, and culture to be essential considerations in weighing the need for obstetric anesthesia.

Unaccustomed by their mode of life to much pain and fatigue, patients in the higher ranks of life are not fitted to endure either of them with the same power or the same impunity as the uncivilized mother, or even as females in the lower and hardier grades of civilized society; and *hence there is the greater propriety and necessity in the physician employing all the means of his art, so as to save them, as far as possible, from their sufferings.*[30]

While Simpson stressed the civilized woman's need for extra pain relief, Samuel Gregory emphasized the superfluity of anesthesia "in cases of childbirth among the humble and healthy classes, and more particularly among the native women of the forest."[31] Lyman repeated identical sentiments more than thirty years later.[32] Such considerations remained extremely important determinants of obstetric anesthesia well into the twentieth century, when they began to assume blatantly eugenic overtones.[33]

Although men and women of the lower orders supposedly needed less protection from pain, they sometimes required anesthesia for purposes of physical control. In a number of cases, ether and the straitjacket were prescribed simultaneously for uncooperative Irishmen in large urban hospitals.[34] But the use of anesthesia to control lower class troublemakers was not generally recommended. For one thing, most nineteenth-century hospitals freely exercised the right to expel miscreant charity patients for almost any reason.[35] Also, forcing anesthesia on a resisting street-wise hooligan could be a chore in itself; and as one young doctor explained in 1860, anesthesia could backfire by making unruly patients even harder to control. A "certain class of navigators, and labourers, whom one occasionally meets with in the several hospitals, having a very small amount of intilect [sic], . . . get into a drunken riotous condition as soon as the inhalation commences."[36]

Class considerations also modified the safety of anesthesia. The same nervous sensitivity that made pain relief so important in the upper classes also made the educated and the rich more susceptible to the effects of anesthetics, according to a report of the Medical Society of New Jersey in 1847. "The judicious physician who knows the effect of powerful stimulants . . . upon persons of high cerebral organization . . . , will be slow to sanction the general use" of anesthetics in such cases.[37] But medical opinion was not unanimous on this point; other physicians advised that anesthesia was safer for "those who have been blessed with education and mental culture, and at the same time are alive to all the refinements of cultivated society."[38]

The Medical Society of Virginia claimed that Negro women were less susceptible to ether than whites were. However, Turnbull and other authorities found blacks to be most susceptible of all "races," followed by the Germans, Americans, and Irish, in that order.[39]

Thus, on the basis of sensitivity and control, anesthetics were especially indicated for rich, cultured, white women and contraindicated for their social opposites. But in considering the relation of social class to safety, opinion was divided.

Similar considerations made nineteenth-century veterinarians slow to employ anesthetics. The belief that brutes were insensitive to suffering, combined with the difficulties of managing their patients during the initial, excitory stage of anesthetization, led most animal surgeons to oppose or ignore anesthesia.[40]

INTEMPERANCE

In anesthetizing the intemperate, the major medical concern was for safety. All forms of intemperance supposedly increased the risks from anesthesia, according to the *American Journal of the Medical Sciences* in 1851. "In smokers—in persons long habituated to the use of opium, or its preparations—in the person of intemperate habits, either large eaters or drinkers, I have often observed that the course of anaesthesia is irregular." The irregularities included "violent convulsions," "hysteria," "vomiting," "extreme debility," and "cerebral oppression." Other writers included "immoderate sexual indulgence" and masturbation as contraindications.[41]

However, drunkenness clearly constituted the main problem. "Alcoholic intoxication, and a condition characterized by *delirium tremens,* should . . . prohibit the use of anaesthetics." "In all such cases there is extreme cardiac debility, and death is liable to occur."[42]

Most medical authorities worried even more about the supposedly dangerous tolerance for anesthesia built up by long-term chronic drinkers than about the acute interactive effects of temporary intoxication. In this view, alcoholics built up a kind of resistance to being anesthetized and thus required enormous, potentially unsafe doses to produce an effect. One doctor estimated that in order to produce insensibility among patients "accustomed to the free use of spirituous liquors" they would have to inhale an anesthetic for up to twice as long as was required for a temperate person.[43] Henry H. Smith's textbook of surgery warned that it would take a minimum dose of four ounces of ether to anesthetize an intemperate man; the comparable dose for a (presumably sober) respectable lady was one-half ounce. "In fact, it has often seemed to me that the amount of ether requisite to induce anaesthesia, might be taken as a good index of the habits of the patient, some having 'stronger heads' than others."[44]

When actually passed out, the drunkard presumably needed no further anesthetic—long after 1846, alcoholic stupor remained an acceptable surgical anodyne. But when sober, the chronic inebriate was exquisitely sensitive. Thus, a medical student in 1860 attributed the fact that drunks required larger doses of anesthesia to their "morbid excess of sensibility in the nerves of common sensation."[45]

Drunks could be unruly patients, of course, but the same considerations that weighed against forcibly anesthetizing disruptive lower class subjects held for alcoholics. The Boston Society for Medical Improvement summed up the best medical opinion of 1861 on both the safety and patient management aspects of the issue, declaring, "Persons of intemperate habits succumb to ether slowly, and with greater reluctance and more opposition than persons unused to intoxication."[46]

THE FEEBLE AND INFIRM

Surgeons generally preferred not to operate at all on people debilitated and exhausted by lingering chronic diseases, for fear the patient would lack the strength to recover.[47] When it was decided to perform surgery on a person enfeebled by age or illness the obvious need to lessen the shock made anesthesia extremely advantageous. Yet with such patients the ability to resist the dangerous effects of anesthesia was presumably minimal as well. The problem was stated most clearly in the *American Journal of the Medical Sciences:* "Jones was of a very peculiar and very sensitive temperament . . . .

It may be said the case was not a subject fit for chloroform, on account of his weak and hectic state. Now, this appears to me to be a question requiring all the experience, and all the observation and judgment, which can be brought to bear upon it. If we are not to use such an agent in the *weak,* the timid, and highly sensitive patient, for what class of patients do we require anaesthetics?[48]

Only a few months later, another surgeon reported an identical dilemma in the same journal.[49]

Many nineteenth-century surgeons considered the anesthetic a greater risk than the shock of surgery in these cases. One of the earliest such warnings against anesthetizing the weak and debilitated came from Alexander Hosack of New York.[50] The Massachusetts General Hospital in 1847 cited "delicacy" as a valid reason for not anesthetizing a surgical patient.[51] A case report printed in 1857 noted matter-of-factly, "I did not think it prudent to submit the patient to the action of chloroform or ether, owing to his feeble condition."[52] The Boston Society for Medical Improvement warned that even with ether, "great caution is demanded in its use with patients who are near death from chronic and exhausting disease.'' Through-out the 1860s, University of Michigan medical students were taught that "debility" contraindicated anesthetization.[53] However, John Collins Warren, Snow, and other eminent authorities disagreed. "The more feeble a patient is, the more quickly and pleasantly does the vapor generally act,'' according to Druitt.[54]

SPECIFIC DISEASE COMPLICATIONS

In addition to general "debility," a wide variety of spe-cific preexisting diseases also altered the balance between the advan-tages and disadvantages of anesthesia. Not surprisingly, diseases of those organs supposed to be most affected by anesthetics were gen-erally cited as indications of greatest danger. The conditions most commonly claimed to increase the risks of anesthesia were nerve and brain diseases, such as "inflammation of the brain," epilepsy, con-vulsions, chorea, apoplexy, fainting, and brain tumors;[55] heart dis-eases, especially valve disease and "fatty degeneration"; and lung diseases, such as consumption, asthma, bronchitis, and emphy-sema.[56]

While these contraindications were very generally ac-cepted in their main points, a wide variety of additional diseases were mentioned by at least some authorities as further barriers to anesthe-tization. These included obesity,[57] kidney disease,[58] aneurism, teta-nus, and many others.[59]

Although the prevention of shock was almost uniformly agreed to be one of anesthesia's greatest advantages, the use of an-esthetics on patients already in a state of severe collapse was a highly controversial issue, because the anesthetic seemingly produced a fur-ther depression of vital energies. As noted previously, mid-nine-teenth-century surgeons were deeply divided over the advisability of operating at all on such patients until they showed signs of "react-ing."[60] Most texts dealing with anesthesia mentioned the problem of anesthetizing those already in shock without providing a definitive ruling, a few prohibited it, a few others claimed the prohibition to be unjustified.[61]

Blood loss often accompanied shock. Many physicians regarded such hemorrhage as precluding the use of anesthetics. A smaller number, however, held the opposite view, that "plethora" and the absence of bleeding made anesthesia more dangerous.[62] The question remained unsettled throughout the century. Clearly, however, most surgeons felt that the risks of anesthesia were least for patients who were neither in shock from an acute injury nor worn out from chronic disease.

SOLDIERS AND BULLET WOUNDS

Between the Mexican and Civil Wars, medical doctrines on the advisability of anesthesia for the armed forces underwent several major changes, reflecting evolution both in attitudes toward soldiers and in the nature of military organization in America. In the war with Mexico, military surgeons like John B. Porter believed soldiers were, or ought to be, impervious to pain. Manly heroism, tempered in the fire of military life and honed by the excitement of battle, made soldiers insensitive to the pain of "almost any operation" and thus made anesthesia superfluous. Porter, chief surgeon of the army hospital at Vera Cruz, concluded, "We do not need the chloroform bottle on the field of battle."[63] Similar arguments were used to justify the use of the lash in the army and navy—hardened troops were impervious to lesser pain. Not only were anesthetics unnecessary in the military, according to Porter, but since gunshot victims were often in shock and highly at risk from infection, anesthesia was also presumed to be particularly dangerous for them.[64]

At the opposite pole from Porter were civilian volunteer physicians like Dr. E. H. Barton of Baltimore. One month after the discovery of anesthesia, Barton began pressuring Army Surgeon General Thomas Lawson to supply ether to the troops. When his efforts became snarled in red tape, Barton simply packed up some ether and headed for Vera Cruz. His "benevolent" efforts were well received and highly publicized at home,[65] though after a few trials, Porter ordered Barton's experiment stopped.[66]

Antebellum military field surgeons like Porter enjoyed almost unlimited control over anesthetic policy. When chloroform became available, Surgeon General Lawson urged Porter to introduce the new painkiller, but Porter simply ignored him.[67] Thus the view that soldiers should not be anesthetized generally prevailed.

By the mid-1850s however, Anglo-American textbooks of surgery and medicine began to reject the notion that soldiers felt less pain or required less anesthesia than did civilians.[68] By the start of the Civil War, both Union and Confederate medical handbooks stipulated as a "humane" duty that anesthesia be administered according to the same general principles governing its use on active young male civilians of equivalent social background and with similar injuries.[69] Of course, most military surgeons still did not expect such hearty young men to require anesthesia as frequently as women or children would. At the Union Hotel Hospital in Georgetown in 1862, "Dr. P.," a veteran of the Crimean War, whose views were reported by Louisa May Alcott, believed that soldiers needed ether only for amputations. Each surgeon at the hospital was still free to follow his own policies; a soldier's chances of receiving anesthesia varied widely depending on the views of the medical officer of the day.[70]

As in the Mexican War, military surgeons enjoyed almost unfettered individual discretion in anesthetization during the early years of the Civil War. And again, civilian volunteers, including William T. G. Morton, traveled through the hospitals, administering anesthesia to whomever they felt needed it, unless actually restrained by the surgeon on duty.[71]

But, by the start of 1863, the Union Army began to standardize and centralize control over anesthetization. As part of an overall plan for hospital organization, Jonathan Letterman, Medical Director of the Army of the Potomac, recommended that each division hospital designate one assistant surgeon to have full authority over the use of anesthesia. The reorganization plan, embodied in a circular letter of October 30, 1862, was first implemented following the Battle of Fredericksburg in December. Responsibility for anesthesia was thus at least nominally delegated to eighteen specified assistant surgeons, instead of being left to each of the Army's more than 162 surgeons and their unnumbered, untrained volunteer helpers.[72] Despite this recommendation, however, civilian volunteers, including Morton, continued to serve as anesthetists in the Army of the Potomac as late as July 1864.[73]

Letterman's plan was a small part of an overall proposal to introduce order and subordination into an individualistic, disorganized medical service. It was both an attempt to bureaucratize benevolence and to coopt bureaucracy for benevolent ends.[74]

The circular letter directed that responsibility for anesthesia be centralized and rationalized but did not explicitly aim at standardizing practice or at limiting the professional discretion of those to whom this responsibility had been delegated. The plan dealt with who would make the decisions about anesthesia, not with what their decisions should be or with how they should make them. But the degree of centralization instituted by Letterman almost certainly did serve to minimize the extreme variations in military anesthetic use, such as those described by Alcott. Under Letterman and Surgeon General William A. Hammond, the Union Army was slowly creating bureaucratic machinery that Hammond hoped eventually might be used to enforce standardized treatment regimens.[75]

There was, however, one use of anesthesia that won immediate acceptance by military surgeons. As early as 1847, American and British anesthetists began using ether to detect malingerers. The pioneer English anesthetist John Snow reported

It is humiliating to the medical officer, and a loss to the country, for him to be deceived by a man who is only pretending illness; yet to charge with feigning a man who is really ill would be a much more serious error; and the difficulties of distinguishing between real and pretended disease are sometimes very great. Lameness and deformities are diseases that are often feigned. Ether has solved the difficulty in which the medical men were placed. . . . In one instance a man was suspected to pretend a deformity . . . . He was put under the influence of ether: his muscles became relaxed, and the deformity disappeared.

American textbooks continued to report such cases throughout the nineteenth century. These early uses of ether marked the birth of so-called "truth serums"; even today, purported truth drugs like sodium pentothal are really simply anesthetics.[76]

MINOR SURGERY
  Modern students of the history of anesthesia have generally noted the fact that by the early 1850s most American surgeons claimed to be using anesthetics in almost all major operations.[77] But most practitioners were equally adamant in barring the use of anesthesia for "minor surgery." Unfortunately, few historians have bothered to look at the fine print to determine what, by midcentury standards, constituted "minor" surgery.[78] Yet most nineteenth-century textbooks on "minor surgery" covered everything except amputation of the limbs; Henry H. Smith's text, *Minor Surgery*, even included a chapter on that subject.[79] A closer look at the nature of minor surgery considerably alters the picture usually presented of midcentury anes-

thesia and provides a startling revelation of what many surgeons considered insignificant pain.

Throughout the nineteenth century, the leading Anglo-American journals and textbooks considered tooth extraction to be the prime example of an operation in which the suffering and shock were generally too minor to justify the dangers of anesthesia. In 1860, young Dr. John Wesley Thompson denounced the "ignorant" public for demanding the improper use of anesthesia "on every trivial occasion," such as, "if a single tooth was to be extracted; an abscess to be opened; . . . or the slightest unpleasant sensation or pain to be felt."[80] Thirty-five years after a dentist introduced anesthesia to the world, Dr. Henry Lyman summed up the conservative physicians' view of dental anesthesia as follows: "The practice of using powerful anaesthetic vapors during the operations of minor surgery should always be discouraged." Chloroform especially should never be used in "operations of a trifling character, such as the extraction of a tooth, the opening of an abscess, and the evulsion of a [toe]nail. If patients about to undergo an insignificant operation *insist* upon insensibility to pain," then a very small dose of ether might be appropriate. However,

When only a single tooth is to be drawn, if ether is employed, it is unnecessary to proceed to the stage of complete unconsciousness. . . . But if the patient be a child, or an adult from whose mouth at least two entire rows of rotten snags must be forcibly removed, it is desirable that complete anaesthesia should be induced. By this means the patient is rendered more easily manageable, and the shock of severe pain is avoided.[81]

In addition to extracting teeth, lancing abscesses, and pulling out infected toenails, another operation usually cited as too minor to warrant anesthesia was the extremely common and ancient procedure of lithotomy—cutting into the bladder for removal of urinary stones. Samuel D. Gross dismissed such surgery as "usually unattended with much pain," and regarded anesthesia as unwarranted, except for children.[82]

In a wide variety of other specific "minor" operations, surgeons felt the use of anesthesia to be unjustified, not only because the pain was too insignificant, but also because insensibility complicated the task of the surgeon or increased the risk to life. In operations on the nose, mouth, throat, tongue, and jaw, many surgeons felt that an unconscious patient ran an unacceptable risk of suffocation.[83] The use of anesthesia to operate on children born with harelip and/or cleft palate proved especially controversial. Despite the tender age and sensitivity of most such patients, surgeons generally opposed their anesthetization.[84]

At the opposite orifice, anesthesia made the painful operations to remove hemorrhoids or close anal fistulae too difficult, because an insensible patient could not maintain the kneeling position deemed most favorable for such procedures.[85] In addition, anesthesia posed problems in that class of operations, discussed above, for which the patient's active help was deemed useful—especially lithotrity (crushing urinary stones) and operations for cataract, crossed-eyes, and hernia.[86]

Turnbull's anesthesia text of 1885 provided the longest listing of operations usually considered too minor for anesthesia. They included amputations of fingers and toes; hydrocele (fluid in the scrotum); removal of dead bone; extirpation of small tumors; urinary catheterization; as well as surgery on the anus and eye.[87] Thus, a wide range of "minor" operations—perhaps the largest part of mid-nineteenth-century surgical practice—were generally held to be more or less unsuitable for the use of anesthetics.

OBSTETRICS

The essence of the new conservatism in medicine was the search for a moderate synthesis of Nature and Art. Yet, in the practice of obstetrics, the ancient distinction between inflicted and natural pains remained firmly rooted.[88] Thus, even many conservative medical authors continued to draw a distinction between "natural" labor and surgical deliveries. The latter included any form of physical intervention, from manual assistance, through forceps manipulation, to the use of hooks, crochets, and the Caesarian section. In these cases of operative obstetrics, where the pain was clearly inflicted by the doctor, the use of anesthesia was subject to the same rules and indications that governed any other surgical operation on a pregnant woman. "In those cases of midwifery where it is necessary to apply the instruments or to turn the child, the ether should be given in the same manner as where a surgical operation is to be performed," Morton stated.[89]

Thus, most obstetrics texts recommended the use of anesthetics for such operations, because the patients were women. Both women's special sensitivity to pain and their greater need to be restrained were cited as reasons for anesthetizing surgical deliveries, based on the same principles as governed other operations on women.[90] The same modifying rules regarding race, ethnicity, class, age, health, and so on, applied to both operative obstetrics and other surgery.[91] And while such deliveries were surgery, they were sometimes considered minor surgery, governed by the rules appropriate for other, less serious operations. Thus, the AMA Committee on Obstetrics declared anesthesia unwise when the utility of having a conscious patient guide the operation counterbalanced the freedom from pain, because, unlike the general surgeon, the obstetrician could not "*see* how and where he is operating."[92] This rule was no different from that governing operations like lithotrity, where the patient's guidance was also deemed useful. However, unlike lithotrity, the reason obstetrical surgery could not be observed directly was not the physical inaccessibility of the organs but their social inaccessibility. In Victorian America, obstetricians sometimes had to work by "touch" only, under a sheet, to protect the patient from the shame of exposure.[93]

While the pain of obstetric surgery was considered "unnatural" because it was inflicted by the doctor, other birth pains could be held "unnatural" in the sense of abnormal or pathological. Physicians who adopted this approach attempted to determine how much birth pain was normal or natural and advocated anesthesia for those women who experienced unnatural, i.e., harmful, levels of suffering.[94]

However, on the subject of what constituted normal birth pain, there was virtually no agreement. While some physicians set a standard so high that "not more than one case in a hundred" could be considered pathological,[95] others considered all pain to be abnormal and hence an indication for anesthesia.[96]

The indications and contraindications a given textbook listed for obstetric anesthesia thus depended in large part on how much (if any) pain the author believed to be natural. If the pain could be defined as unnatural, the same criteria would govern anesthesia in childbirth as in surgery. The nineteenth-century debate over obstetric anesthesia was thus not only a dispute over the merits of "natural" childbirth but also an argument over exactly what "natural" meant.

For some practitioners, any intervention was unnatural and thus prohibited; for others, almost any level of discomfort was unnatural and thus demanded anesthesia.[97]

Only the more heroic interventionists and the most consistent conservatives advocated anesthesia for those birth pains that they considered "natural."[98] Medicine was leading the struggle of human progress to control the forces of nature, the Standing Committee of the Medical Society of New Jersey reported in 1849. "True, it is a natural effort; the pains are not the pains of disease—they are a pure physiological development of a natural law; but the achievements of science in her upward and onward advancement ought not to be arrested by such an objection."[99]

In summary, most nineteenth-century textbooks discouraged anesthesia in "natural" labor—but there was virtually no consensus on what "natural" meant.[100] About the only rules most textbooks could agree on were that anesthetics should be used more often in first births than with more experienced mothers and that the amount administered should be small.[101]

SUMMARY

Nineteenth-century medical authorities urged physicians to consider many different factors in prescribing anesthetics. While few of these specific indications and contraindications won unanimous professional endorsement, anesthetics were generally considered especially appropriate for children; women; educated, upper-class, and white patients; and in major limb amputations, reduction of dislocations, and prolonged tissue dissections. Likewise, the majority of textbooks, journals, and medical schools surveyed felt anesthesia to be contraindicated for lower class, intoxicated, and veterinary patients; those with various specific brain, heart and lung diseases; and those undergoing natural labor, lithotomy (adults), or surgery on abscesses, toenails, teeth, nose, throat, mouth, eye, or anus.

Although there was more disagreement, the balance of medical authority also tilted against anesthesia for strong adult men; nonwhites; the obese, elderly, or chronically sick; menstruating women; those suffering from gunshot wounds or kidney disease; and patients undergoing surgery for hernia or other "minor" operations. Opinion was about evenly divided on the advisability of anesthetizing patients

suffering from shock or hemorrhage. Many individual authors advocated an assortment of other criteria, including some who used Gal-
en's ancient temperaments as a guide to anesthetization.[102]

Despite the inherent formalism of such prescription rules,
most authorities insisted these indications and contraindications not
be applied too mechanically. They urged physicians to weigh the individual pain sensitivity and idiosyncratic drug reactions of each patient, in addition to the textbook criteria.[103] And, while the professional literature emphasized that the doctor should make these decisions,
at least a few physicians advocated a considerable degree of patient
power as well.[104]

Thus, these textbook rules were not generally meant to
be taken in isolation from each other nor as absolutes. A surgery text
of 1854, for example, warned against the use of chloroform in cases
of heart, lung, or neurological weakness, *unless* the patient were also
"so irritable that it is evident that he could not bear the shock." One
student surgeon explained that even in "minor operations," it might
be all right to administer anesthesia to certain patients who had "what
might perhaps be called an ideosyncratic timidity."[105]

Some nineteenth-century physicians denied that "*any* state
of the patient . . . positively contra-indicates the use of ether."[106] A
few seemingly agreed with one Civil War medical manual, which advised using anesthetics as freely as cold water.[107] But, most often,
those who advocated using anesthesia on every type of patient meant
only that no class of patients was *totally* prohibited from receiving
anesthetics, not that all classes should be anesthetized equally often.
While "*any* state of the patient" might be considered for anesthesia,
some states were still clearly better candidates than were others.[108]

CHAPTER NINE

IDEOLOGY AND ACTION: WHO ACTUALLY RECEIVED ANESTHETICS

Thus far, we have seen that in textbooks, journals, and medical schools, nineteenth-century surgeons insisted that the advantages of anesthesia be carefully weighed against the disadvantages. Age, sex, class, ethnicity, general and specific health conditions, compliance with medical authority, and the specific operation to be performed were all factors to be considered in this calculus of suffering. But to what extent did physicians practice such precepts? Is there evidence that such professional rules had any relation to the way anyone actually practiced medicine on a day-to-day basis? To answer this question requires a detailed comparison between what professional leaders said ought to be done and the case records of surgery as actually performed.

This chapter is a first attempt to provide such comparisons, based largely on three sets of midcentury surgical records and other, less complete case histories. I have used the records of the Massachusetts General Hospital (the first hospital to use anesthesia), the Pennsylvania Hospital (probably the last major American hospital to introduce anesthetics), and the private records of Dr. Frank H. Hamilton, a leading spokesman for conservative professionalism in surgery. Geographically and philosophically, Hamilton represented a midpoint between the two hospitals. His practice ranged from rural kitchen tables in upstate New York to the wards of Bellevue, with a stint as Medical Director of the 4th Army Corps in 1862 and 1863. An organizer and leader of the AMA, Hamilton was an acknowledged expert on fractures and amputations.[1]

There are many limitations in these available data, in terms of timespan, completeness, and representativeness.[2] Thus the conclusions presented in this chapter should be regarded as illustrative more than demonstrative. But the evidence available shows that at least some elite East Coast surgeons and institutions behaved in a manner consistent with the ideology we have been discussing.

MASSACHUSETTS GENERAL HOSPITAL (1846–1847)

The precepts of the conservative calculus of suffering provide an extremely accurate description of the actual treatment of patients at the Massachusetts General Hospital in the year 1846–47 immediately following the introduction of anesthesia. Approximately one of every three potentially painful operations performed at the hospital took place without anesthesia.[3] Age, sex, class, ethnicity, patient condition, and type of operation were all correlated with the use of anesthesia in a manner fully consistent with conservative professional ideology.

The single most important factor in anesthetic use, not surprisingly, was the type of operation to be performed. The Boston hospital surgeons performed all major amputations: arm, leg,[4] hand, foot, and all breast removals, on anesthetized patients. But such drastic mutilations accounted for only about one-fifth of all operations done at the hospital.[5] In the remaining cases—including the removal of tumors, toes, fingers, bone sections,[6] bladder stones, polyps, toenails, and burn scars; the opening of abscesses and closing of fistulae; the repair of hernias, dislocations, and cleft palates; and other "minor" operations—more than four of every ten patients faced the knife awake.[7] Furthermore, those specific operations for which anesthesia was contraindicated in the textbooks showed a significantly lower rate of anesthetization than did other types of surgery. For example, none of the seven operations for harelip and/or cleft palate employed anesthetics. Later records indicate that the first such operation to employ ether at Massachusetts General took place in 1855 and that the use of anesthesia remained rare in such cases.[8]

Just as the professional literature recommended, children got anesthesia much more frequently than did adults undergoing noncapital surgery. Children under ten got anesthetics in four out of every five such operations; only half the adolescents and young adults received ether. However, the treatment of older patients diverged from that advocated by most professional authorities. Adults over forty-six got anesthetics in 80 percent of noncapital operations, the same rate as for children (see table 1; this, and all following tables, are in the Appendix), and much more often than the literature indicated. Perhaps the discrepency is due to the fact that no age-based measure can capture the nineteenth-century physicians' primarily functionally based definition of "elderly."[9] Or perhaps the Massachusetts General surgeons took a more solicitous view of pain in the aged than the majority of their colleagues elsewhere did.

Sexual differences at Massachusetts General closely matched the textbook pattern. Women received ether in 69 percent of their minor operations; the "stronger sex" proved their manhood by enduring half of their minor surgery without anesthesia (see table 2). The patient's birthplace was also correlated with the likelihood of undergoing surgery awake. Less than half of foreign-born patients were given anesthetics for minor surgery; Americans got anesthetized in almost two-thirds of such cases (see table 3).

A vast majority of all Massachusetts General patients (like those at all other nineteenth-century American hospitals) came from the poor and working classes, so the connection between economic status and anesthesia use is somewhat obscured in hospital records. But even though almost all Massachusetts General patients were from the lower classes, two occupations in particular seemed to have received special treatment—sailors and "common laborers." The medical and general literature that singled out these two occupations as a kind of nonsentient biological *lumpenproletariat*[10] seems to have been reflected in the daily practice at the Boston hospital. Sailors and laborers were given anesthesia in 43 percent of their noncapital surgery; for all other employed men the corresponding figure was 57 percent (see table 4).

Each of the differences observed in anesthetization according to age, sex, nativity, and type of operation appears to have been strikingly independent of the others. For example, young adults received anesthesia less often than did children and older people, even when the disproportionately male and foreign composition of the young adult population is taken into account (see table 5). In short, the actual treatment of patients at the Massachusetts General Hospital conformed, in almost every particular, to the pattern of anesthetization recommended in the nineteenth-century conservative medical literature.

DR. FRANK H. HAMILTON (1849–1877)

The surgical records of Frank Hamilton reveal the same distinctions of age, sex, occupation, and type of operation, though with some interesting variations. Like the Massachusetts General surgeons, Hamilton varied his use of anesthesia according to the type of operation performed, but unlike the Boston practice there was no class of operation in which Hamilton uniformly gave anesthetics. The New York surgeon anesthetized patients for major limb amputations far more often than for any other type of procedure. But through a quarter century of surgical practice, lasting into the 1870s, he continued to carry out occasional amputations, even of legs and arms, without resort to ether or chloroform (see table 6).[11]

Hamilton, like his Boston colleagues, anesthetized women more frequently than men—but only in the case of amputations. Almost one-quarter of the men recorded as having lost a major limb to Dr. Hamilton's saw faced their ordeal awake. Every woman amputee received an anesthetic (see table 7). On the other hand, in cases of minor surgery, gender made no significant difference in Hamilton's use of anesthesia. Unlike patients at the Massachusetts General, Hamilton's women got anesthetics at an insignificantly lower rate than men did for minor surgery (see table 8).

The age of Hamilton's patients was clearly linked to the likelihood of their being anesthetized. Patients from puberty to middle age suffered through surgery awake far more frequently than did the presumably more sensitive young. And, like the Massachusetts surgeons, Hamilton also disproportionately favored anesthetizing older patients (see table 9). Furthermore, the influence of age was independent of all the other considerations. Male or female, in large or small operations, the young and the old always got anesthetized more frequently than did those in between. The type of operation too was independent of all other factors; regardless of age or sex, amputees were always anesthetized more often than nonamputees. In fact, young adult men comprised the only recorded patients Hamilton ever subjected to amputation without anesthesia (see table 10).

Unlike the antebellum hospitals, Hamilton did not keep very complete records on the occupations or ethnic origins of his patients. However, among the small number of cases for whom Hamilton did see fit to record an occupation, sailors and common laborers once again came out on the short end; they received anesthetics less often (though not significantly less) than did men in any other job (see table 11).

PENNSYLVANIA HOSPITAL (1853–1862)
Unfortunately, the available surgical records of the large and prestigious Pennsylvania Hospital proved of only limited value in testing how well surgeons conformed to the calculus of suffering. The surviving data on pre-1870s anesthetic use deal only with the amputation of limbs following fractures; thus it is not possible to measure the importance of the type of operation as a factor in anesthetic use. Furthermore, the proportion of women, children,[12] and old people subjected to amputation at the Pennsylvania Hospital was incredibly small compared with the practice in Boston and New York. Thus, the Pennsylvania records do not reveal any statistically significant age or sex differences (though these data in turn reveal a great deal about age and sex as factors in the decision to perform operations—see ch. 11).

Despite the lack of adequate numbers for statistical significance, the Pennsylvania Hospital records do follow the familiar pattern with regard to sex—women received anesthetics much more frequently than men did. One-third of male patients lost their limbs while awake; all of the handful of women amputees received anesthesia (see table 12). Among employed men, laborers and sailors once more received anesthesia less frequently than did any other occupational group (see table 13). And, unlike Dr. Hamilton or the Massachusetts General, the Pennsylvania Hospital conformed to the dictates of the professional literature with regard to the elderly; the handful of older patients received anesthesia much less often than did younger adults (see table 14).[13]

OTHER RECORDS

I have not been able to locate any antebellum records relating to the use of anesthesia in childbirth. However, for the last quarter of the nineteenth century, such information has been preserved. A sample of patient records from two Boston hospitals between 1873 and 1899 collected for another study[14] provides an intriguing glimpse of obstetric anesthetization (see table 15). Once again, practice followed the textbook precepts. Women on whom obstetrical forceps were used received anesthetics more than half of the time, but in ''natural'' deliveries, painkillers were very rarely administered. The difference is significant and marked at both hospitals.

In summary, these records of actual patient treatment clearly suggest that antebellum surgeons did differentiate among patients in their use of the new painkillers. The employment of anesthesia appears to have conformed quite closely to the calculus of suffering advocated in professional journals, textbooks, and classrooms. Taken as a whole, these statistics imply that women, children, old people, native-born Americans, skilled workers, and amputees did indeed generally receive anesthesia more frequently than did other medical and social categories of surgical patients.[15] For these types of patients, sex, age, class, and type of operation served as accurate predictors of who would and who would not be anesthetized.[16] But it should also be remembered that women, children, old people, non-manual workers, and amputees all remained small minorities of nineteenth-century hospital patients. In the treatment of the young adult working class men undergoing minor surgery, who comprised the largest group of cases, there was still considerable individual variation in the use of anesthesia, not explained by the broad categories used in the present analysis.

In other words, gender played a larger role in predicting the anesthetization of women than it did in the treatment of men; age played a larger role in predicting the anesthetization of children and older patients than it did in the treatment of young adults; and so on. One hypothetical explanation might be that women, children, and other patient minorities were treated according to broad stereotypes, while young adult men were treated according to more detailed technical considerations.[17] The present analysis indicates that broad social and medical criteria provide excellent predictors of the treatment of unusual patients, without fully explaining much of the variation in the treatment of more typical patients.[18]

CHAPTER TEN

WHY DOCTORS
STILL DIFFERED

Most mid-nineteenth-century surgical authorities called for the anesthetization of some patients and not others. They promulgated and seem to have followed detailed rules by which to calculate the tradeoff between the advantages and disadvantages of anesthesia for many different types of cases.

But within the framework of these common rules, there was still considerable room for differences among practitioners. For example, the textbooks all taught that anesthesia was strongly indicated for amputations, and the available records indicate that all surgeons did in fact anesthetize amputees more frequently than any other type of patient. Yet, whereas the Massachusetts General Hospital etherized virtually all major limb amputees beginning in 1847, the New York Hospital had not yet reached this level by 1854, and the Pennsylvania Hospital not until 1863; Frank Hamilton continued performing unanesthetized limb amputations until the end of his career in the 1870s.[1]

Some of this variation was probably due to differences in the types of patients seen at different institutions, but much of it likely resulted from differences among the physicians. We have seen why most doctors agreed to use anesthesia only some of the time; we must now consider a few of the possible reasons why some still used it earlier or more often than others.

Ideological Differences Within Conservative Medicine

In chapters 3 and 4, we noted the influence of various ideological differences on the differing assessments of anesthesia's advantages and disadvantages. Religion, sexual politics, medical sect, humanitarian beliefs, and similar ideologies all contributed to variations in the assessment of anesthesia's pros and cons. For example, belief that pain was God's punishment for sin did not necessarily preclude the use of anesthetics, but such belief did tip the balance of advantages and disadvantages in a negative direction. Thus, physicians holding such a creed would generally be expected to require a greater potential advantage before using anesthetics in any given case and would thus be expected to use them less often than would others, all else being equal.

Another ideological factor influencing differences among physicians concerned the degree of importance assigned to beliefs whose basic tenets were widely shared. For example, most nineteenth-century physicians believed that blacks felt less pain than did whites, but they varied widely in their assessments of how much less. The many doctors who believed blacks could give birth painlessly shared the same racist ideology as the surgeon who thought "negresses" could be "cut" like "dogs,"[2] but there seems to have been a clear difference in magnitude. Thus, both the ideological differences discussed in chapters 3 and 4 and differences in the intensity of belief in aspects of the shared ideology outlined in chapters 6–8 probably produced a range of individual variation among conservative practitioners, all within the framework of the anesthetic calculus.

Unfortunately, the extent to which any specific ideological position can be correlated with specific differences in the frequency with which individual doctors actually used anesthesia remains an unanswerable question. Quite simply, not enough physicians kept records of their use of anesthesia for us to judge the influence of, say, varying degrees of feminist commitment on varying degrees of anesthetic usage. Even with today's vastly more comprehensive medical records, such studies would be extremely difficult to carry out.

However, it is possible to reach at least tentative conclusions concerning the effect on the use of anesthesia of a number of personal characteristics, such as a doctor's age, sex, and geographic location. The role of time and place is assessed in this chapter; the effect of the physician's gender is discussed in chapter 11.

Soft-Hearted, Innovative Young Students and Reactionary Old Professors

Many observers attributed variations in the use of anesthesia to the age of the surgeon. Younger practitioners supposedly adopted anesthetics much more quickly and employed them more freely than did their older colleagues. Henry J. Bigelow, at age twenty-eight the youngest surgeon on the Massachusetts General Hospital staff, explained that young medical students had not yet become callous to suffering. They still retained some of "that kindly feeling which is generally upon the surface in early youth" and had not yet been hardened by a daily familiarity with pain.[3]

Not only were the young more eager to relieve pain, but they also were more open to all innovations, according to a Confederate medical manual. "Those brought up in the older school, before the days of anaesthetics, in refusing all innovations, still insist on decrying the dangers of this potent remedy, and moralize upon the duty of suffering, as submitting to an express infliction from on high."[4] A brash young student at the University of Pennsylvania Medical College agreed.

As might have been anticipated the subject of anaesthesia was not received with equal favor by all. That portion of the profession, with settled notions and strong prejudices, mostly the older and more routine practitioners, were much incensed at the attempted innovation.[5]

Physiologist Robley Dunglison reminded John Collins Warren that "no physician above 40 years of age at the time of Harvey's great discovery was ever known to embrace it afterwards''; though Dunglison predicted that the opposition to ether would not last quite that long.[6]

However, such claims require verification; they cannot be accepted at face value. After all, Dunglison himself was fifty when he wrote that letter—and ether pioneer Warren had just retired at age seventy.[7] Unfortunately, hospital case records cannot fully resolve the relation between a surgeon's age and the use of anesthetics. At the Massachusetts General Hospital for example, the older surgeons actually used anesthetics somewhat more frequently than their junior colleagues did.[8] But then, at the Massachusetts General and most other hospitals, the really serious operations were generally reserved for the most senior practitioners. In other words, it is likely that the younger surgeons used anesthetics less because they were assigned to perform the less painful, shorter, and less dangerous procedures.[9] It is not possible to know how young surgeons would have used anesthetics if they had performed the same surgery as their elders, since in the institutions whose records are available, they were not in fact given enough such assignments.

However, a variety of indirect evidence indicates that younger surgeons may indeed have been more receptive than their seniors to the use of anesthetics. In the doctoral theses required of antebellum medical students, several recorded their speculations about how they intended to use anesthetics. Nine such dissertations, written between 1849 and 1860, have been preserved at the University of Pennsylvania. All but one of these students advocated a freer use of anesthetics than was approved by their elders at the Pennsylvania Hospital.[10] This willingness to challenge the practice and precepts of their professors is somewhat surprising in a profession where such student independence was traditionally discouraged. There is, of course, no way of proving that these nine students represented the vast majority, who chose to write theses on topics like gout, cholera, or drunkenness. But though not provable, it seems plausible that these surgeons were particularly receptive to the use of anesthetics because of their youth.

Pennsylvania Hospital offers further indirect evidence of a "generation gap" in the frequency with which surgeons used anesthesia. In 1861 and 1863, the hospital replaced senior surgeons George W. Norris and Edward Peace with men trained after 1846. Almost immediately, the use of anesthetics sharply increased. Between October 1852 and October 1861, the Pennsylvania surgeons used anesthetics in 62 percent of the fracture amputations for which information on anesthesia was recorded. There was some fluctuation over this period but in only two individual years did these variations exceed 5 percentage points. However, in 1861 the anesthetization rate jumped suddenly. Between October 1861 and October 1863, 92 percent of fully recorded fracture amputation cases received anesthetics. In calendar year 1863, the hospital first reached the 100 percent rate for such cases.

Any attempt to explain changes over time in anesthetic use must remain highly speculative, given the many limitations of the data and the methodological problems of time-series inferences. However, the change between 1861 and 1863 may well have been linked to the retirement of Norris and Peace. They had been the senior surgeons at the hospital throughout the 1852–1861 period and were the only two of the eight surgeons to serve on the staff between 1852 and 1863 who had been appointed before Morton's 1846 discovery. It is reasonable to speculate that the replacement of these two men led to a change in hospital policy, in favor of allowing a much more liberal use of anesthetics, at least for amputations.[11]

While at any given point in time, older surgeons may have used less anesthesia than their younger colleagues, it seems likely that, over the course of any one surgeon's career, anesthetic usage increased with age. Such individual developments were not, however, always smooth or even unidirectional.

The quarter century record of Hamilton's practice affords an intriguing though highly tentative glimpse of the process of change over the course of one individual career. Between 1850 and 1858, Hamilton gave anesthesia at a fairly even rate—providing it in slightly more than half the operations for which he recorded such data. But in the fall of 1858, when Hamilton moved from Buffalo to Brooklyn, he suddenly increased his recorded use of anesthetics. Between 1859 and 1866, he used anesthesia for every completely reported civilian operation. In 1866, however, Hamilton returned to a policy of selective anesthetization, though at a much higher rate than had been his initial practice. For the remainder of his career, he consistently used anesthetics in about 80 percent of fully recorded cases.[12]

The most notable feature of these changes is that they do not show the steady, progressive increase one might expect would result from a gradual growth in familiarity with and confidence in anesthesia. Instead these records suggest that Hamilton had two rather abrupt changes of policy, in two opposite directions. His move to Brooklyn marked one clear turning point. Perhaps he saw different types of patients in his new position; perhaps he encountered new colleagues who persuaded him to try a new policy. The new pattern did not last long, however. It seems plausible to speculate that Hamilton experimented with universal anesthetization for a few years and found it unsatisfactory. The data suggest, however, that Hamilton did experience something of a growth in confidence in anesthesia between the start and the finish of his career.

Sectionalism, Regional Rivalry, and the Flow of Information

Geographic rivalries figured prominently in mid-nineteenth-century explanations of why some practitioners used anesthetics more than others did. Simpson charged that London physicians avoided chloroform because of its origins in rival Edinburgh. Similarly, many Americans claimed that hostility toward Boston retarded the use of ether, especially among practitioners in Philadelphia. Quaker City dentist J. F. B. Flagg reported that some of his colleagues "repudiate it, because of its Yankee origin!" Morton, like Flagg, blamed the alleged Philadelphia opposition on jealousy of Boston. Dr. Oliver Wendell Holmes agreed. According to both Holmes and Richard Hodges, a Harvard medical student, Philadelphia practitioners avoided ether because they felt their city's traditional medical preeminence was threatened by the growing reputation of their rival on the Charles.[13]

Regional differences clearly did exist both in the speed with which anesthesia was adopted and the extent to which it was used.[14] Furthermore, the differences did seem most marked between Boston and Philadelphia. The Massachusetts General Hospital introduced ether in October 1846. By January 1847, it had been tried in the hospitals of New York, London, and Paris. But at the Pennsylvania Hospital it was not used at all until July 1853.[15] A similar regional pattern appears in the available data on the extent of anesthetic usage. Over any given time period from 1846 to the 1870s, anesthetics appear to have been used most frequently in Boston, less frequently in Philadelphia, with New York practice somewhere in the middle. Between January 1 and October 1, 1847, seventy-nine operations at the Massachusetts General Hospital were performed under anesthesia. At the New York Hospital in the same period, ether was used in only seven cases.[16] The Massachusetts General surgeons anesthetized all amputation cases after 1847. But between 1848 and 1851, the New York Hospital records indicate that anesthetics may have been used in as few as 65 percent of their amputations.[17] In New York City and upstate, Frank H. Hamilton anesthetized 83 percent of his recorded amputation patients in operations between 1849 and 1871.[18] At the Pennsylvania Hospital only 68 percent of amputees received ether or chloroform between 1853 and 1862.[19]

But to what extent were these regional variations actually caused by geographic rivalries? That is a much harder issue to judge. Regional and sectional stereotypes certainly abounded in the rhetoric of the early reactions to Morton's discovery. "Pardon me, we are a little suspicious of our Boston brethren," declared a Baltimore practitioner in December 1846. "They are clever men, very clever, but—some of them—a little credulous." Early attacks on etherization portrayed "Yankees" as fond of foolish innovations and as impractical tinkerers—in philanthropy, technology, and religion, as well as in medicine.[20] The empirical nature of the ether discovery was described as a "Yankee guess."[21] And Morton's patent was almost universally regarded as an example of the "truly Yankee" penchant for sharp trading, speculation, and avarice.[22]

For their part, Bostonians also fit the discovery of anesthesia into preexisting regional stereotypes. However, on the banks of the Charles, Yankee "cleverness" was known as innovation, Yankee "isms" were known as benevolence, and Philadelphia's caution went by the name of timidity. Holmes linked Philadelphia's alleged reluctance to use ether with Benjamin Franklin's opposition to Boston's other great medical first—Cotton Mather's introduction of smallpox inoculation a century and a quarter earlier. Holmes described the Philadelphia reaction to both innovations as "tardy, languid, faint-hearted assent [sweated out] drop by drop from the reluctant pores of those whom many have thought to lead the foremost van of medical improvement."[23] As a result, the glory of anesthesia belonged, not to America, but to Boston. "There are thousands who never heard of the American Revolution, who know not whether an American citizen has the color of a Carib or a Caucasian, to whom the name of Boston is familiar through this discovery."[24] Dr. Isaac Parrish of Philadelphia cautiously concluded that such regional rhetoric really did influence anesthetic usage. "Local pride may have . . . animated its early advocates, and a knowledge of this may, on the other hand, have induced a feeling of distrust in the cautious and timid at a distance."[25]

The medical rivalry between Philadelphia and Boston ran deep and long predated the discovery of ether.[26] Philadelphia had been the acknowledged medical capital of North America since before American independence. The Pennsylvania Hospital was the country's first, sixty years the senior of Massachusetts General. In 1846, it treated far more patients and had larger facilities than did its northern rival. The Philadelphia College of Physicians was the oldest medical association in the country. Even the Philadelphia-based *American Journal of the Medical Sciences* was larger and more prestigious than the *Boston Medical and Surgical Journal*. Philadelphia had more hospitals than Boston, more medical schools, and a haughty medical tradition.[27]

Regional conflict was reinforced by sectionalism in the intense economic rivalry between Boston and Philadelphia to recruit tuition-paying medical students. As the cultural gap between North and South widened in antebellum America, more and more Southerners deserted the Boston school for the more congenial and tolerant climate of Philadelphia—an ironic precursor of their exodus from Philadelphia to Virginia in 1859.[28]

But by the 1840s, Boston medical boosters could pride themselves on having clearly emerged from the shadow of their rival. Expansion of the Massachusetts General Hospital and of Harvard Medical School had added greatly to the size of Boston's establishment. The research of young new physicians, like that of Holmes on puerperal fever, enhanced Boston's scientific stature, while directly challenging the ideas of Philadelphians Meigs and Hodge.[29]

The connection between geography and anesthesia included growing sectional feelings among North, South and West, as well as the continuing economic rivalry among the seaports of the Atlantic. Significantly, Holmes' attack on Philadelphia's opposition to anesthesia came at the conclusion of his notorious diatribe against most medical institutions located southwest of the Charles River. To Holmes, these were *"inferior medical schools,* situated in the wrong places,"[30] such as "on the banks of the Mississippi and Missouri."[31] His sentiments were reciprocated in full by Western and Southern physicians, who argued that the diversity of America's climate (and the biological peculiarities of slaves) required separate sectional medical schools.[32] Sectional and regional jealousies thus colored the rhetoric with which physicians reacted to the news of Morton's discovery.

More importantly, such geographic rivalries shaped both the public communications networks and the private channels of personal influence by which news of medical innovations was diffused. Such information and opinion transmission patterns within the medical community can play an important role in the adoption by individual doctors of a new discovery such as anesthesia.[33]

In the America of 1846, sectional and regional rivalries produced a bi-polar network of contacts among physicians. Boston and Philadelphia each served as the hubs of medical influence for their own regions, but they had much less contact with or influence on each other, except indirectly through England.[34] For example, John Collins Warren played an extremely influential role in the circulation of information among physicians throughout New England and the Midwest. But, judged by his surviving correspondence, his contacts and personal influence fell off south of Staten Island. Interestingly, among the handful of correspondents Warren did have in Philadelphia were William E. Horner and Robley Dunglison—two of the first practitioners in their city to endorse ether.[35] Likewise, J. F. B. Flagg, who claimed to be the first anesthetist among Philadelphia dentists, had an unusual personal information link to Boston in his brother.[36] When the ether discovery was first announced, Warren, Jackson, Bigelow, Morton, Edward Everett, and many other Bostonians rushed to spread the news—not to Philadelphia, but to London and Paris.[37] Thus, by the time word of the discovery reached the Southern and Western states via the European or Philadelphia journals, ether had already been in use for weeks at many European hospitals. Dr. Lunsford P. Yandell of the University of Louisville traced the route by which anesthesia reached Kentucky. "In a few weeks after it was published in Boston, the letheon was tried in London, Paris and Edinburgh, and the results of the practice by the surgeons and physicians of those cities we had here in Louisville long before the winter has passed away."[38]

Patterns of personal trust followed the lines of communication. It was not simply that doctors outside of New England did not get news from Boston—it was rather that they did not fully trust such reports. The most influential source of advice about anesthesia was a physician's personal acquaintances; the second most important influence was European acceptance. Philadelphians and New Yorkers relied on European colleagues more closely than on Bostonians for advice on all medical innovations. The importance of personal communications and the geographic pattern of information flow are both exemplified in a letter written to the *Boston Medical and Surgical Journal* by Dr. F. Willis Fisher from Paris, in February 1847.

In November last I received from a medical friend a letter, in which he informed me of the discovery made by Dr. C. T. Jackson, that the inhalation into the lungs of sulphuric ether would render patients insensible to pain during surgical operations . . . . I should have been cautious in giving credence to this report had it reached me through the pages of a medical or other Journal; but having been communicated to me by my former medical instructer, I could entertain no doubt of its truth.[39]

Although geography thus strongly influenced the initial response of physicians to ether, regional rivalries probably should not be overemphasized in explaining long-term differences in the extent of anesthetic usage. Despite the opposition of the Pennsylvania Hospital, there were doctors in Philadelphia willing to use ether. Both major medical school clinics in Philadelphia began using anesthesia within a year of Morton's demonstration. In all likelihood, this receptivity reflected the relative youth of the clinic surgeons. Thomas D. Mutter, for example, was thirty-six when he introduced anesthesia at the Jefferson Medical School clinic.[40] In addition, the clinics operated on a much larger number of women patients than the Hospital did.[41] It is not possible to tell from the available records whether it was the presence of female patients that spurred the clinics to adopt anesthesia or whether it was the clinics' independent adoption of anesthesia that prompted a sudden upswing in operations on women.[42] But whatever the reason, there were surgeons in Philadelphia who used anesthesia early and frequently.

In addition, while medical sectionalism was intense, it did not quite keep pace with sectional feelings in society at large. The

AMA, for example, was one of the few national institutions in America to survive more or less intact throughout the Civil War.[43] The little available evidence does not indicate any Southern hostility toward the use of Yankee anesthesia. Of the eight surviving antebellum theses written about anesthesia by American students at the University of Pennsylvania, seven were by Southerners (three from Alabama alone). All seven Southerners favored a freer use of anesthetics than did the one Northerner—a Pennsylvanian.[44] By the Civil War, the sectional issue over the use of anesthesia had been transformed into a contest between Georgia and New England for the honor of priority in its discovery.[45]

Factors other than regionalism may also have influenced the differences in anesthetic usage between Philadelphia and Boston. Situated between the Old School Presbyterians at Princeton and the German Reformed sects of Lancaster, Philadelphia was probably the center of orthodox predestinarian religion in antebellum America. In Boston, a more "liberal" brand of theology seemed to prevail.[46] This difference in religious background conceivably might have helped discourage Philadelphia's reception of anesthesia. On the other hand, the City of Brotherly Love's tradition of Quaker benevolence might have served to mitigate Philadelphia's religious hostility toward anesthesia. Quaker physicians such as John D. Griscom, Joseph Pancoast, and Isaac Parrish were among the first Philadelphians to use anesthetics.[47]

However, geography did continue to influence a physician's choice of which anesthetic to use. Once the British introduced chloroform, diehard Yankee-haters could take advantage of anesthesia without having to use a Boston product,[48] while Anglophobes of all sections suddenly found new virtue in the original American article. Thus, for example, the New York *Medical Gazette* of 1870 linked the use of ether with hostility toward England, referring to "the crusade against chloroform, which two or three patriotic periodicals have lately attempted to inaugurate in conjunction with the *Alabama* claims."[49] Philadelphia's *American Journal of the Medical Sciences* proclaimed in 1867 that Boston and Lyons, France, stood alone against the world in advocating ether. An 1862 editorial in the *Buffalo Medical and Surgical Journal* gracefully skirted the dilemma faced by a small city torn between two warring metropolitan hubs. "Boston is for ether; New York is partially at least on the side of chloroform.

We most ardently desire for Buffalo, that it be only on the side of truth.''[50]

Pioneer anesthesia manufacturer Edward R. Squibb of Brooklyn estimated that, of 400,000 anesthesia administrations in the United States in 1870, chloroform accounted for half, ether for forty percent, and other gases and mixtures for the rest.[51] But with the gradual cooling of sectional hostilities and the growing evidence of chloroform's greater danger, the country soon experienced an ether revival, even in formerly solid chloroform country. By the 1860s and 1870s, even the *American Journal of the Medical Sciences* and the Philadelphia *Medical and Surgical Reporter* carried articles favoring ether (most however written by New Yorkers).[52]

Change came suddenly and thoroughly to the students at the University of Michigan. All eight theses on anesthesia written before the end of the Civil War strongly endorsed chloroform. However, the first postwar dissertation on the subject preferred a mixture of alcohol, chloroform, and ether. Thereafter, from 1868 to 1871, all five anesthesia theses emphatically recommended pure ether.[53]

Once again, the students appeared to be ahead of their professors. As late as the winter of 1875, case records from the University of Michigan surgical clinics show that the faculty still used chloroform exclusively.[54] One bold medical student even attacked surgery professor Alpheus Benning Crosby by name in his 1871 thesis, because the instructor continued to use chloroform.[55]

In summary, geography profoundly influenced patterns of communication and personal influence within antebellum American medicine. Over the short run, geography almost certainly affected the speed and extent of anesthetic adoption. Local pride may also account for the long-term tendency of Massachusetts General surgeons to use ether more freely than was the practice elsewhere. Although sectional rivalries and other geographic factors probably did not cause many other long-term differences in the extent of anesthetic usage, they continued to play an important role in the selection of anesthetic agents, at least until the 1870s.

CHAPTER ELEVEN

ANESTHESIA AND THE CALCULUS OF SUFFERING: A CRITICAL EVALUATION

The Calculus of Suffering and the "Furor Operativus"

Since 1847, it has generally been assumed that the discovery of anesthesia greatly increased the frequency of surgical operations. Yet, all previous attempts to document or measure this increase have suffered from serious logical and methodological deficiencies. However, once these difficulties are corrected, it is possible to demonstrate that the use of anesthesia did indeed vastly expand the amount of surgery performed at the Massachusetts General Hospital even more dramatically than previous observers suspected.

From the nineteenth-century cartoonist who portrayed "Furor Operativus" (see plate 1), to the latest histories of nineteenth-century American medicine,[1] most observers have suspected that anesthetics created an enormous boom in surgery. Nineteenth-century surgeons generally shared in this assessment. The *Annual Report* of the Massachusetts General Hospital in January 1848 declared that the discovery of ether "greatly increased the actual number of operations,"[2] a judgment seconded by John Collins Warren.[3] Fear that ether had provoked an irresponsible spree of unnecessary procedures was a major concern of those who felt there was already too much art and not enough nature in surgery. Critics of the supposed epidemic of surgery brought on by anesthesia included natural healers like the hydropaths, as well as influential conservative surgeons like Henry J. Bigelow. Bigelow feared that "the annihilation of pain" would upset the careful conservative balance between benefits and risks.

The balance of surgical responsibility has been shaken to its centre by the extinction of an element whose preponderance may be truly said, in a majority of cases, to have turned the scale; and years must elapse before a standard of expediency can be adjusted. In the mean time, let the burden of proof lie with the patient; let the surgeon avoid operating when he can do so.

As early as March 1847, British surgeon Tyler Smith observed a "general rush towards the operating room" he attributed to ether.[4]

But there is a major conceptual problem in interpreting these charges that anesthesia led to a proliferation of surgery. Do such claims accurately reflect a real increase in surgery, or do they simply reflect the growing hostility of midcentury observers toward an unchanged number of operations? How much did surgery really increase after 1846, and to what extent was anesthesia responsible for this increase? The few attempts to document the actual yield of this surgical harvest have been very inadequate. In one recent effort, William G. Rothstein calculated that, before anesthesia, the Massachusetts General Hospital performed 6.2 amputations annually, while after anesthesia, the figure rose to 20.7. This "much more frequent" resort to the knife, he implied, was due largely to ether.[5]

Such evidence is very inconclusive. First, there is no reason to assume that changes in the tiny number of amputations really reflected changes in the treatment of the overwhelming majority of surgical patients for whom removal of a limb was never contemplated. Second, even in the limited realm of amputations these data are almost worthless because they use 1850 rather than 1846 as the dividing line between the pre-anesthetic and postanesthetic eras and because they are based on the entire timespan from the founding of the hospital in 1821 until the Civil War. Use of such a long time period is highly suspect because any number of other events besides Morton's discovery that occurred in those years might have altered the number of operations performed. Among the changes that might explain a rise in amputations, the most obvious are the rapid growth of Boston's population, especially following the Irish famine migration of 1848; the enormous increase in serious injuries due to the growth of railroads and industry; and the expansion of the hospital with the opening of its new wing in 1847 (an addition planned before Morton's discovery).[6]

On the other hand, developments such as the growing acceptance of conservative professional standards during the 1830s and thereafter may well have helped hold down the total number of amputations performed and thus made Rothstein's estimate of the impact of anesthesia too low.

Nineteenth-century attempts to measure the influence of anesthesia on the rate of surgery suffered from this same inability to control for the effects of other changes. Antebellum surgeons sensed that the conquest of surgical pain had led them to perform an increased number of operations, but they did not know how to measure the extent, if any, to which this rise was actually caused by the availability of anesthesia.[7]

It is possible, however, to distinguish the effects of anesthetics from the effects of other events that might have influenced the number of operations performed at the Massachusetts General Hospital. Table 16 measures the increase in all types of surgery, compared with the increasing number of surgical patients admitted, on a single year basis. By controlling for the total number of patients and by examining only the year before and the year after Morton's discovery, the influence of extraneous variables on the rate of surgery can be minimized. The results show that there was indeed a sharp and sudden increase in surgery at Massachusetts General immediately following the introduction of anesthesia, independent of the simultaneous large increase in the overall number of patients. Before October 16, 1846, less than 16 percent of patients on the surgical wards received any operative treatment. After that date, almost 40 percent of those admitted went under the knife. Thus, the rate of surgery per admission considerably more than doubled.[8] By contrast, at the Pennsylvania Hospital, where anesthesia came into use much more gradually and on a much more limited scale than in Boston, there was no such increase in the operation rate, at least among fracture cases.[9] New York Hospital, which fell between its Boston and Philadelphia counterparts in its adoption of anesthesia, experienced an intermediate upsurge in operations. From June 1845 to May 1846, 18 percent of patients admitted underwent surgery; for 1847–48, the figure increased to almost 22 percent.[10]

Of particular interest, the rate of increase in surgery differed greatly for different types of patients. With one minor exception, the boom in surgery at Massachusetts General was most marked among those patients most likely to receive anesthetics: the aged, women, native-born Americans, nonlaborers, and amputees. For example, the increase in major limb amputations following the discovery of ether far exceeded the increase in any other type of surgery (see table 17). Just before the use of anesthetics, only 1.3 percent of Massachusetts General patients were subjected to the loss of a limb— and the rate of amputation per admission had been *declining* relatively steadily since the 1830s.[11] In the year following the introduction of ether, nearly 7 percent of all patients received amputations, an unprecedented jump of almost five times the previous rate. Put another way, the proportion of amputees among all patients receiving surgery nearly doubled following the introduction of anesthesia. The increase in the frequency of amputations was dramatically larger than that calculated by Rothstein, largely because of his failure to take into account the declining amputation rate and growing conservatism of surgeons between the 1830s and 1846.[12]

Women patients, another group that received anesthetics proportionally more often than other patients, likewise experienced a greater proportional increase in surgery rates following the introduction of ether (see table 18). Before anesthesia, about 16 percent of all patients got operations, with no noticeable difference between the sexes. After ether, one-third of the men but more than one-half of the women were subjected to surgery. Thus, while the rate of surgery for men doubled following the discovery of anesthesia, the rate for women more than tripled. In other words, women received a much larger share of the total number of operations after anesthesia than before (controlling for admissions).

Less dramatic, but still marked, was the proportional rise

in the rate of surgery on native-born Americans (see table 19). Before anesthesia, Massachusetts General surgeons operated on American- and foreign-born patients at roughly the same rate. But following Morton's innovation, surgery became 1.5 times as common on natives as on immigrants. While the rate of surgery for immigrants doubled, the rate for natives almost tripled. Nonlaborers too received slightly more than their share of the increase in surgery (see table 20).

Thus the rate of surgery did increase enormously following the introduction of anesthesia, and the increase was most marked for those types of patients most likely to receive anesthetics. One small exception to this pattern appeared among the very young. Following Morton's discovery, there was actually a slight drop in the rate of operations performed on children below the age of eleven. (Though the actual number of operations on children doubled, the admissions rate rose even more steeply.) But the numbers involved remained quite insignificant—children remained a very minor segment of the hospital population. The elderly, as expected, experienced a proportionally greater increase in rate of surgery than did any other age group (see table 21).

In summary, the introduction of ether was followed by an immediate jump in the rate of surgery at Massachusetts General, an increase not explainable by changes in the number of admissions, the composition of the patient population,[13] or any other outside factors. Furthermore, this rise was most marked among those patients who received anesthetics most frequently—women, the old, the native-born, nonlaborers, and amputees. At the Pennsylvania Hospital, where anesthetics were used much more sparingly and introduced over a two-decade timespan, there was no such dramatic increase in the rate of surgery, while at New York Hospital, the increase was smaller and less sudden than at Massachusetts General.

Nineteenth-century critics and modern historians not only claimed that surgery increased following anesthesia but also that this increase was unjustifiable and unnecessary. Many observers feared that anesthesia had unleashed a horde of knife-happy experimenters, eager for fame and experience, who performed needless and incompetent surgery on their helpless victims. The rise in operations on women in particular seemed to confirm the worst fears of medical nihilists, surgical conservatives, feminists, and moralists, all of whom saw anesthesia as giving vent to the profession's "lust for operating."[14]

Such charges actually contained a number of separate elements; it is best to examine them one at a time. First, to what extent did the use of anesthesia contribute to a rise in experimental or unproven types of operations? In the case of gynecology there is evidence that anesthesia did indeed lead to more new and untested operations. The rise in ovariotomies is perhaps the most dramatic case in point. In this operation, a woman's sex organs were removed, either as the result of a specific physical lesion or for the cure of general systemic and emotional problems.[15] Before 1846, ovariotomy had been done only as an heroic last resort, limited to cases of life-threatening tumors. Perhaps 100 had been performed in the entire history of medicine. With the discovery of anesthesia, the practice of ovariotomy expanded enormously. Between 1849 and 1878, Dr. Washington L. Atlee alone removed the ovaries of 385 women. Many of these were frankly experimental operations, and while most were the result of painful or life-threatening tumors, a few were ventures in "normal ovariotomy." Not surprisingly, Atlee was among the first gynecologists to use surgical anesthetics. His colleague Augustus K. Gardner of New York, an even more outspoken advocate of experimental gynecological surgery, was also a pioneer of anesthesia, who claimed to have been the first New York physician to use chloroform in obstretrics. "I have no doubt that the use of anaesthesia will strip [ovariotomy] of most of its dangers, and render it simple and safe . . . ," Atlee wrote in 1849.[16] Anesthesia itself had been an experiment; thus it is not too surprising that many of its earliest users conducted other experiments as well.

Without anesthesia, the number and scope of surgical experiments undertaken by Atlee, Gardner, and others would have been conceivable only in an extermination camp. One British text of 1859 went so far as to claim that "our large and tedious plastic operations in the female, are all the result directly of the discovery of anaesthetics."[17]

But even with anesthesia, these experiments remained controversial among conservative surgeons, and were infrequently performed by most, before the introduction of antiseptic techniques.[18] At the Massachusetts General Hospital, of the two women diagnosed as having ovarian disease in the year following the discovery of ether, one was dismissed without treatment, even though she demanded an operation. The other was treated by the nonexperimental, noncastrating method of "tapping." After two such treatments, she too requested an ovariotomy; upon its "not being considered prudent" by the surgeons, she was sent home.[19]

In cases of less controversial research, anesthesia also led to a rise in experimentation, even at Massachusetts General. Before 1846, the hospital surgeons had begun to experiment with new techniques in palate, lip, and vaginal fistula repair. Following Morton's discovery, the rate of such experimental surgery increased 1.5 fold (see table 22). George Hayward attributed the increase in his own vesico-vaginal fistula experiments to the availability of ether.[20]

However, the rate of increased experimentation ran considerably behind the overall increase in surgery. While experiments grew 1.5 fold, the overall rate of surgery more than doubled (see table 16). Thus, ether did increase the number of experiments, but not by as much as it increased the frequency of surgery in general. Consequently, minor experimental surgery constituted a smaller share of the total number of operations performed after anesthesia than before (controlling for admissions). The major reason anesthesia did not increase the proportion of such minor experimental surgery may well have been the fact that anesthesia was usually contraindicated for minor surgery in general and for mouth operations in particular.

Thus, while the discovery of anesthesia did lead to a rise in untested operations by some surgeons, the increase in hospital experimentation was less than the increase in routine surgery. Experimental operations remained an insignificant segment of the overall postanesthetic upsurge in hospital surgery.[21]

A second and more subtle criticism of the postanesthetic surgical boom was that painlessness prompted operations on patients who would have recovered equally well without such interference. For example, nineteenth-century critics and some recent historians have pictured a postanesthetic world in which every bruise or fracture was likely to prompt amputation.[22] But before judging whether the increase in surgery after 1846 was "necessary," it is important to remember that the midcentury profession was bitterly divided over the standards by which to judge the legitimacy, value, and "necessity" of surgery. Opponents of surgery, including the more dogmatic hydropaths, homeopaths, and therapeutic nihilists, regarded almost all operations as unnatural and unnecessary. At the opposite pole, heroic surgeons saw the scalpel as a saber with which to lead the charge against the ramparts of disease. Thus, nineteenth-century criticisms must be seen in context; the very same operation that one doctor called legitimate and necessary, might be denounced by another as excessive and irresponsible. Furthermore, by making operations less distasteful and easier to perform, anesthesia probably further muddled the definition of surgical necessity.

This nineteenth-century debate over the standards of surgical legitimacy makes any assessment of the postanesthetic surgical boom more interesting and more difficult for the historian. The task is compounded by the fact that our own standards of what constitutes "necessary" surgery are very controversial; witness our current concern over "second opinions" for elective surgery and over what types of operations ought to be covered by medical insurance.[23]

In one sense, of course, the question is unanswerable—no one can say for sure what would have happened if an operation that was in fact performed had not taken place. But by looking at the experiences of large enough groups of patients with similar medical conditions, it is possible to make some likely inferences. A variety of such evidence indicates that, at the Massachusetts General Hospital, the introduction of ether was followed by a dramatic increase in the proportion of surgery that was performed on those patients who were least likely to recover on their own. In that sense, it may be said that these operations were not unnecessary.

One good indication of this trend is the treatment of emergency and acute injury cases. Through almost all of the nineteenth century, such victims were universally regarded as the single class of patients most likely to die. They generally had the poorest prognosis for recovery regardless of treatment, because they were the most susceptible to infection and to shock.[24] For example, at the Massachusetts General Hospital in the year before Morton's discovery, acute and emergency cases accounted for almost two-thirds of all deaths, though they comprised less than one-third of the patients admitted.[25]

Before the introduction of anesthesia these emergency patients were generally seen as too seriously ill to warrant any surgical treatment.[26] During 1845–46, the Massachusetts General Hospital operated on only 4 of the 66 emergency and acute surgical admissions. Once anesthesia became available, the operation rate on this group of patients jumped to almost 1 in 4. The rate of surgery for emergency cases virtually quadrupled, while the rate for others increased only 2.4 times (see table 23). In other words, emergency cases made up a much larger share of the surgery done after anesthesia (controlling for admissions)[27] than before. Thus, the sharpest increase in the rate of surgery took place on the class of patients generally recognized to be the least likely to recover on their own. And, following ether, these "sickest" patients accounted for a greatly increased proportion of the total number of operations performed.[28]

An unnecessary operation may also be defined as one more extensive in scope than "necessary." In this sense, many nineteenth-century surgeons insisted that ether actually decreased the amount of unnecessary surgery. Anesthesia made more practical the prolonged and intricate conservative procedures required to preserve limbs a pre-anesthetic surgeon would have simply cut off. Many practitioners claimed anesthesia enabled them to substitute bone excisions and resections for amputations, Caesarian section for craniotomy, and so on. But while the conquest of pain made such operations feasible, the available records suggest that they became only slightly more common in practice.[29]

In summary, the development of anesthesia probably increased the proportion of operations done on the sickest patients— those least likely to recover without surgery. In that sense, charges that the increase in surgery was unnecessary are not justified.

But this conclusion is not the same as saying that the increased number of operations did anything to *help* those on whom they were performed. Perhaps, for example, surgeons began to operate more frequently on the sickest patients merely because they regarded such hopeless cases as expendable material for teaching and for practicing their technique. There are two logically separate and distinct issues. Having shown that anesthesia led to a disproportionate increase in operations on people likely to die without aid, we must next judge whether these operations prevented or speeded the deaths of their recipients. Even if postanesthetic surgeons operated only on the sickest patients, their operations may still have been "unjustified" in the sense of worsening rather than improving the recipients' already slim chances for recovery. This possibility is the subject of the next section.

Anesthesia, Industrialization, and the Death Rate from Surgery

The third, and most serious criticism leveled against the additional surgery that followed the introduction of anesthesia was that it increased the surgical death rate. Many mid-nineteenth-century professional and lay periodicals agreed that death resulted from the immediate effects of inhaling chloroform in 1 of every 2,500 to 10,000 cases; ether deaths were variously given in the range of 1 in every 10,000 to 30,000. However, some surgeons suspected the long-term effects of anesthesia might be far more serious. Virtually all the published mid-nineteenth-century American hospital statistics indicated that, following the introduction of anesthesia, more patients died from surgery than ever before. Summarizing printed data on operations performed between 1821 and 1850 at hospitals in Boston, New York, and Philadelphia, Dr. FitzWilliam Sargent placed the death rate at 27.6 percent for nonanesthetized amputations and 32.3 percent for amputees who received an anesthetic—an additional 5 deaths in every 100 operations, due to anesthesia.[30]

Recent historians have accepted such statistics at face value. William Rothstein repeated an 1864 report that claimed to show that the Massachusetts General Hospital amputation mortality rose from 19 percent before ether to 23 percent afterward—that is, an additional 4 deaths in every 100 operations due to the anesthetic.[31] On the basis of similar sources, John Duffy concluded that the increase in surgery following anesthesia ''was not immediately beneficial to patients.''[32]

Nineteenth-century explanations of why anesthesia should have increased surgical mortality varied and have changed further since then. Most observers then and now agreed that the additional deaths were from infection and/or shock, but there the agreement ends. Many antebellum surgeons tended to blame the anesthetic itself for lowering the patients' ''vitality.'' Other midcentury observers, however, claimed that anesthesia had made doctors overeager, careless, and sloppy.[33]

With the gradual acceptance of antiseptic techniques and the germ theory of disease in the late nineteenth century, the explanation for these deaths changed. The modern interpretation, first stated by John Collins Warren's grandson, stresses the fact that antebellum surgeons lacked understanding of the causes of infection. Mid-nineteenth-century surgeons would operate on several patients in a row, using the same instruments, often without even pausing to wash. The more operations done, the less likely it was that even rudimentary sanitary precautions would be taken; thus the opportunity for the spread of germs was greater. By boosting the amount of surgery performed, the development of anesthesia supposedly led to a higher surgical infection rate.[34]

But despite the seeming impressiveness of this explanation, the evidence on which it rests is very thin. None of the figures purporting to show an increase in deaths after anesthesia is statistically significant. Careful reexamination of the data leads to the conclusion that the introduction of anesthesia had little or no effect on the death rate from surgery, and that it actually lowered the overall death rate from serious injuries by making it possible to perform lifesaving operations on patients who would otherwise have died untreated.

As already pointed out, nineteenth-century printed statistics on anesthetic use contain two enormous flaws. First, they cover the entire period from 1821 to the 1850s or 1860s. Second, they make little or no attempt to assess the role of other important changes taking place in those years, inside and outside the hospital. Anesthesia certainly was not the only new development of the 1840s that could have contributed to a higher surgical death rate. The most important of these other considerations was undoubtedly industrialization.

Nineteenth-century surgeons were uniformly horrified by the grisly body count of the industrial revolution. "Everyone who has had frequent occasion to amputate for railroad accidents," knew that "a wheel of a locomotive engine or railway car . . . . in most instances produces a compound and comminuted fracture of the worst kind," according to George Hayward of Massachusetts General.[35] George W. Norris of the Pennsylvania Hospital agreed that "the most desperate kind" of surgery was that "resulting from railroad accidents, machinery, &c." Norris did not know any bacteriology, but he recognized that the extreme tissue damage caused by industrial accidents made infection far more likely in such injuries than in any other type of surgery.[36] Midcentury hospital reports often listed "R. R. accident" and "machinery" as separate categories of disease, distinguished from all other types of accidents and other causes of surgery.[37]

Railroads, factories, and anesthetics appeared at virtually

the same time in American urban history. Noting this coincidence, a few medical observers suspected that ether might be getting the blame for deaths actually the result of industrial accidents. Samuel D. Gross absolved anesthesia and attributed the rise in surgical death rates to the "fearful increase in railway and other terrible accidents, many of which are necessarily fatal, no matter to what treatment they may be subjected." [38] The records of the Massachusetts General Hospital lend strong support to Gross' explanation. If the accident cases are separated from the others, it becomes clear that the introduction of anesthesia made almost no difference in the surgical death rate; indeed there seems to have been a very slight downturn in operative mortality (see table 24). [39]

Both before and after anesthesia, between 1821 and 1850, accident victims died at nearly four times the rate of any other amputees. But, between 1821 and 1846, accidents had caused only one-third of all amputations; after 1846 they accounted for fully half of the limbs lost. Between 1849 and 1854, the percentage of hospital admissions due to accidents more than doubled. Over the entire antebellum era, the proportion of accident victims among patients increased steadily each year (see table 25). [40]

In the most sophisticated nineteenth-century analysis of postanesthetic death rates, Dr. Samuel Fenwick of Newcastle, England, also found that accidents, not anesthesia, explained the rise in surgical mortality. He examined the records of Newcastle Infirmary for 1823 to 1856 and reported that anesthesia lowered the disease-amputation death rate, from 19 to 13 percent and the trauma-amputation death rate from 32 to 31 percent. Fenwick's results were largely unknown in the United States. But his data seem to confirm that it was the growing seriousness of the injuries, and not the use of ether or the growing number of operations per se, that most likely accounts for the rise in surgical mortality. *Punch* was more accurate than he could possibly have realized when he joked, in January 1847, "The establishment of the fact that surgical operations may be performed without pain has been properly described as 'Good News for Travelers by Railway.' "[41]

Table 24 and Dr. Fenwick's study still probably underestimate the life-saving value of postanesthetic surgery. These data cover only deaths following surgery—patients who died after an operation are counted, but those allowed to die without surgery are omitted. As we have seen, however, after the introduction of ether, doctors began to operate more often on people whom they previously had considered too seriously injured for surgery. This new willingness to operate on such high-risk cases probably led to more deaths following *surgery* but fewer deaths overall.[42] Unfortunately, the available evidence is too slim either to confirm this explanation or to rule it out. Among the very worst injuries—compound fractures—the overall death rate for all patients admitted did drop from 40 percent to 32 percent at the Massachusetts General following the introduction of anesthesia, but the number of cases was far too small for statistical significance.[43]

In summary, the evidence examined so far suggests that, following the discovery of anesthesia, operations previously done largely on the strongest and most insensitive patients could now be done on those formerly regarded as too delicate, such as women, old people, and badly injured accident victims. The result was an overall increase in surgery, including some additional experimental operations and some undoubtedly unnecessary interventions.[44] But these latter cases were proportionally rarer after anesthesia than before.

The growing frequency of operations did not cause the rise in the surgical death rate; the more frequent resort to surgery in fact may have saved a number of lives that would otherwise have been lost. It was the industrial revolution, and the growing ability of surgeons to operate on previously hopeless cases, not increased careless or unnecessary surgery, that accounted for the rise in surgical deaths following 1846.

Yet, if anesthesia did improve the ability of surgeons to save lives, the numbers could not have been very great. And while statistics can measure the quantity of life saved, they tell us nothing about the quality of that life. Did the increase in surgery following 1846 enable more people to return to useful happy lives, or did it produce agonized invalids? On this question the records are silent. And while anesthesia may have saved some lives, its major influence was not in the area of life and death but in the removal of pain, an advantage that is not directly measurable.

Despite our conclusions to the contrary, the historical fact remains that many mid-nineteenth-century American physicians thought anesthetic surgery did kill about 5 percent more patients than nonanesthetic operations did. Whereas present-day detective work reveals their conclusions to have been wrong, these original statistical reports are still vital to an understanding of nineteenth-century attitudes toward anesthetics and the importance of pain. Even though their figures may have been erroneous, the early reports provide an invaluable measure of the risk nineteenth-century physicians *thought* they were running by using anesthetics. While a few anti-utilitarians like Meigs considered even 1 death in 10,000 too many to justify anesthesia, Sargent's data indicate that most practitioners considered even a 5 percent increase in the risk of death an acceptable price to pay for avoiding the pain of amputation.[45] Thus, nineteenth-century mortality reports, while inaccurate from our viewpoint, provide an excellent indirect measure of the relative value midcentury surgeons placed on the prevention of pain when weighed against risk to life; they provide a numerical solution to the calculus of suffering.

Anesthesia and Patient Demand for Surgery

Thus far, we have seen that the introduction of anesthesia led to a sudden and dramatic rise in operations on patients admitted to the Massachusetts General Hospital. In other words, more of the people already in the hospital were being operated on after Morton's discovery than before. But contemporary observers also claimed that the elimination of operative pain increased the number of patients coming to the hospital seeking surgical attention. Not only were surgeons choosing to operate on a greater proportion of their patients, noted the *Annual Report* of the Massachusetts General Hospital, but there also were many more patients showing up to request surgery.[46] Private practitioners and dentists likewise reported their business booming. A Boston dentist associated with Morton recalled that within a month of the first announcements, "There was a rush of people to have teeth extracted."[47]

To what extent did anesthesia actually increase patient demand for surgical services? At Massachusetts General, the number of surgical patients jumped from 221 to 293, a sudden and unprecedented one-year increase, seemingly indicating a one-third greater demand for surgery following Morton's discovery.[48]

Unfortunately though, it is not possible to tell how much

of this increase at the Massachusetts General Hospital really represented new demand and how much was simply a result of the hospital's increased capacity to fill preexisting demand, the result of its opening a new wing in July 1847. The hospital reported that, before the expansion, some patients had been treated on an outpatient basis who would have been admitted if space had existed and that, once the new wing was opened, the number of such "out-door" patients seemed to have dropped. However, the hospital did not report the number of outpatients before 1847, and so the exact influence of the new wing cannot be measured against the influence of anesthesia. All that can be said is that it seems unlikely the new facility by itself could have attracted such an enormous increase in surgical patients if the discovery of ether had not substantially lessened patients' fears of operations.[49]

Nineteenth-century surgeons suspected that the increase in surgical patients was proportionally greatest among the chronically ill—those whose fear of pain had caused them to avoid operations for years. Mott and Warren told of patients who had refused surgery for decades, some with tumors that had grown to weigh seven or more pounds, who decided to undergo operations as soon as they learned that it could be done without pain.[50] And at Massachusetts General the greatest increase in demand for surgery did in fact come from people who had been putting off treatment for a long time. Table 26 indicates that the demand for surgery increased most among those who previously had been avoiding treatment the longest; however, the difference is not statistically significant. In fact, the increase in patients seems to have been remarkably uniform among all classes of people (see table 27). Despite the 33 percent rise in the total number of patients, the sex, nativity, occupation, and age ratios remained virtually unchanged.[51]

The great increase in the number of people willing to undergo hospital treatment suggests that anesthesia made surgery and hospitalization less frightening and repulsive experiences. Not only were those operated on spared much pain, but also those awaiting or recuperating from surgery heard fewer blood-curdling screams and thumps from the surgical theater overhead. Yet before and after anesthesia, hospital surgery remained an experience primarily for poor adult men. Anesthesia lessened the dread of surgery among the hospital's traditional clients, but a comfortable middle-class home still remained the medically preferred location for most operations. In fact, immediately following his initial demonstration, Morton himself began administering ether for major surgery in private homes and in a boarding establishment known as the Bromfield House. The equipment usually required for anesthesia was often no more than a bottle and a rag and was easily portable. Well into this century many hospitals provided no special anesthetic equipment; they expected the anesthetist to bring along whatever was needed. A few of the techniques recommended for reviving an overanesthetized patient—hanging by the heels, electric shocks to the heart—might have required some bulky or unusual apparatus best provided in hospitals. But most anesthetists relied on artificial respiration, cold water, smelling salts, or a slap in the face.[52]

Since most of the patients in hospitals were charity cases, the growing demand for hospital operations probably did not enrich the surgeons. While anesthesia dramatically increased the market for hospital operations, it did not expand its narrow social composition. However, if the demand for private surgery at all kept pace with the hospital increase, the additional income for doctors as a result of anesthesia might well have been considerable.

The Calculus of Suffering and the Woman Surgeon

One of the most far-reaching effects of anesthesia was its impact on the recruitment of surgical personnel. A profession whose traditional requirements had included the ability "to cut like an executioner"[53] appealed to a rather small self-selected group of aspiring young recruits. As already noted, otherwise highly qualified practitioners like Haller failed as surgeons because of their inability to inflict pain. The fear of such infliction drove Charles Darwin from medicine altogether.[54] The introduction of anesthesia undoubtedly made possible surgical and dental careers for many persons whose sensibilities would have recoiled from the horrors of the pre-anesthetic art.

Women aspirants in particular stood to benefit from the diminished need to cause pain in surgery. The inability of gentleladies to inflict the requisite pain had long been a key objection raised by practitioners against allowing women to become surgeons. Male doctors insisted that "the practice of surgery hardens the heart and stills those emotions which render the wife, the mother, the sister and the daughter the angels of the home-heaven."[55] Surgeons like Edmund Andrews insisted that the need to remain calm and detached in the face of suffering meant that "the primary requisite for a good surgeon, is *to be a man,*—a man of courage."[56] Obstetrician Walter Channing declared of women, "Their feelings of *sympathy* are too powerful for the cool exercise of judgment"; they lacked the detachment "essential to the practice of the surgeon."[57] The alleged inability of a woman to operate on a struggling, conscious patient while maintaining the proper emotional detachment and the necessary physical control was cited again and again by opponents of women surgeons.[58]

The charge that the agonies of surgery could not be inflicted by a woman came not only from male physicians but also from feminists and women natural healers. "The Past, with the lancet, and poison, and operative surgery, did not insult woman by asking her to become a physician; and the Past has not asked her to become hangman, general, or jailer," Mary Gove Nichols declared in 1851. Hydropaths like Nichols and Ellen Snow, sentimentalist supporters of women physicians like Samuel Gregory, and homeopath-feminists like Elizabeth Cady Stanton all welcomed the woman physician, with her natural, sympathetic, gentle, feminine remedies, as an effective alternative to the masculine, unnatural brutality of operative surgery.[59]

In medicine, as in surgery, Victorian Americans usually assumed that "truly" feminine "ladies" would not be willing or able to practice the harsh and often painful techniques of heroic therapy. Augustus K. Gardner claimed, "Woman has too much kindness of heart, sympathy and sensibility, to properly fulfill this important post."[60] For the very same reason, opponents of painful heroic regimens welcomed the entry of women into the profession. *The Lily,* "A Monthly Journal Devoted to Temperance and Literature," (and to feminism and health reform) hailed the opening of a "Female Medical College," on the grounds that women doctors would be unwilling to inflict heroic therapy. "They must have stronger stomachs and nerves than we, if they can endure the blistering, bleeding, drug dosing system of the old school."[61] Samuel Gregory, founder of Boston's Female Medical College, believed women's greater "sympathy with suffering" would "inculcate generally a milder and less energetic mode of practice."[62]

The conquest of surgical pain thus undermined a major

objection to women as practitioners of surgery—an objection that had been shared by both antifeminists and many feminists. Of course, there were still many other ideological and institutional hurdles in the path of the prospective female surgeon, but, at least in theory, women's supposed tenderness no longer seemed a totally insurmountable obstacle. The first medical school course in surgery for women followed the discovery of etherization by less than five years. When Dr. Elizabeth Blackwell's sister Emily decided to become a surgeon, she chose as her preceptor the pioneer of anesthesia James Simpson.[63] Furthermore, there is fragmentary statistical evidence suggesting that women doctors may actually have resorted to anesthesia in surgery more frequently than their male counterparts did. In the late nineteenth century, in cases of operative obstetrics, the female doctors of the New England Hospital for Women may have used anesthetics in almost 18 percent more cases than did male doctors performing the identical procedures at the Boston Lying-In Hospital (see table 15). The difference is marked, though the sample is too small to be significant.[64]

But while the conquest of surgical pain thus undermined one important objection to women becoming surgeons, many feminists and women physicians remained skeptical of anesthesia. Some feared the loss of patient autonomy, others denounced the intoxicating effects, still others objected to using artificial and unnatural chemical painkillers. And while anesthesia made it possible for gentle Victorian women to practice surgery, many women physicians continued to regard surgery itself as unnatural, unnecessary, and unfeminine. These women practitioners, like Mary Gove Nichols, remained perfectly willing to relinquish such brutal and unnatural fields of endeavor to men. Samuel Gregory implied that if there were more women doctors there would be less need for either surgery or anesthesia.[65] By insisting on the *superiority* of women as gentle natural healers, this feminist ideology wound up abandoning women's claim to *equality* in such unnatural, masculine spheres as surgery and heroic therapy.[66]

Furthermore, whereas the discovery of anesthesia made surgery less painful, the professional calculus still called upon practitioners to inflict a good deal of suffering. Conservative objections to indiscriminate anesthetization meant that women surgeons would still have to witness and perform many painful procedures. Sentimentalists, like the poet Lydia Sigourney, denounced the whole professional calculus as a cold, brutal, inherently masculine approach to pain and suffering. Only a man would stop to weigh the advantages and disadvantages of therapy and to adopt a cost-benefit economic approach to the value of human life. Sigourney denounced men's "measured sympathies." "—And poise ye in the rigid scales/Of calculation, the fond bosom's wealth?"[67]

Thus women surgeons found themselves torn between their intense commitment to a gentler, less painful, more "feminine" style of practice, and their desire to win male professional acceptance and status. The Blackwell sisters, Mary Thompson, and other women who did perform surgery shared the sentimentalist belief that female practitioners should be more gentle and less brutal than men. These women did not simply see themselves as doing a man's job according to masculine standards. They expected that women surgeons would make surgery a more humane and natural art. But at the same time they also felt the desire to harden themselves, to show that they were able to compete with men at any job no matter how painful. "I think I have sufficient hardness to be entirely unaffected by great agony in such a way as to impair the clearness of thought necessary for bringing relief," Elizabeth Blackwell wrote to her mother. "I am sure the warmest sympathy would prompt me to relieve suffering to the extent of my power; though I do not think any case would keep me awake at night."[68] In mid-1849, a leading British surgeon invited Blackwell to witness an amputation. "I noted nothing peculiar in the operation, which was skilfully performed, without chloroform," she coolly recorded.[69]

Sarah Adamson (Dolley) found the conflict more painful. "Yesterday we had at Clinic, a surgical operation," she wrote to her cousin, in 1850.

A boy of five or six years old for hare lip; it was a bad case, and hurt the little fellow very much. They tied his hands and feet, and two held him; it looked very much like butchering, and was unpleasant to see a child, have to be hurt so bad.[70]

But that the child had to be so hurt she never doubted. The tough-minded Marie Zakrzewska repeatedly warned prospective women practitioners that " *'Sympathy'*; sympathy with their fellow mortals of their own sex, with the suffering sisterhood,'' would ''never be the right motive'' for studying medicine.[71]

As a volunteer nurse in the Civil War, Louisa May Alcott experienced the same conflict between her desire to make the practice of surgery more tender and feminine and the need to make herself harder and more masculine. The masculine ''enthusiasm'' of ''Dr. P.,'' ''cutting, sawing, patching and piecing'' without anesthetics in all but the worst cases ''soon convinced me that I was a weaker vessel, though nothing would have induced me to confess it then.'' She served as assistant to Dr. P., ''cherishing the while a strong desire to insinuate a few of his own disagreeable knives and scissors into him, and see how he liked it.'' Yet, Alcott herself had chosen to be this physician's aide, and had volunteered to witness these and similar operations, ''feeling that the sooner I inured myself to trying sights, the more useful I should be.''[72]

The control of surgical pain eliminated a major objection to women becoming operating room nurses, as well as to their becoming surgeons. But feminization of this occupation was not the immediate effect of Morton's discovery. So long as the role of women in nursing was limited to providing tenderness and sympathy rather than technical aid, female operating room nurses seemed even more irrelevant following Morton's discovery than before. As Alcott put it,

> You ask if nurses are obliged to witness amputations and such matters, as a part of their duty? I think not, unless they wish; for the patient is under the effects of ether, and needs no care but such as the surgeons can best give. Our work begins afterward, when the poor soul comes to himself, sick, faint, and wandering; full of strange pains and confused visions, of disagreeable sensations and sights. Then we must sooth and sustain, tend and watch; preaching and practicing patience.[73]

Not until the complicated procedures of antisepsis gained wide acceptance in the 1880s did female nursing emerge as an integral part of operative surgery,[74] and only then did anesthesia actually further the feminization of the field. Beginning at the same time, responsibility for administering the anesthetics themselves began to be transferred from medical to female nursing personnel in the United States.[75]

Thus, the introduction of anesthetics made it possible for

women to enter the operating room in a professional capacity, without abandoning their "feminine sensibilities." But the professional calculus, which still required the moderate infliction of pain, placed severe limits on the extent to which surgery could be feminized and left women surgeons to struggle with an agonizing role conflict.

Anesthesia, Power, and the Patient's Role in Surgical Decisionmaking

Anesthetics conferred unprecedented power to suspend human volition and control people's behavior. Many nineteenth-century surgeons welcomed the additional power the new painkillers provided over their patients. Yet others denounced such authoritarianism and urged that patients' choices be protected.[76] But how did such considerations influence the actual use of anesthesia and with what effect on the relationship between patients and the profession?

In both published and manuscript case records, nineteenth-century doctors matter-of-factly recorded repeated instances in which they used anesthesia to subdue uncooperative patients or to perform unwanted surgery. Such cases were particularly common with patients the doctor judged incompetent to participate in decisions about their treatment, especially children, the retarded, and the insane. In a case of vaginal surgery on a retarded girl, a professor at Indiana Medical College reported using "chloroform, to keep the patient quiet— she being of a refractory disposition." A nine-year-old boy in Brooklyn was reported to be "of an exceedingly wayward disposition and could not be controlled but by main force." A dispensary physician anesthetized him and completed a minor operation without further trouble.[77]

For all his defense of the patient's right to demand anesthesia, even James Simpson was not above using force on a patient who refused chloroform.

CASE I.—"A boy, four or five years old, with necrosis of one of the bones of the fore-arm. Could speak nothing but Gaelic. No means, consequently, of explaining to him what he was required to do. . . . [H]e became frightened, and wrestled to be away. He was held gently, however, by Dr. Simpson, and obliged to inhale . . . . ''

Significantly, when Simpson wanted to satisfy his scientific curiosity about the effects of the anesthetic, he had no trouble in questioning the boy through ''a Gaelic interpreter,'' found among his own medical students. Finding an interpreter could not have been very difficult, considering the operation was done in Edinburgh.[78] The Massachusetts General Hospital's Dr. Samuel Cabot Jr. revealed what he saw to be the central purpose in anesthetizing infants when he noted of one 1854 operation that the young patient had been ''rolled firmly in a sheet as a substitute for ether.''[79]

Anesthetics also found employment in ''tranquilization'' of the insane, both for therapy and for simple control. Dr. Charles Jackson graphically reported his pioneer experiments at the McLean Asylum. Jackson administered over a pint of ether and chloroform to a naked male inmate, a ''furious maniac'' who ''spat at the sponge, tried to bite it, and in every way to prevent the administration of the vapor.'' Though he judged this trial a ''success'' he confined his efforts thereafter exclusively to women inmates.[80] Many nineteenth-century asylums reported using anesthetics to control patients, with varying degrees of success. Although ether and chloroform never became as important a means of institutional control as tranquilizers are today, anesthetics were widely used for that purpose from the first year of their discovery. In fact, modern tranquilizers were first developed as a direct result of research on anesthetics.[81]

Children and the insane were not, however, the only people felt to be incapable of making their own medical decisions. Many nineteenth-century physicians included women in the same category. Textbooks and journals repeatedly urged the use of anesthetics to overcome women's objections to surgery, especially in obstetrics. The practice was justified by explicit analogy to the treatment of children. Women in fact did account for a greatly disproportionate number of involuntary operations.[82]

In some cases, patients' refusal to permit an operation constituted the primary evidence that they were mentally incompetent to make a rational decision. One early but typical example involved an Irish laborer brought to Massachusetts General in 1847 after having been hit by a train. Dr. J. Mason Warren determined that a thigh amputation was essential to save the man's life. The laborer however expressed his intention to die in one piece and became "much excited" at Warren's suggestion of surgery. John Collins Warren attributed the man's "obstinate" refusal to his "ignorance, stupidity, and state of intoxication." The physicians clearly considered the man's position irrational and ordered him put in a straitjacket. When that failed to restrain him enough for surgery, he was forcibly anesthetized and the shattered limb removed. Two days later he died. In an almost identical case from 1855, a "very eccentric" twenty-six-year-old woman author was etherized and operated on "by desire of husband . . . after much resistance on her part."[83]

Nineteenth-century physicians deeply believed that such mental states as fear, worry, depression, or anxiety could directly damage a person's health.[84] Thus, anesthesia also proved useful in performing nonconsensual surgery on patients whom the doctor felt would be physically harmed by the anticipation of an operation. A New Hampshire surgeon reported amputating the leg of a wounded soldier, in 1864.

Not wishing to increase the inevitable shock of the operation by any mental depression, I concealed from him my purpose, and told him I would put him to sleep, and perhaps the ball might yet be extracted . . . and without any suspicion he took the chloroform kindly and was soon sound asleep. The attendants immediately came into the ward with the necessary instruments, &c., and I amputated.

(Contemporary moral philosophers might note that, in this operation, "the femoral artery was admirably compressed by Rev. Mr. Scandlin, Chaplain of the 15th Mass. Vols., a high-toned gentleman.")[85]

In a similar vein, the *Bulletin of the New York Academy of Medicine* presented the case reports of one obstetric surgeon who made it his "unfailing custom" to use anesthetics so that he might operate on the patient "without making known to her the fact that forceps were to be used." "Chloroform is of great advantage . . . to spare the patient the anticipation of the operation . . . : the doctor can come, perform the operation and retire, while the patient is utterly ignorant of what is being done."[86]

Virtually all such uses of anesthesia were justified by reference to the patient's supposed best medical interests. In one extreme example, an Ohio prison surgeon, accused of using anesthesia to perform unwanted operations on convicts, defended himself by claiming that only a doctor could decide what was in the best interests of a prisoner.[87]

Several nineteenth-century medical writers, including at least one homeopath, offered specific suggestions on the best technique for anesthetizing a resisting patient. Perhaps the most outrageous of these was Turnbull's 1885 recommendation that the surgeon cut such troublemakers with his scalpel, to force them to inhale.[88]

Under such circumstances, there were bound to be accidents. At Massachusetts General, the deaths of at least two patients were attributed to involuntary anesthetization by 1860. One patient was a truckman, delirious with fever from an infected leg fracture. The "ward-tender came in to say that patient was growing violent and would have to be confined with straps. House surgeon proceeded to etherize him . . . . The Patient gave 6 or 8 respirations and the pulse suddenly stopped."[89]

According to the ancient common law of battery, a free adult of sound mind could prohibit any unwanted intrusion upon his person and hence had the right to refuse any operation, no matter how medically necessary. In addition, medical malpractice law required that a patient give consent to any surgery, provided that such decision-making constituted good and normal medical practice. Yet, despite the openly acknowledged use of anesthesia for involuntary surgery, almost no such cases found their way into nineteenth-century courts. And, those few that did were decided on the basis of the medically-determined malpractice standard, rather than on the absolute right of self-determination granted by battery law.[90]

One such case was the 1866 British trial of *Absolon v. Stratham*. A seamstress alleged that Mr. Stratham, a surgeon, had forcibly chloroformed her and removed six of her teeth without permission. In his defense, Stratham was allowed to present evidence that his conduct was medically necessary, skillful, and not negligent, as well as that the woman lacked competence to assess her need for surgery. The jury split and the practitioner went free. For most of the nineteenth century, British and American courts held that involuntary surgery could be justified if the lack of consent did not violate good medical practice, that is, if medical authorities found the patient incompetent or likely to be harmed by the stress of decisionmaking.[91]

But "competence" and "harm" are in part value judgments. Nineteenth-century law and medical ethics permitted medical values to govern which patients would be allowed to participate in decisionmaking and which would not. Thus, even though involuntary anesthetization may not have been used very often, the wide discretion granted physicians to use it certainly constituted an expansion of medical authority.

The extent to which anesthesia prompted gross violations of patient autonomy should not, however, be exaggerated. Anesthesia clearly was used to perform operations without the patients' consent, and such surgery had considerable medical and legal sanction. But at least some surgeons opposed these infringements of patients' autonomy.[92] And it is easy to find counterexamples, cases in which a patient who refused anesthesia and/or surgery was allowed to have his or her (but usually his) own way, against medical advice. If the physician concluded that a patient was competent and would not be harmed by the stress of decisionmaking, then the patient's wishes would often prevail, even if it meant foregoing an operation deemed essential.[93]

As isolated instances, these examples do not really tell us whether or not anesthetics led to any increase in the overall amount of involuntary surgery actually performed. The total number of blatantly forcible procedures done at the major nineteenth-century American hospitals remained small, both before and after 1846. Medical journals seemingly published more such cases after anesthesia, but with the possible exception of obstetrics, the rise in reporting seems due to the journalistic novelty of ether, rather than to any sudden epidemic of force. And the victory over pain almost certainly made more patients willing to consent voluntarily to medically indicated operations.

Anesthesia clearly did eliminate the patient's ability to make decisions about those events that might arise during the operation itself. Unanesthetized patients had enjoyed an almost unlimited freedom to express their opinions during surgery and to make known their desires about what should be done to their bodies. However, the practical importance of this freedom was less than it might seem. Once an agreed-upon operation had begun, the professional canons of preanesthetic surgery demanded that the doctor complete the procedure, no matter how strenuously the patient attempted to change his or her mind. The pain-racked patient was assumed to be *non compos mentis* during the operation; the surgeon was no more bound to heed the desires of a patient on the table than he was those of a raving lunatic. Burly assistants were always kept at hand to overcome resistance. Occasionally an agonized sufferer would break free, only to be physically subdued by the attendants. One such escapee, attempting to resist an operation by the eminent British surgeon Robert Liston, locked himself in the lavatory. Liston reportedly forced the door and personally hauled the struggling man back to the table.[94] The use of anesthesia clearly reduced the power of patients to make their wishes heard; it did not necessarily reduce their ability to have their decisions heeded. Not until the 1880s did the inability of anesthetized patients to participate in midoperative deliberations come to be seen as posing either ethical or legal problems.[95]

The long-term effects of anesthesia on the doctor-patient relationship have been the most subtle and the most pervasive. Today, many people rely on painkilling technology to provide a pill or panacea for every discomfort. This modern reliance on medical expertise to provide a "technical fix" for every pain has resulted in a subtle loss of individual autonomy. Painkillers have fostered our dependence on the medical profession. Emily Dickinson elegantly encapsulated the nineteenth-century's medicalization of suffering.

> It Knew no Medicine—
> It was not Sickness—then—
> Nor any need of Surgery—
> And therefore—'twas not Pain—[96]

In addition, the discovery of ether seemingly launched us on an infinitely expanding demand curve—the relief of some pains leaves us more exquisitely sensitive to those pains that remain. As William Lawrence, Episcopal Bishop of Massachusetts, explained in 1904, "The blessing of anesthetics has so released humanity from the awful terrors of pain that we cannot endure even the thought of what our fathers passed through." In a sense, we are addicted.[97]

But our modern dependence on painkillers developed because of lay demands to escape from suffering, not because of a professional plot to medicalize society. Most nineteenth-century Americans seem to have been all too eager to surrender some autonomy in exchange for relief. Conservative physicians complained repeatedly that their patients insisted on pain relief above all else, contrary to professional advice. It was the public, not the medical profession, who insisted that doctors cure every ache and pain, regardless of the price in personal autonomy.[98]

In nineteenth-century America, professional authority expressed itself, not in claims to abolish pain universally, but in the power to eliminate it selectively—not simply a result of anesthesia, but of a professional ideology that gave the physician the right to decide who shall suffer and who shall be relieved. "The discovery and introduction of anaesthetic remedies," declared New Yorker Dr. Peter Van Buren, "places in our hands a new power, . . . enabling us, in many instances, to fix the precise limitation of suffering, and say of pain, so long may it continue, but no longer."[99]

Professionalism and Innovation

Scholars have long debated whether "professionalism" advances or retards "innovation" in medicine. But if the early history of anesthesia is a valid indicator, the question may be misconceived. Professionalism may have divergent, even opposite, effects on the discovery, recognition, diffusion, and application of new therapies; competing varieties of professionalism may produce still further complications.

Anesthesia won acceptance with a speed unprecedented in the history of pre-twentieth-century medical innovation. Yet surgeons used it conservatively and selectively. The rapidity and the caution were likely interrelated. The swift diffusion of anesthetic usage may have resulted in part from the exceptionally strong lay demand for relief from pain, but the willingness of physicians to accommodate themselves to such public pressure probably reflected the availability of a conservative ideology that enabled the profession to limit such patient demands, to retain medical control. Thus, in nineteenth-century America, conservative professionalism both speeded the diffusion, and limited the application, of the new painkillers.[100]

Bureaucracy and Benevolence

The effect of anesthesia on professional benevolence and empathy was enormous but complex. The ability to extinguish pain routinely and automatically made possible what Magendie and other critics had most feared: instead of treating the patient as a feeling human being, the surgeon was now free to carve him like a side of beef.[101] But the development of anesthesia also made possible a freer expression of sensitivity toward patients. With the amount of suffering vastly diminished, the surgeon no longer needed quite so thick a self-protective emotional armor as had Melville's Dr. Cuticle.[102] In other words, anesthesia made possible a greater range of medical sentiment toward patients—both more routine callousness and more benevolent sensitivity.

But the simultaneous emergence of medical bureaucracies restricted that new freedom of expression. By the 1860s, physicians had begun to realize that even the most particularized bureaucracy severely limited the expression of sympathy and full concern for the individual. The organization of the Sanitary Commission and the growing number of large hospitals made possible the efficient technological *treatment* of pain, but they impeded *empathy* with its victims.[103] Many mid-nineteenth-century Americans seemingly preferred this efficient if impersonal relief.

The availability of anesthesia itself played a role in making possible the routinized functioning of large hospitals. Eliminating the wild, disorderly pre-anesthetic scenes of screaming and brutality made possible the eventual emergence of the controlled, efficient, rationalized modern operating room, in which the quiet is broken only by the rhythmic whoosh of the anesthetist's air bag.

Anesthesia also played a large role in the modernization of the American pharmaceutical industry. Ether and chloroform were the first widely used drugs whose obvious and visible effects depended on absolute and reliable purity. The combination of high demand and the need for quality control set the stage for the rapid emergence of large, centralized national drug suppliers. Dr. Edward R. Squibb built his pioneering pharmaceutical company on a reputation for consistent quality and unlimited supply of ether.[104]

And while anesthesia itself expanded the possible range of medical emotions, the conservative ideology limited professional feelings within the measured confines of the calculus of suffering. Emily Dickinson captured the emotional essence of conservative professionalism:

> Bound—a trouble—
> And lives can bear it!
> Limit—how deep a bleeding can go!
> So—many—drops—of vital scarlet—
> Deal with the soul
> As with algebra![105]

Anesthesia and Medical Philosophy

The development of anesthetics also stimulated a reevaluation of several important issues in biomedical philosophy. That a physical substance could so profoundly and directly affect mental processes seemed to call for a rethinking of the strict Cartesian mind-body dichotomy. A number of intellectuals, including Edward Everett and Horace Binney, began to speculate about this problem almost as soon as Morton's discovery had been announced. Yet with the possible exception of William James, few nineteenth-century philosophers were able to incorporate anesthesia into their understanding of the relationship between mind and body.[106]

Anesthesia also raised interesting issues concerning the problem of the accessibility of feelings. The difficulty of deciding whether ether produced true anesthesia or merely amnesia stimulated a revival of interest in the question of whether it is ever possible to tell what someone else is "really" feeling.[107] However, as explained in chapter 7, the social implications of this question in nineteenth-century America led most physicians to assume that they already knew the answer.

The discovery that a drug could completely eliminate a disease symptom such as pain without having any effect whatsoever on the course of the disease itself also led to a profound reevaluation of medical theories on the nature of disease. Many pre-anesthetic physicians of all professional persuasions retained a belief in the ancient concept that a disease was simply a bundle of visible symptoms. This theory is still reflected in the names of many illnesses—"small pox," "yellow fever," and so on.[108] Thus, before anesthesia, most pain relievers, like opium and alcohol, were thought to have therapeutic, as well as analgesic effects. To the extent that pain was considered an integral part of the disease, the removal of pain was felt to be a true cure. In this context, the discovery of anesthesia helped forward a major revolution in medical philosophy underway throughout the nineteenth century—the concept that diseases were discrete specific entities with an existence of their own apart from any symptoms. Walter Channing carefully explained to the Boston Society for Medical Improvement in 1852 that the use of chloroform "abolishes pain—we do not say cures disease."[109]

Finally, anesthesia made possible the later introduction of antisepsis and the eventual control of surgical infection. The hyperhygienic rituals of modern aseptic surgery would be inconceivable in a world where a struggling, convulsed patient still had to be wrestled to the table and where every second of delay was an eternity of pain.[110]

The End of An Era

The calculus of suffering dominated the first generations of professional anesthesia, from the 1840s through the 1880s. But during the late nineteenth century, the era of selective anesthetization gradually drew to a close. One important cause was the development of new anesthetic drugs and techniques. As early as 1878, Turnbull listed thirty different substances known to have anesthetic effects. The real expansion of the anesthetic menu began with Carl Koller's 1884 introduction of cocaine drop local anesthesia and William Halsted's 1885 use of a hypodermic cocaine nerve block.[111] From then on, anesthetists began to concentrate more on tailoring the choice of anesthetic to suit the patient, instead of selecting those patients best suited to anesthesia. The development had been predicted by Samuel H. Dickson as early as 1860. Dickson noted "there are many well-known objections" to "promiscuous" anesthetization, "but it is equally clear that as their number and variety are augmented we shall be more likely, upon a careful study of their peculiar influences, to find some one among them which shall be adapted in each particular case to our immediate purpose."[112]

The gradual adoption of antiseptic surgery also helped end selective anesthetization. The complex rituals of Lister's technique virtually demanded that all patients be immobilized with anesthesia. And the resulting ability of practitioners to open the body cavity without causing infection in turn led to a new, less conservative surgical outlook. Finally, the discovery of infectious microbes, new vaccines, and "magic bullet" drugs in the turn-of-the-century decades diminished professional concern for individualized prescriptions. These breakthroughs revolutionized medicine, not the least because of their seeming universality and disease-specificity. One result was a new professional insistence that prescriptions be tailored to the disease rather than to the patient.[113]

The practice of selective anesthetization may have ended before 1900, but the issues it raised still confront physicians today: the need to balance life saving and painkilling, the need to reconcile a universal science with human variability. To the extent that today's doctors and patients alike seem to be questioning the magic bullets of recent decades and returning to supposedly more "holistic" concern with people, as well as diseases, many of these problems are even reappearing in something remarkably close to their nineteenth-century trappings.[114]

Suffering, Human Variation, and the Ideal of Equality

Nineteenth-century physicians discriminated among patients on the basis of age, sex, race, class, ethnicity, and similar variables in their use of anesthetics. But how are we to judge such discrimination? For example, the calculus of suffering resulted in men being anesthetized less often than women. Was that good or bad? The calculus of suffering likewise seems to have made possible more experimental surgery on women than on men. Was that good or bad? To the extent that such differences represented adjustments to "real" individual variations in human "needs," it seems we ought to approve. To the extent that they reflected and reinforced vicious racial, sexual, and similar dehumanizing antiegalitarian stereotypes, it seems we ought to disapprove.

But assessing individual "needs" is not always simple. Whereas medicine should ideally meet each individual's specific "needs," it is surely unrealistic to expect physicians or anyone else to judge objectively and dispassionately what the differences in human "needs" really are, especially in such personal and nonobjective areas as pain. Any human system of medical decisionmaking is bound to lead to some errors in judging "need." The goal should be to minimize all errors, but it is not clear that erring on the side of overuniformity is morally equivalent to erring on the side of overdiscrimination. Assuming that mistakes are going to be made either way, is it better to overlook a "real" difference in medical needs or to act upon a "spurious" difference? Is it better to make a mistake on the side of equality or on the side of individuality? The answer depends on a value judgment, not on objective science. One who believes that egalitarianism is at least marginally more valuable than individualism might therefore find it somewhat preferable for his physician to err by following universal rules that turn out not to apply to him than to err by mistakenly assuming to know what is "best" for him personally or for "people like him."

Most nineteenth-century American doctors sought to personalize their therapies; they adopted highly particularized rules by which the physician could determine the different "needs" of many different "types" of patients. A few even insisted on complete individualization. Yet some nineteenth-century Americans realized that such particularity could be purchased only by the loss of equality.

Speaking the language of the conservative physician, Walt Whitman reassured the woman he embraced, "I do not hurt you anymore than is necessary for you."[115] As if in direct reply, Lydia Maria Child pointed out that the power to make such distinctions reduced the woman to slavery. "The most inveterate slaveholders are probably those who . . . would be most ashamed to have the name of being *unnecessarily* cruel."[116]

AFTERWORD

PROFESSIONALISM AND CHANGE: HISTORY AND SOCIAL THEORY

The practice of most professions in eighteenth-century America was a harsh and grim business. Educators, from school masters to college presidents, plied the rattan and ferule. Jurists sentenced criminals to the gallows or the lash. Physicians bled, blistered, and purged, while dentists and surgeons performed their operations on screaming, struggling patients. The need to inflict great physical pain on clients pervaded daily professional life. It constituted an integral part of the self-image, ideology, and organization of most eighteenth-century professions.

But, by the mid-nineteenth century, a variety of separate social, ideological, and technological innovations made it possible to soften some of the more brutal inflictions of professional practice. The introduction of anesthesia in 1846, the evolution of alternatives to physical punishments, and the growing skepticism toward heroic medicine all lessened the amount of physical suffering that practitioners were expected to inflict. This declining need to hurt clients resulted in part from simple improvements in technology. But it also both affected and reflected changes in social values and professional ideology.

Even today, most professions require practitioners to inflict some form of suffering to gain some future benefit. Establishing and enforcing standards to balance painful means against worthwhile ends still constitutes an extremely important function of a professional ideology. Professionalism protects the practitioner from the twin sirens of sadism and timidity. While no sane person would want to inflict more pain than "necessary," one vital function of professionalism has been to provide criteria by which to determine how much is "necessary" and for what purposes.[1]

But the content of professionalism can change greatly over time, as a result both of innovations in technology and of alterations in social values. Practices sanctioned or demanded by professionalism two centuries ago would be considered barbaric today. Mid-nineteenth-century America witnessed great changes both in public attitudes toward suffering and in the technical capacity to eliminate pain. This era also produced great internal upheaval in most American professions. These changes converged to produce a revolution in professional attitudes toward suffering and the relief of pain.

Professionalism thus is a changing ideology, one that demands very different attitudes and behavior from practitioners at different times. Yet this conclusion runs directly counter to the basic assumptions of most previous scholarly work on the professions. The literature on professionalism is vast, and yet, with a few notable exceptions, none of these studies takes any notice of the fact that the meaning of "professionalism" has *changed* over time. Too often, social scientists have focused on the detailed values of the present-day professions (usually just medicine) as if these occupations constituted the only (or at least the purest) form of professionalism. Even those sociologists who have employed historical evidence have used the past to search out a few common denominators that then could be taken as universal and timeless characteristics of all professions, rather than regarding the changeable features as valuable objects of study in their own right.[2] Once all the historically variable aspects have been winnowed away, a few common attributes, such as autonomy and monopoly, are supposedly left as the universal elements of professionalism. But is this remainder the true kernel or merely the chaff left over after the real germ of the idea has been stripped away? A feature could conceivably have been *common* to all past professions, yet *central* to none. The problem can be resolved only by contextual historical research; the answer cannot be deduced or assumed.

Sociological definitions generally fall into two schools: those listing a specific set of attributes that allegedly constitute the hallmarks of a ''profession'' and those outlining the functionally necessary ideological content of ''professionalism.'' The ''attributes-listing'' school usually describes a profession as an occupation that requires mastery of a systematic body of esoteric knowledge, knowledge that is applied to serve other people. Less laudatory definitions focus on the power of autonomous self-regulation and the monopolization of skills.[3] Other features commonly listed include full-time employment, specialized functions, formal organization, esprit de corps, codes of ethics, and training requirements. Few occupations have ever met all the many criteria, but to the extent that they do, they are placed on a scale ranging from most to least professional.[4]

One difficulty in defining the professions by enumerating their attributes is that the criteria on most lists conflict with one another. Thus, raising training requirements may reduce the supply of services. Increasing specialization may fragment esprit de corps. Serving the needs of one client may be incompatible with serving the needs of other clients. Adding more attributes only increases the likelihood that they will conflict.[5]

Most importantly, defining a profession in terms of any fixed list of criteria does not allow for the possibility that the attributes have changed over time. Yet the available evidence indicates that many of the features most commonly cited as characteristic of professions today were either absent from, or even antithetical to, past ideals of professionalism.[6] Today, for example, specialization is often cited as a hallmark of professionalism in medicine; conversely, a doctor who claims expertise in too many fields of practice is sure to arouse hostility or suspicion.[7] But, for most of American history, quite the opposite was true. A physician who claimed specialized knowledge of any specific disease or specific organ would have been branded a quack.[8] Nineteenth-century hostility to specialization was not unprofessional, protoprofessional, or a deviant case. Nineteenth-century professions were simply different from modern professions. While past views of specialization differed markedly from more recent standards, neither is *inherently* ''more professional'' than the other.

Likewise, formal organizations and institutions are often mentioned as features that make an occupation a profession. The relative weakness of such institutions in mid-nineteenth-century America thus becomes, by definition, proof that medicine, law, divinity, etc., were not very professional in that era. But such a definition rules out the possibility of asking whether these occupations may have been unorganized in part because some of their members regarded bureaucratic institutions as either irrelevant to, or a violation of, *their* concept of professionalism. There is evidence that at least a few nineteenth-century physicians regarded the American Medical Association as an unprofessional conspiracy to limit the individual freedom of action that, for them, characterized a free, liberal profession.[9] Any definition of a profession ought to permit us to distinguish between those who may have opposed organization because they were against all forms of professionalism and those who may have done so because they regarded organization as itself unprofessional—even though it may turn out that most nineteenth-century Americans still fell into the former category. Similarly, monopoly, self-regulation, and virtually all the other alleged characteristics of the contemporary professions have, at one time or another, been regarded as antithetical to some past concept of professionalism.[10]

Functionalist accounts take a different tack. Rather than listing the supposed characteristics of a profession, they attempt to specify what values are necessary in order for practitioners of a given occupation to fulfill their socially assigned roles. Talcott Parsons, who pioneered this approach, described five basic ideological orientations that he thought necessary for a physician to hold in order to fulfill the duties assigned by society to a healer. These included values like emotional neutrality as opposed to empathy and universalism as opposed to particularism.[11]

But there are difficulties with Parsons' approach as well. One problem is that, in the real world, such lopsided values do not really turn out to be "functional," because society and fellow practitioners each make a variety of different, even conflicting, demands in their role expectations for physicians. Some of these conflicts arise in professional-client relations. For example, a physician is expected to show empathy and concern for patients while at the same time maintaining cool-headed unemotional detachment.[12] Professionals are also expected to combine technical manual skills with broad academic theory.[13]

Even the most basic functions of a profession may be in conflict. Physicians are asked to prevent disease, study disease, cure disease, relieve suffering, and save lives, but in some cases, carrying out any one of these duties may preclude success in the others. An effective cure may destroy the opportunity to do further research or may undermine the commitment to preventive measures. Curing a disease or doing research may each require the performance of painful or life-threatening procedures. Prolonging life may require prolonging vast suffering, and, as we have seen, relieving pain often requires risk to life or limb. Without some means of setting priorities among such conflicting demands, the occupation of physician would be untenable. To be truly "functional," professionalism must be an ideology that provides practitioners with behavioral values to help resolve such conflicting role demands.[14]

Parsons' approach also minimized the role of historical change by assuming both that the social functions of the professions were fixed and that only one set of values could best meet these timeless demands. But both the expected functions and the technical capabilities of the professions have changed dramatically over time. Furthermore, several different sets of professional values have often existed simultaneously, either symbiotically or in competition. Even among contemporary American professions such differences remain important. For example, medical professionalism in America today places much more emphasis on practitioner autonomy than does legal professionalism, while many religious denominations severely restrict autonomous action by individual clergymen. But in themselves, none of these ideologies is intrinsically more professional than the other. Likewise, no one value system can provide one universally correct professional balance between empathy and detachment, nor between technical and academic knowledge, nor between doing research and serving clients. No one point on the continuum between caring and aloofness is *inherently* more "professional" than the other.

Too often, historians have adopted uncritically one or another sociological model of professionalism, most commonly one of the "attribute-listing" variety. The anachronism inherent in using such presentist definitions to describe the past is illustrated by one recent historian's assertion that, because nineteenth-century medicine did not meet several twentieth-century criteria of professionhood, "medicine in 1858 was not truly a profession."[15] If the word "profession" is reserved for jobs that fully meet our present criteria of professionalism, then *no* occupation before 1890 was "truly a profession," although people had been using that word to describe their vocations at least since the Middle Ages.[16]

Although historians generally use such presentist definitions, most have sensed something amiss. Thus, Burton Bledstein modified his obligatory recital of the timeless attributes of a profession by focusing his study on a vague but temporally unique nineteenth-century professional "culture." Thomas Haskell also attempted a "contextualist" aproach, cautioning against assuming that "professional" is better than "amateur." But, like Bledstein, Haskell still relied on a fixed list of presentist attributes to define a "profession."[17] Since both books concentrate on the late nineteenth-century emergence of *modern* professionalism, their presentist definitions are more appropriate than they would be for earlier periods.

However, a few historians have made the changes and conflicts in past concepts of professionalism their objects of study. Thomas Bender's essay on the shift from "civic"- to "disciplinary"-based professionalism in medicine and academia; Merle Borrowman's classic study of the trend from "liberal" to "technical" professionalism among teachers; and Monte Calvert's evocative portrayal of the triumph of "school" over "shop" culture in engineering each demonstrated one dimension of the complex evolution in the concept of professionalism during the nineteenth century.[18]

In this study, I did not seek to impose a preconceived definition of professionalism on the past but rather to discover through historical research what ideals and practices actually characterized those occupations mid-nineteenth-century Americans called professions, to determine in particular what values and ideals governed the midcentury surgeon's attitudes toward pain and how those values changed over time. Thus, instead of referring to "professions" or "professionalism" in general, I discussed the similarities and differences among "eighteenth-century genteel professionalism," "heroic professionalism," "conservative professionalism," and so on. I have treated nineteenth-century professionalism not as the primitive precursor of modern professional values, but as an ideology with which nineteenth-century practitioners attempted to resolve nineteenth-century occupational problems.

Approaching "professionalism" in this manner makes it possible to distinguish between two often blurred but very different meanings of "professionalization." "Professionalization" may mean either "the process by which a past occupation attempted to achieve the professional ideals of that past era," or "the process by which a past occupation came to resemble present-day professions." Each definition has its uses, but the two ought not to be used interchangeably. The first provides a measure of how well past practitioners succeeded in formulating and following *their* own professional values; the second provides a measure of how different their past values were from those of *our* times.[19]

This unabashedly empirical-historical approach does not rule out the theoretical study of professionalism. Rather, it is simply returning the horse to the front of the cart—by insisting that any theory of professionalism be based on, rather than imposed on, historical and crosscultural empirical data.

What theoretical considerations, then, might be suggested by my empirical findings? This study found that the occupational self-image and professional ideals of nineteenth-century surgeons were profoundly shaped by conflicting expectations of professional function, such as the demand that doctors should both save lives and relieve pain. This ancient role conflict had been resolved in a variety of reasonably functional ways by various earlier professional ideologies. But a combination of social, ideological, and technological changes rendered these earlier resolutions obsolete in mid-nineteenth-century America and thus exacerbated the intensity and significance of the conflict. In creating a new set of occupational values to reconcile their competing duties, nineteenth-century surgeons deeply altered their concept of how a professional should react to suffering and, to that extent, changed the meaning of professionalism.

On the basis of this study, it seems plausible to hypothesize that other similar role conflicts have played a corresponding part in shaping the professional values of other occupations in other times and places. Indeed, those few historians who have studied changes in the concept of professionalism have found specific role conflicts central to the process.[20] These divergent occupational demands may have originated with changes in the economic structure, ideology, or technology of society. They may also have been provoked by ideological or technical changes within the profession itself. But, whatever the source of the conflict, the attempt to resolve incompatible job demands may well prove to have been one hitherto overlooked critically important driving force in explaining the historical evolution of professionalism.[21]

APPENDIX OF STATISTICAL TABLES

Table 1 Use of Anesthetics in Nonamputations, by Age of Patient, MGH, 1846–47

Age in Years	0–10	11–20	21–46	47+	Unknown	Total
Operations with anesthetic	4	6	35	14	0	59
Operations without anesthetic	1	8	29	4	1	43
Percent with anesthetic	80.0	42.9	54.7	77.8	0	57.8

SOURCE: MGH Records, November 7, 1846–October 15, 1847.
    Notes: Omitted are amputations of major limbs and breasts. Selection of age brackets was based in part on secondary literature concerning the history of the life cycle in antebellum America; however, brackets had to be modified to ensure enough cases per cell to be statistically meaningful. Dichotomizing the data, the age group 11–46 differed significantly from all other ages, at the .02 level.

Table 2 Use of Anesthetics in Nonamputations, by Sex of Patient, MGH, 1846–47

	Operations With Anesthetic	Operations Without Anesthetic	Percent With Anesthetic
Men	32	31	50.8
Women	27	12	69.2
Total	59	43	57.8

SOURCE: MGH Records, November 7, 1846–October 15, 1847.

Notes: Omitted are amputations of major limbs and breast. Difference of proportions significant at .05 level.

Table 3 Use of Anesthetics in Nonamputations, by Nativity of Patient, MGH, 1846–47

	Operations With Anesthetic	Operations Without Anesthetic	Percent With Anesthetic
American born	42	23	64.6
Foreign born	17	20	45.9
Total	59	43	57.8

SOURCE: MGH Records, November 7, 1846–October 15, 1847.

Notes: Omitted are amputations of major limbs and breast. American born refers to United States of America only; Canadians are counted as foreign born. Difference of proportions significant at .05 level.

Table 4 Use of Anesthetics in Nonamputations, by Occupation, for Employed Male Patients, MGH, 1846–47

	Operations With Anesthetic	Operations Without Anesthetic	Percent With Anesthetic
Seamen and laborers	10	13	43.5
All other occupations	21	16	56.8
Total	31	29	51.7

SOURCE: MGH Records, November 7, 1846–October 15, 1847.

Notes: Omitted are major limb amputations. Difference of proportions *not* significant at .05 level. Since these data are based on a complete tabulation rather than a random sample, the difference in treatment between laborers and other workers is real, but it is not possible to rule out the hypothesis that this difference happened by sheer chance.

Table 5 Use of Anesthetics in Nonamputations, Controlling for Age, Sex, and Nativity of Patient, MGH, 1846–47; Fraction and Percentage of Operations With Anesthetics

	Age	*11–46*	*All Other Ages*
A Men	Foreign born	$8/21 = 38\%$	$2/3 = 67\%$
	American born	$14/27 = 52\%$	$8/11 = 73\%$
B Women	Foreign born	$6/12 = 50\%$	$1/1 = 100\%$
	American born	$13/18 = 72\%$	$7/8 = 88\%$

SOURCE: MGH Records, November 7, 1846–October 15, 1847.

Notes: Omitted are amputations of major limbs and breast. Patients for whom the data were incomplete were omitted. One American man of unknown age did not receive anesthetic. Cells are too small for meaningful significance tests; however, note that the influence of each variable is very independent of the others.

Table 6 Use of Anesthetics, by Type of Procedure, Frank H. Hamilton, 1849–1877

	Operations With Anesthetic	*Operations Without Anesthetic*	*Percent With Anesthetic*
Major limb amputations	38	8	82.6
All other operations	56	35	61.5
Total	94	43	68.6

SOURCE: Hamilton Case Books.

Note: Difference of proportions significant at .01 level. Since Hamilton, unlike the hospitals, did not record all his cases, significance tests in tables 6–14 refer only to the significance of differences among the *recorded* population, not the total patient population. Unfortunately, the criteria by which Hamilton selected cases for recording are unknown.

Table 7 Use of Anesthetics in Major Limb Amputations, by Sex of Patient, Frank H. Hamilton, 1849–1877

	Operations With Anesthetic	Operations Without Anesthetic	Percent With Anesthetic
Men	28	8	77.8
Women	10	0	100.0
Total	38	8	82.6

SOURCE: Hamilton Case Books.
  Notes: Difference of proportions just barely not significant at .05 level.

Table 8 Use of Anesthetics in Operations Other Than Major Limb Amputations, by Sex of Patient, Frank H. Hamilton, 1849–1877

	Operations With Anesthetic	Operations Without Anesthetic	Percent With Anesthetic
Men	38	21	64.4
Women	15	14	51.7
Total	53	35	60.2

SOURCE: Hamilton Case Books.
  Notes: Patients for whom the data were incomplete were omitted. Three operations with anesthetic were performed on patients of unrecorded gender. Difference of proportions between men and women not significant at .05.

Table 9 Use of Anesthetics, by Age of Patient, Frank H. Hamilton, 1849–1877

Age in Years	Operations With Anesthetic	Operations Without Anesthetic	Percent With Anesthetic
0–10	11	1	91.7
11–46	54	33	62.1
47+	13	4	76.5
Unknown	16	5	76.2
Total	94	43	68.6

SOURCE: Hamilton Case Books.
  Notes: Dichotomizing the data, the age group 11–46 differed significantly from all other known ages, at the .02 level. See note, table 1, for explanation of selection of age brackets.

Table 10 Use of Anesthetics, Controlling for Type of Procedure, Age, and Sex of Patient; Frank H. Hamilton, 1849–1877; Fraction and Percentage of Operations With Anesthetic

Age If Known		*11–46*	*All Other Ages*
A			
Major limb	Men	20/27 = 74%	2/2 = 100%
amputations	Women	5/5 = 100%	4/4 = 100%
B			
All other	Men	19/36 = 53%	13/17 = 76%
operations	Women	8/19 = 42%	5/6 = 83%

SOURCE: Hamilton Case Books.
Note: Cells are too small for meaningful significance tests. See text for interpretation. Three cases in which sex was not recorded and twenty-one in which age was not recorded have been omitted from this table.

Table 11 Use of Anesthetics, by Occupation, Among Employed Men Patients, Frank H. Hamilton, 1849–1877

	Operations With Anesthetic	*Operations Without Anesthetic*	*Percent With Anesthetic*
Sailors and laborers	6	3	66.7
All other occupations	8	2	80.0
Total	14	5	73.7

SOURCE: Hamilton Case Books.
Note: Difference of proportions not significant at .05 level.

Table 12 Use of Anesthetics in Fracture Amputations, by Sex of Patient, Pa. H., 1853–1862

	Amputations With Anesthetic	*Amputations Without Anesthetic*	*Percent With Anesthetic*
Men	44	22	66.7
Women	3	0	100.0
Total	47	22	68.1

SOURCE: Pa. H. Fracture Books, October 16, 1853–October 15, 1862.
Notes: Difference of proportions not significant at .05 level.

Table 13 Use of Anesthetics in Fracture Amputations, by Occupation of Employed Men Patients, Pa. H., 1853–1862

	Amputations With Anesthetic	Amputations Without Anesthetic	Percent With Anesthetic
Sailors and laborers	12	6	66.7
Other unskilled trades	15	6	71.4
Skilled trades	14	5	73.7

SOURCE: Pa. H. Fracture Books, October 16, 1853–October 15, 1862.

Notes: Difference of proportions *not* significant at .05 level. Unlike the MGH data, the Pa. H. recorded a large number of unskilled workers who were not simply called "laborers." These included factory boy, quarryman, errand boy, brakesman, huckster, fireman, foundryman, carter, miner, teamster, and boatman. Skilled trades were assumed to be sashmaker, saddler, farmer, machinist, bricklayer, blacksmith, printer, weaver, cooper, carpenter, gardener, baker, conductor, stonecutter, iron worker, skinner, coachman, listmaker. (A listmaker is a tax assessor.)

Table 14 Use of Anesthetics in Fracture Amputations, by Age of Patient, Pa. H., 1853–1862

Age	Amputations With Anesthetic	Amputations Without Anesthetic	Percent With Anesthetic
0–11	0	3	0
12–45	40	17	70.2
46+	1	2	33.3
Total	41	22	65.1

SOURCE: Pa. H. Fracture Books, October 16, 1853–October 15, 1862.

Notes: Age brackets were altered slightly from MGH and Hamilton data, because of the dearth of cases at either end of the age spectrum, see note table 1 above. Dichotomizing the data, the difference of proportions between 0–11 and all other ages is significant at .05 level.

Table 15 Use of Anesthetics in Natural and Forceps-Assisted Childbirth, Two Boston Hospitals, 1873–1899; Fraction and Percent Anesthetized

	Forceps Deliveries	*Natural Deliveries*
Boston Lying-In 1887–1899	21/41 = 51.2%	20/244 = 8.2%
New England Hospital for Women 1873–1899	11/16 = 68.8%	15/139 = 10.8%
Total, both hospitals	32/57 = 56.1%	35/383 = 9.1%

SOURCE: Sample of hospital records drawn by Gina Morantz, see ch. 9 note 14, in the text.

Notes: Difference of proportions between natural and operative cases is significant at .01 level at each hospital. Difference of proportions between hospitals is not significant, at .05 level.

Table 16 Increase in Rate of Surgery per Admission, MGH, 1845–47

1845–46			*1846–47*			
Total Surgical Patients Admitted	*Number of Patients Operated on*	*Percent of Patients Operated on*	*Total Surgical Patients Admitted*	*Number of Patients Operated on*	*Percent of Patients Operated on*	*Increase in Rate of Surgery*
221	35	15.8	293	116	39.6	2.5 times

SOURCE: MGH Records, October 16, 1845–October 15, 1847.

Notes: In tables 16–23, 26, 27: A patient operated on is counted only once per admission, regardless of how many operations he or she received. A patient discharged and readmitted later is counted as a new admission and if operated upon again is counted as a new operation. These tables also include the seven cases omitted from tables 1–5; see ch. 9, note 2. They also include cases operated on during the October 16–November 7 period, not included in tables 1–5 above. Patients for whom data were lacking for a single social variable were omitted from the tabulations for that variable only. The difference of proportions in surgical rates between 1845–46 and 1846–47 is significant at the .05 level.

Table 17 Increase in Rate of Surgery per Admission, by Type of Procedure, MGH, 1845–47

Type of Procedure	1845–46			1846–47			Increase in Rate of Surgery
	Total Surgical Patients Admitted	Number of Patients Operated on	Percent of Patients Operated on	Total Surgical Patients Admitted	Number of Patients Operated on	Percent of Patients Operated on	
Major limb amputations	221	3	1.4	293	20	6.8	4.9 times
All other operations	221	32	14.5	293	96	32.8	2.3 times

SOURCE: MGH Records, October 16, 1845–October 15, 1847.

Table 18 Increase in Rate of Surgery per Admission, by Sex of Patient, MGH, 1845–47

Sex	1845–46			1846–47			Increase in Rate of Surgery
	Number of Surgical Patients Admitted	Number of Patients Operated on	Percent of Patients Operated on	Number of Surgical Patients Admitted	Number of Patients Operated on	Percent of Patients Operated on	
Men	150	25	16.7	208	71	34.1	2.0 times
Women	66	10	15.2	85	45	52.9	3.5 times

SOURCE: MGH Records, October 16, 1845–October 15, 1847.

Table 19 Increase in Rate of Surgery per Admission, by Nativity of Patient, MGH, 1845–47

Nativity	1845–46			1846–47			
	Number of Surgical Patients Admitted	Number of Patients Operated on	Percent of Patients Operated on	Number of Surgical Patients Admitted	Number of Patients Operated on	Percent of Patients Operated on	Increase in Rate of Surgery
Foreign born	104	16	15.4	139	43	30.9	2.0 times
American born	110	19	17.3	153	73	47.7	2.8 times

SOURCE: MGH Records, October 16, 1845–October 15, 1847.

Table 20 Increase in Rate of Surgery per Admission, by Occupation of Employed Men Patients, MGH, 1845–47

Occupation	1845–46			1846–47			
	Number of Surgical Patients Admitted	Number of Patients Operated on	Percent of Patients Operated on	Number of Surgical Patients Admitted	Number of Patients Operated on	Percent of Patients Operated on	Increase in Rate of Surgery
Sailors and laborers	65	8	12.3	89	23	25.8	2.1 times
All other occupations	72	14	19.4	98	45	45.9	2.4 times

SOURCE: MGH Records, October 16, 1845–October 15, 1847.

Table 21 Increase in Rate of Surgery per Admission, by Age of Patient, MGH, 1845–47

Age	1845–46			1846–47			Increase in Rate of Surgery
	Number of Surgical Patients Admitted	Number of Patients Operated on	Percent of Patients Operated on	Number of Surgical Patients Admitted	Number of Patients Operated on	Percent of Patients Operated on	
0–10	5	2	40.0	13	4	30.8	.8 times
11–46	168	25	14.9	234	88	37.6	2.5 times
47+	31	6	19.4	43	23	53.5	2.7 times

SOURCE: MGH Records, October 16, 1845–October 15, 1847.

Table 22 Increase in Rate of Experimental Surgery per Suitably Ill Patient Admitted, Minor Procedures, MGH, 1845–47

1845–46			1846–47			Proportional Increase in Rate of Surgery
Number of Suitably Ill Patients Admitted	Number of Patients Operated on	Percent of Patients Operated on	Number of Suitable Ill Patients Admitted	Number of Patients Operated on	Percent of Patients Operated on	
10	6	60.0	13	12	92.3	1.5 times

SOURCE: MGH Records, October 16, 1845–October 15, 1847.

Notes: Minor experimental surgery consisted of palate, lip, and vaginal surgery; suitably ill patients were those diagnosed as hare lip, cleft palate, lip cancer, and vesico-vaginal fistula. The difference of proportions between 1845–46 and 1846–47 is significant at the .05 level.

Table 23 Increase in Rate of Surgery per Admission, by Previous Duration of Illness, MGH, 1845–47

	1845–46			1846–47			
Previous Duration of Illness	*Number of Surgical Patients Admitted*	*Number of Patients Operated on*	*Percent of Patients Operated on*	*Number of Surgical Patients Admitted*	*Number of Patients Operated on*	*Percent of Patients Operated on*	*Increase in Rate of Surgery*
Emergency and acute (less than one week)	66	4	6.1	89	21	23.6	3.9 times
Intermediate and chronic (one week or longer)	155	31	20.0	202	95	47.0	2.4 times

SOURCE: MGH Records, October 16, 1845–October 15, 1847.

Table 24 Relation of Anesthesia to the Death Rate in Major Limb Amputations, Controlling for the Increasing Number of Accident Cases, MGH, 1821–1850

	Without Anesthesia			With Anesthesia		
Type of Case	*Number of Amputations*	*Deaths*	*Percentage Deaths Per Amputation*	*Number of Amputations*	*Deaths*	*Percentage Deaths Per Amputation*
Accident	30	12	40.0	26	10	38.5
Other	59	7	11.9	26	3	11.5

SOURCES: *AJMS* (1851), 21:178–83; *AJMS* (1852), 23:453; *Trans AMA* (1848), 1:215–17.

Notes: The decline in death rates is not a significant difference of proportions for either accidents or other amputations between anesthetic and nonanesthetic operations, at the .05 level. This table includes *all* accidents, industrial and nonindustrial. Industrial accidents were far more deadly. For the postanesthetic period, all the accidents listed were industrial; for the earlier period this was probably not the case. Thus these figures probably still underestimate the improvement in amputation survival following anesthesia when specifically *industrial* accidents are controlled for.

Table 25 Accidents as a Percentage of Total Medical and Surgical Admissions, MGH, 1844–1861

Year	Total Admissions	Accidents	Percent Accidents
1844	435	55	12.6
1845	453	62	13.6
1846	459	59	12.9
1847	674	74	11.0
1848	804	103	12.8
1849	870	97	11.1
1850	746	98	13.1
1851	839	123	14.7
1852	826	132	16.0
1853	925	159	17.2
1854	922	212	23.0
1855	915	157	17.2
1856	976	189	19.4
1857	920	163	17.7
1858	1,015	186	18.3
1859	1,240	212	17.1
1860	1,240	233	18.8
1861	1,416	297	21.0

SOURCE: Bowditch, *History of Massachusetts General Hospital* (2nd ed.), p. 702.

Notes: This rise in hospital admissions due to accidents might have been caused by increased overcrowding in the hospital, as well as by a rise in the accident rate in Boston, because accident and emergency cases had priority for admission when beds were in short supply. The rank order correlation, Spearman's rho, is .83. (Perfect correlation would be 1.00.) The correlation is significant at better than the .001 level.

Table 26 Composition of Patient Population, by Previous Duration of Disease, MGH, 1845–47

Type of Case	1845–46		1846–47		Magnitude of Change in Share of Patient Population (In Percentage Points)
	Number of Admissions	Percent of Total Admissions	Number of Admissions	Percent of Total Admissions	
Emergency and acute (less than one week)	66	29.9	89	30.6	+ .7
Intermediate (one week to one year)	89	40.3	100	34.4	− 5.9
Chronic (more than one year)	66	29.9	102	35.1	+ 5.2
Total	221	100.1	291	100.1	0

SOURCE: MGH Records, October 16, 1845–October 15, 1847.

Notes: There are *no* significant differences of proportions in patient population composition between the pre-anesthetic and postanesthetic years, at the .05 level.

Table 27 Stability of Composition of Patient Population MGH, 1845–47

Type of Patient	1845–46		1846–47		Magnitude of Change in Share of Patient Population (In Percentage Points)
	Number of Admissions	Percent of Total Recorded Admissions	Number of Admissions	Percent of Total Recorded Admissions	
Men	150	69.4	208	71.0	+1.6
Women	66	30.6	85	29.0	−1.6
Foreign born	104	48.6	139	47.6	−1.0
American born	110	51.4	153	52.4	+1.0
Laborers/sailors	65	47.4	89	47.6	+.2
Other employed men	72	52.6	98	52.4	−.2
0–10 years old	5	2.5	13	4.5	+2.0
11–46 years old	168	82.4	234	80.7	−1.7
47+ years old	31	15.2	43	14.8	−.4

SOURCE: MGH Records, October 16, 1845–October 15, 1847.

Notes: There are *no* significant differences in patient population composition before and after anesthesia, at the .05 level. Cases for which some data were not recorded were omitted from the tabulation of that particular variable. Occupation was calculated as a percentage of the total number of men whose jobs were recorded.

NOTES

To conserve space, only authors, titles, pages, and dates of cited works are listed in the notes. Full publication information for all sources used is provided in the complete bibliography.

1. THE CASE OF MCGONIGLE'S FOOT

1. Surgical Records of the Massachusetts General Hospital (hereafter cited as MGH Records), vol. 30, case admitted September 25, 1846. This volume of the records was located in the vault of the hospital. All volumes of the records are now in the Countway Library of Medicine, Boston. As per my agreement with the library and the hospital, full names of patients are not mentioned in this book, even though the institution's nineteenth-century surgeons did not believe that charitable hospital cases were entitled to such confidentiality; see John Collins Warren, *Etherization; With Surgical Remarks* (1848), p. iv. Since the volumes of records are mostly unpaginated, specific references are to the admitting date.

2. *New York Herald,* July 9, 1847, p. 1. *Westminster Review* (1871), 96:92. The history of the ether discovery has been told and retold. Some typical accounts are: René Fülöp-Miller, *Triumph Over Pain* (1938); Bernard Seeman, *Man Against Pain: 3,000 Years of Effort to Understand and Relieve Physical Suffering* (1962); Betty MacQuitty, *The Battle for Oblivion: The Discovery of Anaesthesia* (1969); Victor Robinson, *Victory Over Pain* (1946); Virginia Sarah Thatcher, *History of Anesthesia, With Emphasis on the Nurse Specialist* (1953); Thomas E. Keys, *The History of Surgical Anesthesia* (1963, 1945); Howard Riley Raper, *Man Against Pain: The Epic of Anesthesia* (1945); George Bankoff, *Conquest of Pain: The Story of Anaesthesia* ([1946]); Barbara M. Duncum, *The Development of Inhalation Anaesthesia* (1947); Grace

S. Woodward, *The Man Who Conquered Surgical Pain: A Biography of William Thomas Green Morton* (1962); *Journal of the History of Medicine and Allied Sciences* (October, 1946), vol. 1.

However the two most useful histories remain Richard M. Hodges, *A Narrative of Events Connected with the Introduction of Sulphuric Ether into Surgical Use* (1891), and, for Morton's viewpoint, Nathan P. Rice, *Trials of a Public Benefactor* (1859). For Britain, see A. J. Youngson, *The Scientific Revolution in Victorian Medicine* (1979).

3. See, for example, John B. Blake, *Benjamin Waterhouse and the Introduction of Vaccination* (1957); Martin Kaufman, "The American Anti-Vaccinationists and Their Arguments," *Bulletin of the History of Medicine,* (September 1967), 41:463–478; William G. Rothstein, *American Physicians in the Nineteenth Century: From Sects to Science* (1972), pp. 253–79.

4. Fracture Book, 1853, case admitted April 11, 1853, Records of the Pennsylvania Hospital, Historical Library of the Pennsylvania Hospital, Philadelphia (hereafter cited as Pa. H. Fracture Books). As per my agreement with the hospital, patient names are not given in full, and identification of citations is by admission date.

The earliest use of anesthetics for surgery mentioned in the available records dates from July 28, 1853. The surgeon was Dr. John Neill. See also James E. Eckenhoff, *Anesthesia from Colonial Times: A History of Anesthesia at the University of Pennsylvania* (1966); and the comments by J. T. Metcalfe in the *Transactions of the New York Academy of Medicine* (1847–1857), 1:140–41.

5. Pa H. Fracture Books, case admitted July 15, 1862.

6. Pa. H. Fracture Books, October 16, 1853–October 15, 1862. These dates were selected to cover the same months per year as the Massachusetts General data. Major limbs were defined as arms, legs, hands, and feet. Two cases of amputation of digits that were included in the amputation records were also counted; both involved complications and both patients received anesthetics.

A total of sixty-nine cases were counted. Fifteen in which the space for recording anesthetic use was left blank were omitted from the data (ordinarily, "no anaesthetic" was written in when none was used). There is apparently a gap in the data for parts of 1860–61; otherwise they appear complete when checked against printed accounts.

7. MGH Records, vols. 30–33, November 7, 1846–October 15, 1847. The dates were from the resumption of ether administration to the first anniversary of its use. The index of operations at the back of each volume was not used, for it was found to omit many smaller procedures (such as finger and toe amputations). These case records were also checked against printed reports that listed only the anesthetized operations: *Transactions of the American Medical Association* (1848), 1:215–17 (hereafter cited as *Trans AMA*); *American Journal of the Medical Sciences* (1851), 21:179–83 (hereafter cited as *AJMS*). One hundred thirty cases were counted; seven cases for which the manuscript and printed records conflicted were omitted from the data. Unlike the Pa. H. Fracture Book, these records did not ordinarily write in "no anesthetic" when none was used; hence the necessity of cross-checking with the printed cases in which all cases of anesthetization supposedly were recorded. Furthermore, many of the case records contained comments such as "pat. was very little disturbed by the operation," and "pain was moderate," confirming the impression that no anesthetic had been given; see MGH Records, vol. 31, cases admitted January 27, and February 10, 1847.

The failure to record anesthetic usage systematically continued through at least 1860; unfortunately for these years published data were not available for cross-checking the missing cases. For example, in the year October 16, 1854–October 15, 1855, almost half (47.9 percent) of the 376 operations recorded lacked data on anesthesia. However, of the fully reported cases, 11.1 percent were recorded as nonanesthetic.

8. *AJMS* (1852), 23:452. One-third of the case records indicated nothing concerning anesthesia.

Examination of the actual case records revealed an even higher rate of missing data, because the published cases omit "minor" procedures. For the years 1847–48, 1854–55, and 1859–60, more than three-fourths of the 1,312 operation records omit any reference to anesthesia. However, of the fully recorded operations, 34/243 or 14.0 percent stated that no anesthetic had been used. (Data based on June 1–May 31; 1854–55 includes information for First Surgical Division only.) For an example, see patient number 545, discharged June 18, 1854, following nonanesthetized amputation of the arm, Surgical Casebooks, vol. 18, First Surgical Division, Surgical Records of the New York Hospital (hereafter cited as NYH Records), New York Hospital Archives, New York.

A large-scale multivariate analysis of case records from both MGH and NYH, 1840–60, in which I am currently engaged, may reveal ways in which the fully reported operations differed from the others and thus perhaps may indicate approximately how many of the unrecorded cases might have received anesthesia. However, since those patients and procedures considered too medically or socially insignificant to require anesthetics (see chapter 8 below) were also the cases likely to have been considered too insignificant for careful recording of data, the puzzle may never be fully resolvable.

9. Morris J. Vogel, *The Invention of the Modern Hospital: Boston 1870–1930* (1980); Vogel, "Patrons, Practitioners, and Patients: The Voluntary Hospital in Mid-Victorian Boston," in *Victorian America*, ed. by Daniel Walker Howe (1976), pp. 120–38.

10. *Buffalo Medical Journal* (August 1847), 3:152–53; Case Books of Frank H. Hamilton, 3:18; 6:126–44, in Frank H. Hamilton Papers, National Library of Medicine, Bethesda, Md. (hereafter cited as Hamilton Case Books). A total of 46 amputations were counted. Military cases were excluded from this count because of the possibility that the military imposed restraints on Hamilton's practice not encountered in civilian surgery. I would have tabulated the military cases separately, but there were too few of them to reach any meaningful conclusions. For a brief biography, see Howard A. Kelly and Walter L. Burrage, *American Medical Biographies* (1920), pp. 483–84.

11. John Lynck, "Alcohol as an Anaesthetic," *Cincinnati Lancet and Observer* (May 1876), 37:409–16. For a random assortment of such accounts, see the following: S. R. Adamson [Sarah Adamson Dolley] to Elijah F. Pennypacker, February 3, 1850, typescript of letter in Archives of the Medical College of Pennsylvania, Philadelphia; Elizabeth Blackwell, *Pioneer Work in Opening the Medical Profession to Women* (1895; reprinted 1977), p. 102; *Trans AMA* (1848), 1:176–77; Rothstein, *American Physicians*, p. 253. A large number of individual nonanesthetic cases are mentioned in the medical journals. See, for example, *AJMS* (1851), 21:76; *Philadelphia Medical Examiner* (hereafter cited as *Phil Med Ex*) (July 1847), n.s. 3:395–98; and other cases mentioned throughout the rest of this book.

Many such reports came from the American Civil War, and many were clearly *not* simply the result of wartime shortages, see Bell Irvin Wiley, *The Life of Johnny Reb, The Common Soldier of the Confederacy* (1943), pp. 265–66; Walt Whitman, *Memoranda During the War* (1962, reprint of 1875 edition), pp. 9–10; Louisa May Alcott, *Hospital Sketches*, ed. by Bessie Z. Jones (1960, reprint of 1863 edition), pp. 37–38, 87–88; Mark DeWolfe Howe, *Justice Oliver Wendell Holmes: The Shaping Years, 1841–1870*, (1957), 1:104. Joseph Stafford Redding and John Carter Matthews, "Anesthesia During the American Civil War," *Clinical Anesthesia*, No. 2 (1968), p. 9, cites 254 cases of nonanesthetic amputation during the Civil War.

For similar British examples, see Charles Kidd, *A Manual of Anaesthetics*, (1859), p. 244, and W. Stanley Sykes, *Essays on the First Hundred Years of Anaesthesia* (1960) 1:166; 2:73.

12. Reuben Maurits, "Individualized Anesthesia," *Journal of the Michigan State Medical Society* (August 1935), 34:463–68.

13. Martin S. Pernick, "Medical Professionalism," *Encyclopedia of Bioethics*, ed. by Warren T. Reich (1978) 3:1028–34. Thomas L. Haskell, *The Emergence of Professional Social Science: The American Social Science Association and the Nineteenth-Century Crisis of Authority* (1977).

2. A HOUSE DIVIDED

1. Charles E. Rosenberg, *The Cholera Years: The United States in 1832, 1849, and 1866* (1962); Richard H. Shryock, *Medicine and Society in America, 1660–1860* (1960); Judith Walzer Leavitt and Ronald L. Numbers, "Sickness and Health in America: An Overview," in *Sickness and Health in America* (1978) pp. 3–10; Martin S. Pernick, "Politics, Parties, and Pestilence: Epidemic Yellow Fever in Philadelphia and the Rise of the First Party System," *William and Mary Quarterly* (October, 1972), 3d ser. 29:559–86.

2. René Dubos and Jean Dubos, *The White Plague: Tuberculosis, Man, and Society* (1952); Leavitt and Numbers, "Sickness and Health." Estimates are derived primarily from Massachusetts data.

3. Such causes of disease included Galen's classic formulation of the "non-naturals," see Owsei Temkin, *Galenism: The Rise and Decline of a Medical Philosophy* (1973).

4. Pernick, "Politics, Parties, and Pestilence"; Richard H. Shryock, *The Development of Modern Medicine: An Interpretation of the Social and Scientific Factors Involved* (1947), ch. 12.

5. Erwin H. Ackerknecht, "Anticontagionism Between 1821 and 1867," *Bulletin of the History of Medicine* (September–October 1948), 22:562–93; George Rosen, "Political Order and Human Health in Jeffersonian Thought," *Bulletin of the History of Medicine* (January–February 1952), 26:32–44; Pernick, "Politics, Parties, and Pestilence."

6. For a few widely known examples of this literature, see: [Lemuel Shattuck], *Report of the Sanitary Commission of Massachusetts, 1850* (1850, reprinted 1948); John H. Griscom, *The Uses and Abuses of Air . . .* (1850, reprinted 1970); Catherine Beecher, *Letters to the People on Sickness and Happiness* (1855); and such journals as William A. Alcott's *The Teacher of Health and the Laws of the Human Constitution*, 1 (1843); William Cornell's fascinating *The Practical Educator and Journal of Health*, 2 (1847).

For Britain, see John M. Eyler, *Victorian Social Medicine: The Ideas and Methods of William Farr* (1979). In general, see notes 5, 7, and 8, this chapter.

7. Barbara Gutmann Rosenkrantz, *Public Health and the State: Changing Views in Massachusetts, 1842–1936* (1972); James C. Mohr, *The Radical Republicans and Reform in New York during Reconstruction* (1973), pp. 61–114; Rosenberg, *Cholera Years;* John Duffy, *A History of Public Health in New York City, 1625–1866* (1968); Howard D. Kramer, "Early Municipal and State Boards of Health," *Bulletin of the History of Medicine* (November–December 1950), 24:503–29. For the effect on other reforms, see Gerald N. Grob, *Edward Jarvis and the Medical World of Nineteenth-Century America* (1978); and notes 28, 29, this chapter.

8. Barbara Gutmann Rosenkrantz, "Causal Thinking in Erewhon and Elsewhere," *Journal of Medicine and Philosophy* (December 1976), 1:372–84; Rosenberg, *Cholera Years*. See also Charles E. Rosenberg and Carroll Smith Rosenberg, "Pietism and the Origins of the American Public Health Movement: A Note on John H. Griscom and Robert M. Hartley," *Journal of the History of Medicine and Allied Sciences* (January 1968), 23:16–35. For a modern discussion of the same issues, see Rob Crawford, "Sickness as Sin," *Health/PAC Bulletin* (January–February 1978), pp. 10–16.

The degree of social and individual responsibility for disease is a product of social ideology, but it also varies depending on the epidemiology of the particular diseases most prevalent at any particular time; see Pernick, "Politics, Parties, and Pestilence," p. 571. For a closely related discussion of causality and blame, see Thomas L. Haskell, *The Emergence of Professional Social Science: The American Social Science Association and the Nineteenth-Century Crisis of Authority* (1977); and C. S. Griffin, *The Ferment of Reform, 1830–1860* (1967), pp. 54–55.

9. Temkin, *Galenism*.

10. John Harley Warner, "Physiological Theory and Therapeutic Explanation in the 1860s: The British Debate on the Medical Use of Alcohol," *Bulletin of the History of Medicine* (Summer, 1980), 54:235–57.

11. Charles E. Rosenberg, "The Therapeutic Revolution: Medicine, Meaning, and Social Change in Nineteenth-Century America," *Perspectives in Biology and Medicine* (Summer, 1977), 20:485–506.

12. Dale C. Smith, "Quinine and Fever: The Development of the Effective Dosage," *Journal of the History of Medicine and Allied Sciences* (July 1976), 31:343–67; J. Worth Estes, *Hall Jackson and the Purple Foxglove: Medical Practice and Research in Revolutionary America, 1760–1820* (1980), esp. ch. 5.

13. Rosenberg, "Therapeutic Revolution."

14. Peter H. Niebyl, "The English Bloodletting Revolution, or Modern Medicine Before 1850," *Bulletin of the History of Medicine* (Fall, 1977), 51:464–83.

15. Shryock, *Development of Modern Medicine*, p. 31.

16. Benjamin Rush, "The Progress of Medicine: A Lecture," (1801) in Dagobert D. Runes, ed., *The Selected Writings of Benjamin Rush* (1947), pp. 236–38; Alex Berman, "The Heroic Approach in Nineteenth Century Therapeutics," *Bulletin of the American Society of Hospital Pharmacists* (September–October 1954), 11:321–27; Harris L. Coulter, *Science and Ethics in American Medicine* (1973), p. 38; Rosenberg, "Therapeutic Revolution"; Shryock, *Development of Modern Medicine*, p. 31.

17. On Louis and his methods, see Erwin H. Ackerknecht, *Medicine at the Paris Hospital, 1794–1848* (1967); William Osler, "The Influence of Louis on American Medicine," in *An Alabama Student and Other Essays* (1908), pp. 189–210; Ackerknecht, "Elisha Bartlett and the Philosophy of the Paris Clinical School," *Bulletin of the History of Medicine* (January–February 1950), 24:43–60. For early-nineteenth-century opposition to Rush, see ch. 6, notes 53–55 below.

18. This nineteenth-century terminology was meant to draw an explicit parallel between the growth of divisiveness within religion and within medicine. In both cases, the "orthodox" called their opponents "sects," as a way of blaming the disintegration of consensus solely on them. For the similar disputes over the blame for the rise of political opposition, see Richard Hofstadter, *The Idea of a Party System: The Rise of Legitimate Opposition in the United States, 1780–1840* (1969).

Rothstein, *American Physicians*, pp. 21–24 adopts a version of the homeopathic terminology by calling all systems "sects." He coins the self-contradictory term "regular sect" to refer to users of "orthodox" therapies. Homeopaths called orthodox medicine "allopathy."

19. On medical sects in general, see Rothstein, *American Physicians*, pp. 125–73, 217–43. On homeopathy, see Coulter, *Science and Ethics;* and Martin Kaufman, *Homeopathy in America: The Rise and Fall of A Medical Heresy* (1971).

In addition, I have examined the following: American Institute of Homeopathy, *Proceedings* (1847); *North American Journal of Homeopathy* 1 (1851); *Hahnemannian Monthly* 4 (1869); Homoeopathic Medical Society of New York, *Transactions* (1864–67); William Harvey King, *History of Homeopathy and Its Institutions in America* (1905). Especially useful were the manuscript M.D. theses in the Hahnemann University Archives, Philadelphia, for the years 1857–1885.

20. Ronald L. Numbers, *Prophetess of Health: A Study of Ellen G. White* (1976); Marshall Scott Legan, "Hydropathy in America: A Nineteenth Century Panacea," *Bulletin of the History of Medicine* (May–June 1971), 45:267–80; Richard H. Shryock, "Sylvester Graham and the Popular Health Movement," in *Medicine in America: Historical Essays* (1966); Stephen Nissenbaum, *Sex, Diet, and Debility in Jacksonian America: Sylvester Graham and Health Reform* (1980); James C. Whorton, "Tempest in a Flesh-Pot: The Formulation of a Physiological Rationale for Vegetarianism," *Journal of the History of Medicine and Allied Sciences* (April 1977), 32:115–39; Richard W. Schwarz, *John Harvey Kellogg, M.D.* (1970); Edwin Scott Gaustad, ed., *The Rise of Adventism: Religion and Society in Mid-Nineteenth-Century America* (1974).

21. Alex Berman, "The Impact of the Nineteenth-Century Botanico-Medical Movement on American Pharmacy and Medicine" (unpublished Ph. D. dissertation, University of Wisconsin, Madison, 1954). See also Berman's published articles, including: "The Thomsonian Movement and its Relation to American Pharmacy and Medicine," *Bulletin of the History of Medicine* (September–October 1951) and (November–December 1951), 25:405–28, and 519–38; "Social Roots of the Nineteenth-Century Botanico-Medical Movement in the United States," *Actes du VIIIe Congres International d'Histoire des Sciences* (Florence, Italy, 1956), 2:561–65; "A Striving for Scientific Respectability: Some American Botanics and the Nineteenth-Century Plant Materia Medica," *Bulletin of the History of Medicine* (January–February 1956), 30:7–31; and "Neo-Thomsonianism in the United States," *Journal of the History of Medicine and Allied Sciences* (April 1956), 11:133–55. Also see Ronald L. Numbers, "The Making of an Eclectic Physician," *Bulletin of the History of Medicine* (March–April 1973), 47:155–66.

In addition, I have examined the following: *Eclectic Medical Journal* n.s. 1–2 (1849–1850); Massachusetts Eclectic Medical Society, *Publications* (1860–72); John King, *American Eclectic Obstetrics* (1855); Benjamin L. Hill, *Lectures on the American Eclectic System of Surgery* (1850); and W. Beach, *The American Practice Condensed* (1847).

22. Rosenberg, "Therapeutic Revolution;" John Harley Warner, " 'The Nature-Trusting Heresy': American Physicians and the Concept of the Healing Power of Nature," *Perspectives in American History* (1977–78), 11:303–08, 310–13; Guenter B. Risse, "Epidemics and Medicine: The Influence of Disease on Medical Thought and Practice," *Bulletin of the History of Medicine* (Winter, 1979), 53:515. See also Leon S. Bryan, Jr., "Blood-Letting in American Medicine, 1830–1892," *Bulletin of the History of Medicine* (November–December 1964), 38:516–29; Erwin H. Ackerknecht, "Aspects of the History of Therapeutics," *Bulletin of the History of Medicine* (September–October 1962), 36:389–419.

In addition, some physicians switched from heroic use of depleting drugs to heroic use of tonics, see chapter 5, notes 10–16, 73.

23. Charles E. Rosenberg, "Florence Nightingale on Contagion: The Hospital as Moral Universe," in *Healing and History* (1979), pp. 116–136; Dubos, *White Plague*. For a typical example of the transition from environmental causes to environmental cures, see Jacob Bigelow, *Brief Expositions of Rational Medicine* (1858), pp. 63, 67.

24. Worthington Hooker, *Physician and Patient; or, a Practical View of the Mutual Duties, Relations, and Interests of the Medical Profession and the Community* (1849), ch. 14.

25. Charles Rosenberg, "And Heal the Sick: The Hospital and the Patient in the 19th Century America [sic]," *Journal of Social History* (June 1977), 20:428–47; David J. Rothman, *The Discovery of the Asylum: Social Order and Disorder in the New Republic* (1971), pp. 3–56; Brian Abel-Smith, *The Hospitals, 1800–1948: A Study in Social Administration in*

England and Wales (1964); John Woodward, *To Do the Sick No Harm: A Study of the British Voluntary Hospital System to 1875* (1974); William H. Williams, *America's First Hospital: The Pennsylvania Hospital 1751–1841* (1976); Leonard K. Eaton, *New England Hospitals, 1790–1833* (1957); John E. Ransom, "The Beginnings of Hospitals in the United States," *Bulletin of the History of Medicine* (May 1943), 13:514–39; Henry E. Sigerest, "An Outline of the Development of the Hospital," *Bulletin of the History of Medicine* (July 1936), 4:573–81.

26. In addition to the sources in note 25 this chapter, see Rosenberg, "Florence Nightingale"; Rosenberg, "The Hospital in America: A Century's Perspective," in *Medicine and Society: Contemporary Medical Problems in Historical Perspective* (1971), pp. 181–94; George Rosen, "The Hospital: Historical Sociology of a Community Institution," in Elliot Freidson, ed. *The Hospital in Modern Society*, (1963), pp. 1–36; David B. Lovejoy, Jr., "The Hospital and Society: Growth of Hospitals in Rochester, New York, in the Nineteenth Century," *Bulletin of the History of Medicine* (Winter, 1975), 49:536–55; John D. Thompson and Grace Goldin, *The Hospital: A Social and Architectural History* (1975).

For an early (1832) example of "residence therapy" for the poor, see Lovejoy, "The Hospital and Society," p. 539.

27. Rosenberg, "And Heal the Sick;" Morris J. Vogel, *The Invention of the Modern Hospital: Boston, 1870–1930* (1980); David Rosner, *A Once Charitable Enterprise: Hospitals and Health Care in Brooklyn and New York, 1885–1915* (1982).

28. On asylums, see Rothman, *Discovery of the Asylum*, pp. 109–54, 206–95; Norman Dain, *Disordered Minds: The First Century of Eastern State Hospital in Williamsburg, Virginia, 1766–1866* (1971); Gerald Grob, *The State and the Mentally Ill: A History of Worcester State Hospital in Massachusetts, 1830–1920* (1966); Grob, *Mental Institutions in America: Social Policy to 1875* (1973); William L. Parry Jones, *The Trade in Lunacy: A Study of Private Madhouses in England in the Eighteenth and Nineteenth Centuries* (1972); Andrew Scull, ed., *Madhouses, Mad-Doctors, and Madmen: The Social History of Psychiatry in the Victorian Era* (1981), part 2.

For analyses of Rothman's approach, of varying insight and criticism, see: Christopher Lasch, "The Origins of the Asylum," in *The World of Nations: Reflections on American History, Politics, and Culture* (1974), pp. 3–17; and Gerald N. Grob, "Rediscovering Asylums: The Unhistorical History of the Mental Hospital," *Hastings Center Report* (August 1977), 7:33–41.

For a sample of the impact of asylums on public schools, see the letters to Horace Mann by Edwin Chadwick (June 8, 1844), Samuel B. Woodward (June 6, 1845), and Andrew Combe (April 30, 1846), and many similar items in the Horace Mann Papers, Massachusetts Historical Society, Boston.

For the influence on Utopian communities, see: Philip R. Wyatt, "John Humphrey Noyes and the Stirpicultural Experiment," *Journal of the History of Medicine and Allied Sciences* (January 1976), 31:55–66; Robert D. Thomas, *The Man Who Would Be Perfect: John Humphrey Noyes and the Utopian Impulse* (1977).

29. The intimate connection between medicine and social reform in the mid-nineteenth century has never been fully examined. As just one small example, William Cornell's *Journal of Health* served as the first official organ of the Massachusetts *Teachers'* Association. A recent study that does stress the interconnections of medical thought and many varieties of social reform is Ronald G. Walters, *American Reformers 1815–1860* (1978). Yet even this book totally overlooks the role of orthodox physicians in public health reform. See Rosenberg and Rosenberg, "Pietism and Public Health." For other pieces of the story, see Ronald G. Walters, *The Antislavery Appeal: American Abolitionism After 1830* (1977); Rothman, *Discovery of the Asylum;* and Bernard Wishy, *The Child and the Republic: The Dawn of Modern American Child Nurture* (1968).

30. Mohr, *Radical Republicans*, pp. 86–114.

31. American Medical Association, *Transactions* (1848), 1:30; hereafter cited as *Trans AMA;* also quoted in Barbara Gutmann Rosenkrantz, "The Search for Professional Order in 19th Century American Medicine," *Proceedings of the XIVth International Congress of the History of Science* (1975), no. 4, pp. 113–24.

32. For a complaint against the narrowing of the grounds on which physicians participated in social policy, see Stephen Smith, "The Physician as Citizen," in *Doctor in Medicine; and Other Papers on Professional Subjects* (1872), pp. 149–53. See also *Trans. AMA* (1848), 1:328.

Of course, *immoderate* zeal in reform could also cause disease. See, for example, Amariah Brigham, *Observations on the Influence of Religion Upon the Health and Physical Welfare of Mankind* (1835). For Oliver Wendell Holmes' skepticism about reform, see Eleanor M. Tilton, *Amiable Autocrat: A Biography of Dr. Oliver Wendell Holmes* (1947), p. 167; for the less amiable comments of Alfred Stillé, see *AJMS* (1852), 23:163–64; and Stillé's acerbic letters to George C. Shattuck, e.g., letters of July 8, 1848, and September 28, 1851 in George C. Shattuck Papers, vols. 21 and 22, Massachusetts Historical Society, Boston. See also Barbara Sicherman, "The Paradox of Prudence: Mental Health in the Gilded Age," *Journal of American History* (March 1976), 62:890–912.

33. Grob, "Rediscovering Asylums."

34. Ackerknecht, *Paris Hospital*, p. 154. See Martin S. Pernick, "The Patient's Role in Medical Decisionmaking: A Social History of Informed Consent in Medical Therapy," in *Making Health Care Decisions: A Report on the Ethical and Legal Implications of Informed Consent in the Patient-Practitioner Relationship*, vol. 3, *Studies on the Foundations of Informed Consent*, President's Commission for the Study of Ethical Problems in Medicine (1982), pp. 1–35.

35. NYH Surgical Records, 2 S.D., case number 901, discharged February 28, 1846, entry of January 12, 1846. MGH Surgical Records, vol. 67, East Ward, p. 128, admitted September 11, 1855.

The specific moral prescriptions often harkened back to the agrarian virtues of the Founding Fathers: country air, self-sufficiency, Protestant morality, and hard work. But, in addition, physicians advised the adoption of new routines more in harmony with the needs of urban commercial life. For an example of the combination of morality, agrarian virtue, commercial virtue, and public order in health reform literature, see Shattuck, *Report,* pp. 241–78.

36. Lasch, "Origins of the Asylum."

37. Sorting out conflicting claims about the cure rates of nineteenth-century asylums is one goal of the massive computer analysis of mental hospital patient records now being conducted by Barbara Rosenkrantz and Maris Vinovskis.

38. Grob, "Rediscovering Asylums"; Scull, *Madhouses;* Michel Foucault, *Madness and Civilization: A History of Insanity in the Age of Reason* (1965).

39. Aldous Huxley, *Brave New World* (1932).

40. My conceptualization of the Art-Nature dichotomy was greatly enhanced by Perry Miller, *The Life of the Mind in America* (1965), and Miller, "The Romantic Dilemma in American Nationalism and the Concept of Nature," *Harvard Theological Review* (October 1955), 48:239–53, reprinted in *Nature's Nation* (1967), pp. 197–207. See also Leo Marx, *The Machine in the Garden: Technology and the Pastoral Ideal in America* (1964).

41. *Oxford English Dictionary*, hereafter cited as *OED*. "Art" meant anything manmade, including both the humanistic arts and technology but excluding the "natural" sciences.

42. Jacob Bigelow, *Nature in Disease, and Other Writings.* (1854). However, he accepted medical art as assisting this natural healing force.

43. For an historical overview, see Warner, "Nature-Trusting Heresy."

44. Coulter, *Science and Ethics*, pp. 56, 38. See also Pernick, "Politics, Parties, and Pestilence," esp. p. 575; Rush, "The Progress of Medicine," in *Selected Writings*, pp. 236–38; Berman, "Heroic Approach."

45. Hooker attributed this latter formulation to A.-F. Cholmel, Pierre Louis' preceptor; Hooker, *Physician and Patient*, p. 219. For typical attacks on "nihilism," see Oliver Wendell Holmes, *Medical Essays, 1842–1882* (1891).

On the classical roots, see Albert Jonsen, "Do No Harm: Axiom of Medical Ethics," *Philosophical Medical Ethics*, edited by Stuart F. Spicker and H. Tristram Engelhardt, Jr. Philosophy and Medicine, vol. 3 (1977), pp. 27–42; René Dubos, *Mirage of Health* (1959); and Harris L. Coulter, *The Patterns Emerge: Hippocrates to Paracelsus* (1975).

46. For a typical homeopathic example, see Charles Henry Giles, "The Origin Nature and Use of Pain," unpublished M.D. thesis, Hahnemann Medical College, 1883, Hahnemann Medical College, Hahnemann University Archives, Philadelphia, p. 11. For hydropathic examples, see ch. 3 below.

47. Hooker, *Physician and Patient*, p. 219; also Holmes, "The Medical Profession in Massachusetts," in *Medical Essays*.

48. For the history and philosophy of the distinction between acts of omission and commission in medicine, a good place to begin is K. Danner Clouser and Arthur Zucker, *Abortion & Euthanasia: An Annotated Bibliography* (1974). For further discussion of the ethical issues, see Clouser, "Allowing or Causing: Another Look," *Annals of Internal Medicine* (1977), 87:622–24.

For a nineteenth-century example of the distinction, see Bigelow, *Nature in Disease*, p. 35.

49. For examples of heroic hydrotherapy, see Edmund Wilson, *Patriotic Gore: Studies in the Literature of the American Civil War* (1977), p. 673; Thomas L. Nichols, *Forty Years of American Life*, (1864), 1:364.

50. Austin Flint, "Conservative Medicine," *American Medical Monthly* (1862), 18:1–24, reprinted in Gert H. Brieger, ed. *Medical America in the Nineteenth Century: Readings from the Literature* (1972), pp. 134–42; Bigelow, *Nature in Disease;* Bigelow, *Rational Medicine;* Hooker, *Physician and Patient*. The best general account is Rosenberg, "Therapeutic Revolution," but see also Warner, "Nature-Trusting Heresy."

51. Thomas Percival, *Percival's Medical Ethics*, edited by Chauncey D. Leake (1927).

52. For typical examples of the incorporation of such views into everyday medical writing, see *AJMS* (1850), 19:96, 473.

53. On this particular point, see the comments of Samuel Phillips, Jr., founder of an elite New England academy of the 1770s, as quoted by James McLachlan, *American Boarding Schools: A Historical Study* (1970), p. 41:

. . . the happiness of such a child (a rich one) is of as great consequence as that of a poor child, his opportunity of doing good greater. His disinterestedness is a great argument in favor of his honest intentions in following the profession of a minister, that he does it from principles, and not from *a lucrative view;* but [charity] scholars must purse this; they speak because they are hired to; it is their living.

See also Fridolf Kudlien, "Medicine as a 'Liberal Art' and the Question of the Physician's Income," *Journal of the History of Medicine and Allied Sciences* (October 1976), 31:448–59, which deals mostly with classical antiquity.

54. The preceding paragraphs are based on William Joseph Reader, *Professional Men: The Rise of the Professional Classes in Nineteenth-Century England* (1966); Samuel Haber, "The Professions and Higher Education in America: A Historical View," in Margaret S.

Gordon, ed. *Higher Education and the Labor Market*, (1974), pp. 237–80; and Jeffrey L. Berlant, *Profession and Monopoly: A Study of Medicine in the United States and Great Britain* (1975).

See also Merle Borrowman, *The Liberal and the Technical in Teacher Education* (1956); Charles D. Aring, "Gentility and Professionalism," *Journal of the American Medical Association* (February 4, 1974), 227:512.

The tension between liberal gentility and technical skill is similar to but not identical with Talcott Person's well-known "achieved-ascribed" dichotomy. Gentlemen were born, not made, and were thus an ascribed category; however, the lack of achieved skill could *un-make* a professional gentleman.

55. On the level of animosity, see Shryock, *Development of Modern Medicine*, pp. 31–32. Some provocative explanations are suggested in David Hackett Fischer, *The Revolution of American Conservatism: The Federalist Party in the Era of Jeffersonian Democracy* (1965), pp. 206, 208, 354, 360.

56. Haber, "Professions and Higher Education"; David C. Humphrey, "The King's College Medical School and the Professionalization of Medicine in Pre-Revolutionary New York," *Bulletin of the History of Medicine* (Summer 1975), 49:206–34. Less useful, but with some general information on the colonial period, is Martin Kaufman, *American Medical Education: The Formative Years, 1765–1910* (1976), pp. 3–35; Nathan Smith Davis, *History of Medical Education and Institutions in the United States from the First Settlement of the British Colonies to the Year 1850* (1851).

57. "Duties of a Physician: A Closing Lecture to Medical Students," in *Selected Writings*, pp. 308–309, 321. For Rush's acerbic critique of the gentleman as a professional model, see his "Commonplace Book" for July 21, 1792, in George W. Corner, ed., *The Autobiography of Benjamin Rush* (1948), pp. 224–25.

58. Rush, "The Progress of Medicine," in *Selected Writings*, pp. 236–38.

59. Richard Harrison Shryock, *Medical Licensing in America, 1650–1965* (1967), pp. 3–30; Haber, "Professions and Higher Education"; Berlant, *Profession and Monopoly;* Humphrey, "King's College Medical School." At one time New York banned only those unlicensed practitioners who prescribed drugs "as a profession"—thus seemingly making *professional pretensions* rather than the *practice* of healing itself the subject of restriction.

60. The best study of nineteenth-century licensing is Matthew Ramsey, "The Politics of Professional Monopoly in Nineteenth-Century Medicine: The French Model and Its Rivals," in Gerald L. Geison, ed., *Professions and the French State* (1984), pp. 225–305.

For the ideological aspects of anti-licensing, see Walter Hugins, *Jacksonian Democracy and the Working Class: A Study of the New York Workingmen's Movement, 1829–1837* (1960), pp. 112–28, 148–71. I have also examined the course of the anti-licensing movement in New York State; the following are particularly useful in understanding the ideological basis of the movement: New York State Assembly, *Documents*, 53d sess., 1830, vol. 3, no. 217; 55th sess., 1832, vol. 3, nos. 185, 244, 246, 249, 250, 251, 261, 272; 63d sess., 1840, vol. 8, no. 346; 67th sess., 1844, vol. 3, no. 60; 82nd sess., 1859, vol. 3, no. 157; New York State, Assembly, *Journal*, 55th sess., 1832, pp. 108, 173, 319, 509, 564, 570; 67th sess., 1844, pp. 1042, 1162; New York State, Senate, *Documents*, 67th sess., 1844, vol. 1, no. 31; vol. 2, no. 55; 73d sess., 1850, vol. 3, no. 80; New York State, Senate, *Journal*, 67th sess., 1844, pp. 219, 634–35. See also the account in the *New York Post* of March 8, 1844.

For the general background of medical deregulation see: Shryock, *Medical Licensing in America*, pp. 30–43; Rothstein, *American Physicians*, pp. 63–84, 104–108, 145–46; Joseph F. Kett, *The Formation of the American Medical Profession: The Role of Institutions, 1780–1860* (1968), esp. pp. 115, 168, 181–83. See also Reginald H. Fitz, "The Rise and Fall of the Licensed Physician in Massachusetts, 1781–1860," *Transactions of the Association of American Physicians* (1894), 9:1–18.

61. Rothstein, *American Physicians*, pp. 131–33, 142.

62. For the practitioners' takeover of Thomsonianism, see Berman, "Neo-Thomsonianism." For the survival of self-help among lay sectarians, see Ronald L. Numbers, "Do-It-Yourself the Sectarian Way," in Leavitt and Numbers, *Sickness and Health*, pp. 87–95. Rothstein, *American Physicians*, p. 231.

63. Rothstein, *American Physicians*, chs. 7–12, and pp. 221, 287; Berman, "Social Roots of the Botanico-Medical Movement"; Kaufman, *Homeopathy in America*, p. 29; Rosenberg, "The Therapeutic Revolution"; Bryan, "Blood-Letting in American Medicine."

64. Kett, *Formation of the American Medical Profession;* James G. Burrow, *AMA: Voice of American Medicine* (1963), pp. 1–26; *Trans. AMA*, (1848) vol. 1; Philip Van Ingen, *The New York Academy of Medicine: Its First Hundred Years* (1949). See also Nathan Smith Davis, *History of the American Medical Association from Its Organization up to January, 1855* (1855); Morris Fishbein, *A History of the American Medical Association, 1847–1947* (1947); and Byron Stookey, "Origins of the First National Medical Convention: 1826–1846," *Journal of the American Medical Association* (July 15, 1961), 177:123–30.

65. Daniel H. Calhoun, *Professional Lives in America: Structure and Aspiration, 1750–1850* (1965), ch. 2.

66. Hooker's *Physician and Patient*, the major statement of conservative professional ethics, reprinted the AMA code in its entirety.

67. Rothstein, *American Physicians*, p. 93; Kaufman, *American Medical Education*.

68. Hooker, *Physician and Patient*, chs. 8, 10, 11. Also see *Trans. AMA* (1848), 1:8, 239–40; Stephen Smith, "Doctor in Medicine," in *Doctor in Medicine*, pp. 1–5; and Kett, *Formation of the American Medical Profession*, pp. 161–74.

69. Davis, *History of Medical Education;* Davis, *History of the American Medical Association; Trans. AMA* (1848), 1:244. For the economic basis of the school-preceptorship conflict, see Rothstein, *American Physicians*, ch. 6. For similar conflicts in other professions, see Borrowman, *Liberal and Technical in Teacher Education;* and especially Monte A. Calvert, *The Mechanical Engineer in America, 1830–1910: Professional Cultures in Conflict* (1967) on the ideological basis of the "school versus shop" conflict. As late as 1888 Henry I. Bowditch continued to support Hooker's position against restrictive membership criteria for the profession; see Vincent Y. Bowditch, *Life and Correspondence of Henry Ingersoll Bowditch* (1902), 2:254–57.

70. Shryock, *Medical Licensing in America*, p. 51; Shryock "Women in American Medicine," in *Medicine in America*, pp. 177–202. There are several studies of the entry of women into professional medicine, including John B. Blake, "Women and Medicine in Ante-Bellum America," *Bulletin of the History of Medicine* (March–April 1965), 39:99–123; Mary Roth Walsh, *"Doctors Wanted: No Women Need Apply": Sexual Barriers in the Medical Profession, 1835–1975* (1977); Regina Markell Morantz, "The 'Connecting Link': The Case for the Woman Doctor," in *Sickness and Health*, edited by Leavitt and Numbers, pp. 117–28.

71. Herbert M. Morais, *The History of the Negro in Medicine* (1967). W. Montague Cobb, "A Medical Bibliography," *Negro History Bulletin* (November 1973), 36:162, provides a brief introduction to the available literature. See in particular M. O. Bousfield, "An Account of Physicians of Color in the United States," *Bulletin of the History of Medicine* (January 1945), 17:61–84.

72. Stewart H. Holbrook, *The Golden Age of Quackery* (1962), pp. 79–87.

73. George Rosen, *The Specialization of Medicine, with Particular Reference to Ophthalmology* (1944); Rosemary Stevens, *American Medicine and the Public Interest* (1971), pp. 44–54; Haber, "Professions and Higher Education," p. 254. For examples, see *Trans AMA* (1859), 12:30; Edward Warren, *The Life of John Collins Warren* (1860), 2:95.

74. Shryock, *Development of Modern Medicine*, pp. 172 ff.

75. Rosenberg, *Cholera Years,* p. 157.

76. For hydropaths, M[ary] S. Gove Nichols, "Woman the Physician," *Water-Cure Journal* (October 1851), 12:3. For homeopaths, Rothstein, *American Physicians,* p. 231 n. 3. For Eclectics, W. Beach, *American Practice Condensed,* pp. 150–55.

77. Flint, "Conservative Medicine," in *Medical America,* p. 135. See also ch. 11 below for analysis of hospital case records.

78. The rise of sectarian surgery has received virtually no sustained historical study. Silas Gleason's introduction of surgery at the Elmira, New York, Water-Cure provoked a schism within hydropathy; see Jane Gastineau, "Healing the Sick and Suffering Sisterhood: Dr. Rachel Brooks Gleason and the Care of Female Patients, 1852–98," unpublished paper, North of 40 Midwest Historians of Medicine Conference, March 27, 1982, Bloomington, Indiana. John Harvey Kellogg surmounted his hydropathic scruples to become a prolific surgeon at Battle Creek; see Schwarz, *Kellogg.*

For botanic surgery, see *Buffalo Medical Journal* (March 1859), 14:583–84. For Eclectics, see Hill, *Lectures.*

For homeopaths, see Rothstein, *American Physicians,* p. 231; Bushrod W. James, "An Essay on The Progress of Surgery," unpublished M.D. thesis, Homoeopathic Medical College of Pennsylvania, February 1, 1857, Hahnemann University Archives, Philadelphia; J. G. Gilchrist, *A Syllabus of Lectures on Surgery* (1877). At the University of Michigan, the homeopathic hospital built an operating room before the orthodox hospital had such a facility; see Wilfred B. Shaw, ed., *The University of Michigan: An Encyclopedic Survey* (1951) 2, (part V):959, 1010.

3. THE DRAWBACKS OF ANESTHESIA

1. Some criticisms applied to all anesthetics; others applied to some agents more than other ones. Distinctions among chloroform, ether, and nitrous oxide will be noted wherever relevant.

2. *New York Journal of Medicine and the Collateral Sciences* (January 1847), 8:122 (hereafter cited as *NYJ Med*); *Medical Examiner* [Philadelphia] (April 1847), n.s. 3:229 (hereafter cited as *Phil Med Ex*); Richard Manning Hodges, *A Narrative of Events Connected with the Introduction of Sulphuric Ether into Surgical Use* (1891), pp. 59–60. See also Edward Everett to Henry Holland, December 31, 1846, Edward Everett Papers, vol. 70, reel 27, items 159–60, Massachusetts Historical Society, Boston (hereafter cited as Everett Papers).

3. Henry Jacob Bigelow, "Insensibility During Surgical Operations Produced by Inhalation," *Boston Medical and Surgical Journal* (1846), 35:311; *Phil Med Ex,* (January 1847), n.s. 3:19; J. F. B. Flagg, *Ether and Chloroform: Their Employment in Surgery, Dentistry, Midwifery, Therapeutics, Etc.* (1851), p. 22.

4. John B. Porter, "Medical and Surgical Notes of Campaigns in the War With Mexico," *AJMS* (1852), 23:33; (1852), 24:30. See also *AJMS* (1850), 20:96.

5. *Trans AMA* (1848), 1:189–96.

6. *Western Lancet and Hospital Reporter* (1847), 6:54 (hereafter cited as *Western Lancet*); Mayo G. Smith to John Collins Warren, October 22, 1848, John Collins Warren Papers, vol. 23, item 22, Massachusetts Historical Society, Boston (hereafter cited as John C. Warren Papers).

7. Samuel Gregory, *Man-Midwifery Exposed and Corrected; . . . Together With Remarks on the Use and Abuse of Ether, and Dr. Channing's "Cases of Inhalation of Ether in Labor,"* (1848), p. 42.

8. John Erichsen, *The Science and Art of Surgery* (1860), p. 30; William T. G.

Morton, *Morton's Letheon Circular* 5th ed. ([1847]), p. 23; Porter, "Medical and Surgical Notes," *AJMS* (1852), 24:29–30.

9. Gregory, *Man-Midwifery,* p. 43.

10. Smith to Warren, October 22, 1848, John C. Warren Papers.

11. *Western Lancet* (1848), 7:363.

12. *AJMS* (1849), 18:90–95.

13. *Boston Medical and Surgical Journal* (1847), 36:183, hereafter abbreviated *B Med Surg J; AJMS* (1850), 19:529; (1850), 20:250; A. D. Farr, "Early Opposition to Obstetric Anaesthesia," *Anaesthesia* (1980), 35:898.

14. *AJMS* (1850), 20:96; in addition, many case reports of anesthesia death did not speculate on a causal mechanism.

15. Letter of J. F. Flagg in *B Med Surg J* (1847), 37:522. J. F. Flagg of Boston was the brother of J. F. B. Flagg of Philadelphia, see *Dictionary of American Biography* (hereafter cited as *DAB*).

16. *AJMS* (1851), 21:254. See also Francis Henry Ramsbotham to James Y. Simpson, January 23, 1852, Ramsbotham Papers, National Library of Medicine, Bethesda, Md. (hereafter cited as Ramsbotham Papers); S. H. Dickson, "An Introductory Lecture, delivered before the Medical Class of Jefferson College, Philadelphia, October 13th, 1859; on Pain and Death," *Charleston Medical Journal and Review* (1860), 15:63.

This concern reflected philosophical debate over whether one person can tell what another is "really" feeling and over the related question of whether true suffering could exist in the absence of memory. See chs. 7 and 11 below.

Anesthetics have the ability to separately suspend pain sensation, other sensations, mobility, consciousness, and memory, depending on the agent used, the dosage, and the psychological state of the individual patient. This phenomenon, well-known to nineteenth-century surgeons, is only just being rediscovered and researched today. See Jacobus W. Mostert, "States of Awareness During General Anesthesia," *Perspectives in Biology and Medicine* (Autumn, 1975), 19:75. For my assessment and further nineteenth-century citations, see the section on medical philosophy in ch. 11 below.

17. John Collins Warren to George W. Norris, March 6, 1848, John C. Warren Papers, vol. 26; Flagg, *Ether and Chloroform,* pp. 32, 35; for similar claims, see William T. G. Morton, "Comparative Value of Sulphuric Ether and Chloroform," *B Med Surg J* (1850), 43:110–19.

Chloroform advocates sometimes claimed ether could also produce sudden death; see: *B Med Surg J* (1850), 42:538; *AJMS* (1867), 52:183; *Ohio Medical and Surgical Journal* (1849), 2:35–36; *American Medical Times,* (September 1, 1860), p. 160, reprinted from a British journal, clipping of article in Hamilton Case Books, 3:214; for a typical tabulation of chloroform deaths see "Homicides by Chloroform," *B Med Surg J,* (February 17, 1870), n.s. 5:113–14.

18. J. H. Clark, "On the Constitutional Effects of Anaesthetic Agents," *New York Journal of Medicine* (1856), 3d ser., 1:181–89; F. D. Lente, "The Remote Effects of Anaesthesia on the System," *ibid.* pp. 354–57. *The American Journal of Insanity* (1865), 22:58–61, 76–81, summarized and debated the literature to that date.

19. *Bulletin of the New York Academy of Medicine* (1864), 2:327–45, contains a full debate on the issue to that date. Frank Hastings Hamilton, *A Treatise on Military Surgery and Hygiene* (1865), pp. 622–23; *Dental Cosmos* (1869), 11:166.

20. *Bulletin of the New York Academy of Medicine* (1864), 2:327–45; *AJMS* (1867), 52:176–79; *B Med Surg J* (1888), 119:293–94; Peter C. English, *Shock, Physiological Surgery, and George Washington Crile: Medical Innovation in the Progressive Era* (1980), p. 9.

21. *B Med Surg J* (1870), n.s., 5:113–14.

22. Martha Coffin Wright to Ellen Wright Garrison, October 31, 1869, Sophia Smith Collection, Smith College, Northampton, Massachusetts, reprinted in *The Female Experience: An American Documentary,* edited by Gerda Lerner, (1977), p. 80. For similar cases of patients objecting to the danger of anesthesia, see MGH Records, vol. 31, case of James D., admitted March 12, 1847; *Buffalo Medical Journal* (1857), 13:215.

My analysis of the records of 2,037 operations performed between 1846 and 1877 found only 8 cases (0.4 percent) in which the patient refused a prescribed anesthetic. Unfortunately, the patient's reasons were rarely recorded. MGH, NYH, Pa. H. Surgical Records, Hamilton Casebooks.

But in 1868 Michigan, popular fears were reportedly so great "that it is almost impossible in country practice to induce a patient to take an anaesthetic, no matter how painful the operation may be," according to Stillman Hiram Smith, "Anaesthetics," unpublished M.D. thesis, University of Michigan, 1868, p. 33, Bentley Library, Michigan Historical Collections, Ann Arbor, Michigan.

23. On this debate, see J. H. M'Quillen, "Action of Anaesthetics on the Blood Corpuscles," *Dental Cosmos* (1869), 11:113–19; Laurence Turnbull, *The Advantages and Accidents of Artificial Anaesthesia: A Manual of Anaesthetic Agents,* (1885), p. 180; Henry M. Lyman, *Artificial Anaesthesia and Anaesthetics* (1881), pp. 14–29.

24. See notes 135–139, this chapter.

25. See notes 55–56, this chapter.

26. Ellen M. Snow, "Duties of Physicians," *Water-Cure Journal* (1856), 21:56; T. L. Nichols, *The Curse Removed: A Statement of Facts Respecting the Efficacy of Water Cure in the Treatment of Uterine Diseases, and the Removal of the Pains and Perils of Pregnancy and Childbirth* (1850), pp. 13–14. I am indebted to Gina Morantz for these citations.

27. For a good summary of the dangers, written by an anesthesiologist for lay readers, see Ronald Woolmer, *The Conquest of Pain: Achievements of Modern Anaesthesia* (1961), pp. 27, 60–71. For a witty, judicious account of newly discovered dangers, see Paul Brodeur, "Annals of Chemistry," *The New Yorker,* November 24, 1975, pp. 122–48. I am indebted to Nancy Reed for this reference.

For the most recent moderate appraisal of the very controversial issue of obstetric anesthesia side effects, see G. B. Kolata, "Scientists Attack Report That Obstetric Medications Endanger Children," *Science* (April 27, 1979), 204:391–2.

28. For aspects of the curare story, see Richard D. French, *Antivivisection and Medical Science in Victorian Society* (1975), pp. 70, 108, 127, 143, 302–3; Woolmer, *Conquest of Pain.*

29. Henry K. Beecher, *Research and the Individual* (1970), p. 128. See also Beecher and Donald P. Todd, *A Study of the Deaths Associated with Anesthesia and Surgery* (1954). For my assessment of these dangers see ch. 11.

30. For anesthesia and statistics, see *Western Lancet* (1847), 6:53–56; and ch. 6 below. For the general development of therapeutic statistics, see Richard H. Shryock, "The History of Quantification in Medical Science," *Isis* (June 1961), 52:215–37.

31. Porter, "Medical and Surgical Notes," *AJMS* (1852), 24:20.

32. For the AMA role, see Paul F. Eve, "Report of Operations performed under Anaesthetic Agents," *Southern Medical and Surgical Journal,* (1849), n.s. 5:278–79; and note 43 below. For the New York Academy of Medicine, see Van Ingen, *New York Academy of Medicine,* p. 17. *B Med Surg J* (1847), 36:126. For similar deference to European opinion on anesthesia, see Sir James Paget, "The Discovery of Anesthesia," *Eclectic Magazine* (1880), 94:222; *Summary of the Transactions of the College of Physicians of Philadelphia* (1846–1849), 2:166-68; Charles F. Henry, "Etherization, As a Surgical Remedy," unpublished M.D. thesis, University of Pennsylvania, February 1853, p. 1, located in the Library of the University of

Pennsylvania, Philadelphia. For my assessment of the role of geography in the diffusion of anesthesia, see ch. 10 below.

33. For my assessment of the role of hospital experimentation, see ch. 11 below.

34. The other alternatives were experimentation on one's self and on one's pets, both of which were seen as obligatory phases of mid-nineteenth-century research. For the obligation to perform auto-experimentation with anesthesia before administering it to patients, see "Report of the Committee of the Medical Society of Virginia, On the Utility and Safety of Anaesthetic Agents," *The Stethoscope and Virginia Medical Gazette* (April 1851), 1:188. For Morton's progression from the family goldfish to the family dog, to himself, in his experimentation, see Fülöp-Miller, *Triumph Over Pain,* pp. 119–22. For Simpson's auto-experimentation, see Fülöp-Miller, pp. 332–33. For opposition to animal experimentation, see French, *Antivivisection.*

For other animal trials of anesthesia, see: Turnbull, *Artificial Anaesthesia,* pp. 128–29; Charles T. Jackson, *A Manual of Etherization* (1861), p. 75; *Buffalo Medical Journal* (1847–48), 3:710–12. For the general background, see L. K. Altman, "Auto-Experimentation: An Unappreciated Tradition in Medical Science," *New England Journal of Medicine* (1972), 286:346–52.

35. For an early and influential study, see Beecher, *Research and the Individual.* The most comprehensive work is Jay Katz, ed., *Experimentation with Human Beings* (1972).

36. For the threats against McDowell, see the popularized account in James Thomas Flexner, *Doctors on Horseback: Pioneers of American Medicine* (1969), pp. 115–20. For nineteenth-century American attitudes toward research, see Richard H. Shryock, *American Medical Research: Past and Present* (1947); Shryock, "American Indifference to Basic Science During the Nineteenth Century," in *Medicine in America,* pp. 71–89. For attitudes toward autopsies, see John B. Blake, "The Development of American Anatomy Acts," *Journal of Medical Education* (August 1955), 30:431–39; Linden F. Edwards, "Resurrection Riots During the Heroic Age of Anatomy in America," *Bulletin of the History of Medicine* (March–April 1951), 25:178–84. For the greater freedom of French physiologists to experiment with anesthesia, see Jackson, *Manual,* p. 75.

37. For the threats against Morton, see Fülöp-Miller, *Triumph Over Pain,* p. 123.

38. See the comments of Judge T. J. Mackey in his introduction to J. Marion Sims, *The Story of My Life* (1884, reprinted 1968), p. 10; Chester R. Burns, "Professional Ethics and the Development of American Law as Applied to Medicine," in *Legacies in Law and Medicine* (1977), pp. 299–310.

39. For the suit against Morton, see Rice, *Trials of a Public Benefactor,* p. 121; the *Phil Med Ex* is quoted in Flexner, *Doctors on Horseback,* p. 281; S. W. Barker, "Anesthesia," *Harper's* (1865), 31:457–58.

40. *The Annalist; A Record of Practical Medicine* (1846–1847), 1:167 (hereafter cited as *Annalist*); *B Med Surg J* (1846), 35:472.

41. Rosenberg, "Therapeutic Revolution."

42. *Trans AMA* (1848), 1:32, 101–102.

43. Calhoun, *Professional Lives,* ch. 2. For a very perceptive comment on the role of medical societies in legitimating anesthesia, see Fülöp-Miller, *Triumph Over Pain,* p. 210. For a charge that the AMA in general was "manifesting a squeamishness, which, if carried out in practice, cannot but retard individual advancement, and consequently individual usefulness," see *B Med Surg J* (1847), 37:33. Joseph Ben-David has argued that medical societies fostered innovation, "Scientific Productivity and Academic Organization in Nineteenth Century Medicine," *American Sociological Review* (December 1960), 25:828–43. For my assessment, see ch. 11, note 100 below.

44. MGH Records, vol. 30, case admitted September 25, 1846. The reference to

anesthesia is phrased in a way to indicate the passage of time, it is in a different handwriting from the rest of the case record, and it is pasted in.

45. Whiggish historians of medicine have been almost uniformly unsympathetic to the belief in the value of pain. For a typical dismissal of such criticism as religious fanaticism, see Flexner, *Doctors on Horseback*, p. 304. See also Philip Rhodes' review of Ivan Illich's *Medical Nemesis* in the *British Medical Journal*, December 7, 1974, p. 577, for the automatic assumption that any defense of suffering must spring from theology. In this section, I am attempting to defend the logic and rationality of those critics of anesthesia who saw value in pain—however, as will become clear, I myself do not share such views. Two studies that present both sides of the issue for obstetrics are Farr, "Early Opposition," and Youngson, *Scientific Revolution*, pp. 94–124.

46. Sir James Paget, "The Discovery of Anesthesia," *Eclectic Magazine* (1880), 94:219–20; for related insightful comments, see Lloyd G. Stevenson, "Suspended Animation and the History of Anesthesia," *Bulletin of the History of Medicine* (Winter 1975), 49:482–511. Also related is the marvelous tale by Edgar Allan Poe, "The Facts in the Case of M. Valdemar," in which the common Victorian association of mesmerism, suspended animation, and death receives terrifying treatment, *American Whig Review*, December 1845, in *The Complete Works of Edgar Allan Poe*, James A. Harrison, ed. (1902), 5:154–66.

47. Eugene H. Pool and Frank J. McGowan, *Surgery at the New York Hospital One Hundred Years Ago* (1930), p. 46. The exact date is not given, but on the basis of case numbers, the operation was done between 1826 (p. 76) and 1831 (p. 144).

The immensely popular preacher Henry Ward Beecher summarized the argument in 1872: "The less pain, the less life-capacity. The less pain-power, the less life-power," "The Ministration of Pain," *The Sermons of Henry Ward Beecher in Plymouth Church, Brooklyn, "Plymouth Pulpit,"* Fifth Series (1872), p. 120.

48. Felix Pascalis, "Remarks on the Theory of Pain," *American Medical and Surgical Journal* (1826), 1:80. Pascalis, a French refugee resident in New York, was an eminent follower of Benjamin Rush. See also *AJMS* (1850), 19:88–89.

49. J. M. D. Olmsted, *François Magendie* (1944), pp. 244–47; Fülöp-Miller, *Triumph Over Pain*, p. 211.

See also Charles Lamb to Bernard Barton, January 9, 1824, "Pain is life,—the sharper, the more evidence of life," *The Best Letters of Charles Lamb*, edited by Edward Gilpin Johnson (1892), p. 269.

50. Turnbull, *Artificial Anaesthesia*, p. 275. Born in Scotland, Turnbull was a Philadelphia eye and ear specialist.

51. "Deaths From the Administration of Ether," *The Medical Gazette* of New York, August 20, 1870, clipping located in the Hamilton Case Books, 8:44. See also *Bulletin of the New York Academy of Medicine* (1864), 2:330.

52. Raper, *Man Against Pain*, p. 105. The terminology used reflects the continued importance of vitalism as opposed to materialism in medical philosophy. There were at least three related vitalist viewpoints on the functional necessity of pain: (1) pain itself is the vital force; (2) pain is a spur to the vital force; (3) pain is separate from the vital force, but anything strong enough to overcome one would also overpower the other. Vitalists opposed anesthesia for other reasons as well, especially because they feared the materialist implications of a physical substance that could directly control mental processes. For a perceptive guess on this point, see Stephen Kern, *Anatomy and Destiny: A Cultural History of the Human Body* (1975), pp. 69, 78. For my assessment, and for further documentation, see the section on medical philosophy in ch. 11 below. Additional opposition to anesthesia as causing "failure of the life force" is noted in John Wesley Thompson, "Anaesthesia," unpublished M.D. thesis, University of Pennsylvania, January 1860, p. 5; Howard Haggard, *Devils, Drugs, and Doctors: The Story of*

the Science of Healing from Medicine-Man to Doctor (1929), p. 112; *Phil. Med. Ex.* (December 1846), n.s. 2:719–20; Youngson, *Scientific Revolution,* p. 107; Augustin Prichard, "Death From Chloroform," *British Medical Journal* (1858), 252, as quoted in R. M. Weller, "Death in Bristol: An Exchange of Views Between Augustin Prichard and John Snow," *Anaesthesia* (1976), 31:90–96.

For general comments expressing concern about the similarity between anesthesia and death, see also "Report of Medical Society of Virginia," p. 182; *Trans AMA* (1848), 1:222. General belief in the similarity of death and sleep was of course very widespread (see, e.g., *Hamlet*).

For vitalist arguments in favor of anesthesia, see ch. 4.

53. *Bulletin of the New York Academy of Medicine* (1864), 2:336. For ancient usage, see Galen, *On the Natural Faculties,* trans. by Arthur John Brock (1963), p. xxxviii. Bailey's dictionary of 1721 defined "anaesthesia" as "a Defect of Sensation, as in Paralytic and blasted Persons," according to the *Oxford English Dictionary* (hereafter cited as *OED*). For a nineteenth-century American example of such usage, see *AJMS* (1850), 20:164.

54. Mayo G. Smith to John Collins Warren, October 22, 1848, John C. Warren Papers, vol. 23, item 22; John P. Harrison, "On the Physiology, Pathology, and Therapeutics of Pain," *Western Lancet* (1849), 9:352.

55. The theory is similar to that by which a slap in the face may revive an unconscious person (or a swift kick may revive a balky piece of machinery). For a late nineteenth-century variant, see Henry M. Lyman, *Artificial Anaesthesia and Anaesthetics* (1881), p. 49. The best explanation is in Thompson, "Anaesthesia," pp. 5, 12–14. For discussion of the relation of shock, anesthesia, and reaction, see also Erichsen, *Science and Art of Surgery* (1860), p. 32; Porter, "Medical and Surgical Notes," *AJMS* (1852), 24:29.

Whether or not to wait for "reaction" before performing surgery, that is, whether operations should be "primary" or "secondary," was an extremely controversial topic in nineteenth-century medicine, in which the role of pain was only one of several issues. For other comments on the similarity between the state of anesthetization and the state of shock, see *Trans AMA* (1848), 1:213, also 190; *AJMS* (1851), 21:254–55. For more on this subject, see chs. 8 and 11 below.

56. S. Roodhouse Gloyne, *John Hunter* (1950), p. 51; Flint, "Conservative Medicine," in *Medical America in the Nineteenth Century,* edited by Brieger, p. 51. The doctrine of counterirritation was related to the larger theory of "sympathy," by which stimuli affecting one part of the body could influence other parts of the body not directly touched by the stimulus. "Sympathy" was the key integrating force in the holistic, vitalistic concept of the body held by many nineteenth-century healers of all schools.

57. Benjamin Rush, "Commonplace Book," in *The Autobiography of Benjamin Rush, His "Travels Through Life," together with his* Commonplace Book *for 1789–1813,* edited by George W. Corner (1948), entry of August 5, 1793, p. 231. "The Author of nature seems to have had a design in making medicines unpalatable," Rush opined, "Duties of a Physician," *Selected Works,* p. 312.

58. For the survival of belief that one disease could drive out another during the 1849 cholera epidemic, see Rosenberg, *Cholera Years,* pp. 166–67. For use of anesthetics as counterirritants, see *AJMS* (1851), 22:112. For more on anesthesia and counterirritation, see ch. 5 below.

59. King, *Eclectic Obstetrics,* p. 506, emphasis in original.

60. *OED;* for Victorian America, see Leonard N. Neufeldt, "The Science of Power: Emerson's Views on Science and Technology in America," *Journal of the History of Ideas* (April–June 1977), 38:339; Herbert Marcuse, *Eros and Civilization* (1955). "Suffering . . . is universally accepted as the measure of value . . . ," according to Henry Ward Beecher, "Suf-

fering, The Measure of Worth," *The Sermons of Henry Ward Beecher in Plymouth Church, Brooklyn, "Plymouth Pulpit," First Series* (1870), p. 327.

61. Rosenberg, "Therapeutic Revolution"; Bigelow, *Rational Medicine,* p. 64.

62. [Frederick Adolphus Packard] A Citizen of Pennsylvania, *An Inquiry into the Alleged Tendency of the Separation of Convicts, One from the Other, to Produce Disease and Derangement* (1849), p. 144. Packard was recording secretary of the American Sunday School Union.

63. J. Julian Chisholm, *A Manual of Military Surgery for the Use of Surgeons in the Confederate States Army* (1862), p. 433; Edward Clarke, "Anaesthesia in Surgery," unpublished M.D. thesis, University of Pennsylvania, January 1860, pp. 4–5 (this was *not* Edward H. Clarke, the writer on medicine and sex in education); *NYJ Med* (1847), 9:122–25, also quoted in Duffy, *History of Public Health in New York City 1625–1866,* p. 463, emphasis in original.

The quotation from Hall may be found in Farr, "Opposition to Anaesthesia," p. 906. For the similar views of British surgeons Bransby Cooper, R. Nunn, James Pickford, and others, see *ibid.* p. 897; *Westminster Review* (1859), 71:67; Kidd, *Manual of Anaesthetics,* p. 22; J[ames] Y. Simpson, *Anaesthesia, Or the Employment of Chloroform and Ether in Surgery, Midwifery, Etc.* (1849), pp. 38–39. For another American Civil War expression of such views, see George Worthington Adams, *Doctors in Blue: The Medical History of the Union Army in the Civil War* (1961), p. 107. The appeal of such opinions to military surgeons was due in part to the extremely high rates of infection and shock produced by nineteenth-century weaponry, not simply a display of manly endurance.

The argument that *pain* itself is vital to healing is logically distinct from the view that anesthetic substances chemically blocked the process of healing.

64. *OED;* see also I Samuel 4:19. For nineteenth-century comment on this usage, see Simpson, *Anaesthesia,* p. 233; *AJMS* (1852), 24:126; William Potts Dewees, "An Examination of Dr. Osburn's Opinion, of the Physical Necessity of Pain and Difficulty in Human Parturition," *Philadelphia Medical Museum* (1805), 1:272.

65. *AJMS* (1851), 21:252–53.

66. *AJMS* (1851), 21:252–53; Gregory, *Man-Midwifery,* p. 43; see also Simpson, *Anaesthesia,* p. 232, for further citations. For refutation of this idea, see William Potts Dewees, *An Essay on the Means of Lessening Pain, and Facilitating Certain Cases of Difficult Parturition* (1806), p. 23.

67. Chisholm, *Manual,* p. 433; Porter, "Notes," *AJMS* (1852), 24:29. See also Francis R. Packard, *A History of Medicine in the United States* (1901), 1:639; Hodges, *Introduction of Ether,* p. 126; Rice, *Trials of a Public Benefactor,* p. 123; Thompson, "Anaesthesia," p. 12.

68. N. I. Bowditch, *History of Massachusetts General Hospital* (1851), p. 217 for "enthusiasm"; Edward Warren, review of *A Treatise on Etherization in Childbirth,* by Walter Channing, in *North American Review* (April 1849), 68:313, for "zeal." For the military view of anesthesia as "philanthropy," see *Western Lancet* (1848), 7:128. See also George M. Fredrickson, *The Inner Civil War: Northern Intellectuals and the Crisis of the Union* (1971).

69. Hill, *Eclectic Surgery,* p. 209.

70. Gregory, *Man-Midwifery,* p. 43; N. M. Greene, "Anesthesia and the Development of Surgery, 1846–1896," *Anesthesia and Analgesia* (1979), 58:5–12.

71. Josiah Gilbert Holland, *Bitter-Sweet; A Poem,* 15th edition (1863), p. 72. Augustus K. Gardner, *Our Children* (Hartford: Belknap and Bliss, 1872), pp. 25–51, quoted in G[raham] J. Barker-Benfield, *The Horrors of the Half-Known Life* (1976), p. 283. For childbirth pains as "interesting," see Nichols, *The Curse Removed,* pp. 13–14; Emerson's essay on "Compensation" is in *Essays, First Series,* (1888), pp. 89–122; for a critique, see Paul F. Boller, Jr., *American Transcendentalism 1830–1860: An Intellectual Inquiry* (1974), pp. 145–

57. See also Dubos and Dubos, *The White Plague,* for a good analysis of Victorian infatuation with ethereal, sickly women.

72. Haggard, *Devils, Drugs, Doctors,* p. 116.

73. Edward R. Mordecai, "The Effects of Chloroform on the System and Its Therapeutical Applications," unpublished M.D. thesis, University of Pennsylvania, February 1849, pp. 18–19. See also Harrison, "Physiology of Pain," *Western Lancet* (1849), 9:352; Gunning S. Bedford, *The Principles and Practice of Obstetrics* (1863), p. 733; Rev. Henry Hayman, "The Economy of Pain," *Bibliotheca Sacra* (1888), 45:8.

74. Gail Parker, ed., *The Oven Birds: American Women on Womanhood 1820–1920* (1972), p. 20; for the general concept of "domestic feminism," see Daniel Scott Smith, "Family Limitation, Sexual Control, and Domestic Feminism in Victorian America," in *Clio's Consciousness Raised: New Perspectives on the History of Women,* edited by Mary S. Hartman and Lois W. Banner (1974), pp. 119–36; Youngson, *Scientific Revolution,* pp. 111–12.

75. Fülöp-Miller, *Triumph Over Pain,* p. 91. Others regarded not painlessness but loss of rationality as the brutalizing, dehumanizing aspect of anesthesia: *Westminster Review* (1859), 71:68; John Duns, *Memoir of Sir James Y. Simpson, Bart.* (1873), pp. 221–22; see notes 114–124, 130, this chapter.

76. Laird W. Nevius, *The Discovery of Modern Anaesthesia: By Whom Was it Made? A Brief Statement of Facts* (1894), p. 107. In a letter to Simpson in 1848, Meigs disclaimed any professional familiarity with surgical anesthesia but went on to attack it anyway, *Buffalo Medical Journal* (1848), 3:674–78.

77. Edward H. Horner, "Anaesthetics," unpublished M.D. thesis, University of Pennsylvania, February 1855, p. 28. For the belief that pain, as part of God's creation, must have some purpose, even if presently undiscovered, see Youngson, *Scientific Revolution,* pp. 104, 111.

78. Gregory, *Man-Midwifery,* p. 43; Francis Henry Ramsbotham to James Y. Simpson, August 10, 1853, Ramsbotham Papers; see also Porter, "Medical and Surgical Notes," *AJMS* (1852), 23:33. But such lapses into the naturalistic fallacy were *not* the major grounds for believing pain to be functional.

79. Turnbull, *Artificial Anaesthesia* (1885), p. 275.

80. The claim that birth pain is essential to female emotional health has retained supporters, from 1847 to the present. "Childbearing is so essential an experience for a woman that the thwarting of its normal course by the excessive use of analgesics may cause great damage to her personality. If she is carried through delivery in an unconscious state, she is deprived of the experience of giving birth to her child and in some cases will pay for this escape from reality with nervous disorders," a psychologist told the 1936 convention of the AMA. And in January 1978, a woman in Denver filed suit against her doctor, claiming that the use of obstetric anesthesia had left her incapable of forming an emotional attachment to her daughter.

Flexner, *Doctors on Horseback,* p. 304; "CBS Evening News," radio broadcast by Stephanie Shelton, January 3, 1978, 8 p.m. See also Richard W. Wertz and Dorothy C. Wertz, *Lying-In: A History of Childbirth in America* (1977), p. 117.

81. John Duffy, "Anglo-American Reaction to Obstetrical Anesthesia," *Bulletin of the History of Medicine* (January–February 1964), 38:32–44. Although Duffy dismissed most defenses of pain as theological or cryptotheological, he was one of the first historians to attempt to seriously assess the opposition arguments.

82. Genesis 3:13–16.

83. *Western Lancet* (1848), 7:363, the views of A. C. Castle, M.D., of New York, emphasis in original. W. Tyler Smith, *Parturition, and the Principles and Practice of Obstetrics* (Philadelphia: Lea & Blanchard, 1849), summarized in *AJMS* (1849), 18:182; Ramsbotham to Simpson, November 29, 1852, Ramsbotham Papers.

For the charge that anesthesia robbed God of the prayers of parturient sufferers, see

Rice, *Trials of a Public Benefactor;* MacQuitty, *Battle for Oblivion,* p. 104; Haggard, *Devils, Drugs, Doctors,* p. 108. For other accounts of fundamentalist opposition to obstetric anesthesia, see Fülöp-Miller, *Triumph Over Pain,* pp. 335–39; Edward Warren, review of *Etherization in Childbirth,* p. 311.

Dr. Hugh L. Hodge, obstetrician at the University of Pennsylvania (whose brother Charles was Moderator of the General Assembly of the rigidly predestinarian Old School Presbyterians and editor of their *Princeton Review*), opposed anesthesia in normal labor, though he did not mention any religious motives, Hodge, *The Principles and Practice of Obstetrics* (1864), p. 429.

For a judicious assessment of Old School Presbyterianism in the antebellum North, see Theodore Dwight Bozeman, "Inductive and Deductive Politics: Science and Society in Antebellum Presbyterian Thought," *Journal of American History* (December 1977), 64:704–22.

84. Nichols, *The Curse Removed,* p. 8.

85. *Ibid.,* p. 7.

86. This question forms the heart of the problem of "theodicy." For a few helpful introductory sources, see John Bowker, *Problems of Suffering in the Religions of the World* (1970); Dorothee Soelle, *Suffering,* trans. by Everett Kalin (1975); C. S. Lewis, *The Problem of Pain* (1962); David Bakan, *Disease, Pain, Sacrifice* (1968); and the idiosyncratic but wide-ranging and provocative treatment by John Ferguson, *The Place of Suffering* (1972). I am indebted to Robert Sevensky for suggestions in exploring this literature.

87. J. B. F. Walker, M.D., "Is It Wicked To Be Sick?" *The Water-Cure Journal* (1861), 31:60. I am indebted to Gina Morantz for this citation. Walker was not as strong an advocate for mechanical natural laws as this selection makes him sound; he tried to reconcile these views with a personal, wrathful God.

88. Nichols, *The Curse Removed,* pp. 13–14. William A. Alcott, "Healing Wounds," *The Teacher of Health and the Laws of the Human Constitution* (1843), 1:180–84, makes the same point, from the viewpoint of a pre-anesthetic natural-healing physician.

89. Snow, "Duties of Physicians," p. 56.

90. For nineteenth-century survival of the belief in collective punishments, see George M. Marsden, *The Evangelical Mind and the New School Presbyterian Experience* (1970), p. 23. The collectivist view of suffering is contained in Jeremiah 2:29–35. Another especially important source was Jonah 1. The sailors were all subject to the ravages of the storm merely because of the presence of Jonah in their midst. Even a well-behaved civil sinner could bring down God's wrath on the community. The only protection against such a person was to heave him overboard (hence one source for the Puritan practice of "warning out"). For recent discussions of Puritan concepts of communal responsibility and their decline, see Joseph A. Conforti, "Samuel Hopkins and the New Divinity: Theology, Ethics, and Social Reform in Eighteenth-Century New England," *William and Mary Quarterly,* (October 1977), 3d ser. 34:572–89; see also Richard Bushman, *From Puritan to Yankee: Character and the Social Order in Connecticut, 1690–1765* (1970).

The decline of eighteenth-century belief in communal punishments sprang from the growing social diversity of America, as well as such intellectual trends as Romanticism and Arminianism. While eighteenth-century religious commentators from Cotton Mather to Benjamin Rush portrayed the era's smallpox, diphtheria, and yellow fever epidemics as God's judgment against the entire community, by 1832 many church leaders regarded the cholera epidemic as punishment exclusively of the afflicted individuals. (Differences in the epidemiology of the specific diseases must also, however, be considered.) Rosenberg, *Cholera Years,* ch. 2; Wertz and Wertz, *Lying-In,* pp. 115–16.

91. Walker, "Is It Wicked To Be Sick?" p. 60. See also Barbara Gutmann Rosenkrantz, "Causal Thinking in Erewhon and Elsewhere," *Journal of Medicine and Philosophy* (December 1976), 1:372–84.

92. Harold Schwartz, *Samuel Gridley Howe, Social Reformer, 1801–1876* (1956), pp. 140, 93, emphasis in original. For the identical views of Rev. Henry Ward Beecher, see "The Ministration of Pain," *"Plymouth Pulpit," Fifth Series*, pp. 123, 127, 129.

93. For criticism of similar trends in Transcendentalism, see Boller, *American Transcendentalism*, ch. 5. The book of Job in particular rejects this simplistic equation of suffering and sin.

94. For examples, see Shattuck, *Report*, pp. 293–94; *AJMS* (1850), 19:96.

95. Giles, "Origin of Pain," p. 11.

96. Quoted in Wertz and Wertz, *Lying-In*, p. 115.

97. Coulter, *Science and Ethics*, pp. 364–65. See also J. Arthur Bullard, "Some Thoughts About Doctors and Homeopathic Doctors and Homeopathy," *The Medical Counselor* (November 1903), 22:353–55.

98. James H. Ridings, "An Essay on Anaesthetics," unpublished M.D. thesis, Homoeopathic Medical College of Pennsylvania, January 30, 1868, pp. 27–28; Clarence T. Campbell, "A Thesis on Anaesthesia," unpublished M.D. thesis, Homoeopathic Medical College of Pennsylvania, February 1866, pp. 31 on medicine, 28 on obstetrics; both in Hahnemann University Archives, Philadelphia.

99. Campbell, "Thesis on Anaesthesia," p. 29; James H. McClelland, "An Inaugural Dissertation on Anaesthesia in Labor," unpublished M.D. thesis, Homoeopathic Medical College of Pennsylvania, February 1, 1867, pp. 12, 15, in Hahnemann University Archives, Philadelphia.

100. John Jolliffe Mulheron, "Pain," unpublished M.D. thesis, University of Michigan, 1869, Michigan Historical Collections, Bentley Historical Library, Ann Arbor, Mich., pp. 89–90.

101. Gregory, *Man-Midwifery*, p. 43.

102. Although Hamilton was a "specialist" in bone surgery, he performed enough deliveries to fill an entire casebook on obstetrics—a good example of the point that midcentury professionalism sanctioned special interests but not *exclusive* specialization. Vol. 13 of the Hamilton Case Books contains all obstetric cases; see also 3:134; 12:83. Although Hamilton did not think anesthesia warranted in most obstetric cases, his records indicate that he did use it at least a dozen times. For more information on Hamilton's view of natural healing and therapeutic conservatism, see his 1877 address, "Abuse of Drugs," pasted in the back of Case Book 12.

103. The clipping is in 10:39. The only attribution is to "*—Temple Bar.*" It seems clear from the placement of the clipping that Hamilton intended to base a lecture on it. This is virtually the only clipping in Hamilton's Case Books on which he did not carefully note down the exact citation. *Temple Bar* was a London magazine, founded in 1861. The clipping appears, however, to be from an American periodical.

104. S. W. Barker, "Anesthesia," *Harper's* (1865), 31:456–57. I have been unable to verify this claim. For an alternative account of the Zurich action, which claims the ban was limited to "minor surgical operations," see *Western Lancet* (1847), 6:182. For the claim that surgeons called ether "damnable," see Robley Dunglison to John Collins Warren, January 29, 1848, John C. Warren Papers, vol. 23, item 40. For a general discussion of the doctor as part of the punishment for sin, and much else on the relation of medicine to the transformation of New England theology, see Oliver Wendell Holmes, *Elsie Venner: A Romance of Destiny* (1891, 1861). For cases of patients refusing *surgical* anesthesia on predestinarian grounds, see Rice, *Trials of a Public Benefactor;* MacQuitty, *Battle for Oblivion*, p. 106; see also the Cockney dialect joke about its being "wicked" to use ether, sent to John Collins Warren by S. B. Green, May 26, 1846 [1849], John C. Warren Papers, vol. 23, item 81; and the allegation that such views survived among some women in 1898, William Barry, "The Ethics of Pain," *The Living Age* (1898), 219:861–64.

105. Atkinson quoted in Raper, *Man Against Pain*, p. 105. Atkinson, who called himself a Spiritualist, was the son of a Methodist preacher and a Quaker "doctoress." See Charles R. E. Koch, ed., *History of Dental Surgery* (1909) 2:177–83.

106. Proverbs 13:11–12; Job 5:17; Job 6:10; quote paraphrases Proverbs 13:24. See Sidney E. Ahlstrom, *A Religious History of the American People* (1972), pp. 321, 463–65, 721–23.

107. Luke 12:33–59; Mark 14:7. C. S. Griffin, *Their Brothers' Keepers: Moral Stewardship in the United States, 1800–1865* (1960).

Belief that anesthesia deprived God's stewards of the opportunity to soothe and empathize with the suffering went far beyond the theologically orthodox. Louisa May Alcott sensed a genuine loss in the role of the nurse once anesthesia had robbed nurses of the chance to sympathize with surgical pain, see Louisa May Alcott, *Hospital Sketches*, ed. by Bessie Z. Jones, (1960), p. 86. For general comments on the preference of some nineteenth-century romantics to *empathize* with pain rather than to *relieve* it, see Bowditch, *Life and Correspondence of Henry Ingersoll Bowditch*, 2:207–11; Parker, *Over Birds*, p. 20; Miller, *Life of the Mind*, pp. 78–84; John L. Thomas, "Romantic Reform in America, 1815–1865," *American Quarterly* 17 (Winter, 1965) reprinted in *Intellectual History in America*, edited by Cushing Strout, (1968), 1:200; Fredrickson, *Inner Civil War*, p. 82; Silvan S. Tomkins, "The Psychology of Commitment: The Constructive Role of Violence and Suffering for the Individual and for His Society," in *The Antislavery Vanguard: New Essays on the Abolitionists*, edited by Martin Duberman (1965), pp. 270–98; Anne L. Kuhn, *The Mother's Role in Childhood Education: New England Concepts, 1830–1860* (1947), p. 22. For more on romantic attitudes toward empathy as contrasted with relief of pain, see ch. 5 below.

108. The Old School *Presbyterian* of Philadelphia reprinted a number of European and American news accounts unfavorable to anesthesia between 1846 and 1848; however, I could find no explicitly theological discussion of the issue (1847), 17:52, 120, 123; (1848), 18:208. See also Farr, "Opposition to Obstetric Anaesthesia," in which a search for predestinarian opposition proved fruitless.

109. M[ary] S. Gove Nichols, "Woman the Physician," *Water-Cure Journal* (October 1851), 12:3.

110. "To take one's medicine" as a metaphor for accepting a deserved punishment appears to have originated in nineteenth-century American usage, Mitford M. Mathews, *A Dictionary of Americanisms* (1951). However, the basic idea, that painful medicine is the punishment for unhealthy living, can be traced back to Plato, *Gorgias*, 479a; Temkin, *Double Face of Janus*, p. 53. The word "pain" itself is derived from the Latin for "punishment," *OED*.

The Philadelphia *Presbyterian* printed a favorable report of Sir Charles Napier's plan to have British military surgeons administer painful medical blisters, instead of flogging, to punish drunken soldiers (1847), 17:96.

111. Benjamin Rush, *The Autobiography of Benjamin Rush, His "Travels Through Life," together with His* Commonplace Book *for 1789–1813*, edited by George W. Corner (1948), pp. 231, 229. For use of this argument against anesthesia, see Hill, *Eclectic Surgery*, pp. 208–209.

112. *An Extract from the Report of the Directors of Massachusetts State Prison, . . . Reviewing Certain Parts of the Second Annual Report of the Prison Discipline Society, to which is Added, the Report of the Physician of Massachusetts State Prison* (1827), pp. 25, 23–24 (hereafter cited as *Report of the Physician*). For Kant's critique of the rationalist, utilitarian equation of surgery with punishment, see the *Critique of Practical Reason*, part 1, book 1, ch. 2, as reprinted in *Philosophical Perspectives on Punishment*, edited by Gertrude Ezorsky (1972), p. 102.

This view that all pain, including surgery, is a valuable *punishment* closely parallels the view that all pain is a valuable *discipline;* that every pain has something to *teach* us, and that only through suffering can we learn. For many examples, from classical times to the present, see Ferguson, *The Place of Suffering,* pp. 36, 52, 91, 97, 129, 134. For nineteenth-century examples, see Elizabeth Barrett Browning, "knowledge by suffering entereth," in "A Vision of Poets," (1844), *The Complete Works of Elizabeth Barrett Browning,* edited by Charlotte Porter and Helen A. Clarke (1900), 2:345, 348; see also similar sentiments in *Massachusetts Teacher* (1850), 3:206, 273; Rush, *Selected Works, p. 197.* For a brief discussion of this point in the context of surgical anesthesia, see Kern, *Anatomy and Destiny,* p. 78. For the converse, that education and mental discipline create extreme sensitivity to pain, see ch. 7 below.

113. Horace Mann, *Twelfth Annual Report* (1848) as reprinted in *The Republic and The School: Horace Mann on the Education of Free Men,* edited by Lawrence A. Cremin, (1957), p. 99.

114. Alcott, *Hospital Sketches,* pp. 87–88; Charles F. Henry, "Etherization, As a Surgical Remedy," unpublished M.D. thesis, University of Pennsylvania, February 1853, p. 10.

115. *Western Lancet* (1848), 7:365; see also "Chloroform in Surgical Operations, the Cases in which it Should Not be Applied," *Lancet,* October 20, 1855, clipping in Hamilton Case Books, 15:58.

116. *Trans AMA* (1848), 1:230; (1849), 2:248–49. For other specific diseases in which this objection was raised, see ch. 8 below, and *AJMS* (1851), 22:140, 426, 490. The development of local anesthesia combined with the increasing level of surgical dexterity has lessened the force of such arguments today.

117. *Trans AMA* (1849), 2:249.

118. *Western Lancet* (1848), 7:365.

119. Reprinted in the *Journal of the History of Medicine and Allied Sciences* (October 1946), 1:611. The doctor who "amputated the healthy limb, and left the fractured one to recover," was already proverbial by 1851, see Flagg, *Ether and Chloroform,* p. 32. For an 1847 version, see Beach, *American Practice Condensed,* p. 151.

Such charges were not unfounded. Shocking mistakes still do occur in surgery today, as a result of the anesthetized patient's inability to protest the surgeon's error. See *New York Times,* March 23, 1980, p. 28, col. 6; *ibid.,* April 6, 1980, p. 20, col. 6; William A. Kelly, "The Physician, The Patient, and the Consent," *University of Kansas Law Review* (March 1960), 8:422.

120. Philippe Ariès, "Death Inside Out," *Hastings Center Studies* (May 1974), 2:3–18; Maris A. Vinovskis, "Angels' Heads and Weeping Willows: Death in Early America," *Proceedings of the American Antiquarian Society* (1977), 86:273–302; David E. Stannard, "Death and Dying in Puritan New England," *American Historical Review* (December 1973), 78:1305–30; Stannard, *The Puritan Way of Death* (1977).

121. For Magendie, see Fülöp-Miller, *Triumph Over Pain,* p. 211; Olmsted, *Magendie,* pp. 244–47. For Iowa quote, see Duffy, "Obstetrical Anesthesia," p. 43.

"The thing I really dread, Doctor, is being 'put out,' . . . having my mind and my will taken away," one modern anesthesiologist quotes a patient as saying, see Woolmer, *Conquest of Pain,* p. 27.

122. Henry J. Bigelow, "Inaugural Lecture, Introductory to the Course on Surgery, Delivered Before the Medical School of Harvard University, Boston, 1849," in *Surgical Anaesthesia: Addresses and Other Papers* (1900), p. 240. For a barrage of similar charges, and my attempt to define and assess the actual extent of "unnecessary" surgery, see ch. 11 below.

123. Plate 1 is taken from Otto L. Bettmann, *The Good Old Days—They Were Terrible!* (1974), p. 145, used with permission of the Bettmann Archive. Unfortunately, in or-

der to assure themselves royalties, the Bettmann Archive does not reveal the sources of their collection and even cropped the name of the artist from the print. Such conduct greatly diminishes the historical worth of their materials. The artist was Fernando Miranda, whose work often appeared in the New York *Daily Graphic*, c. 1875. I am grateful to Elizabeth E. Roth, Keeper of Prints, New York Public Library, for this attribution.

124. *AJMS* (1851), 22:495; see also Nathaniel Friend, "Anaesthesia in Labour," unpublished M.D. thesis, University of Pennsylvania, January 1857, pp. 9–10. Popular fears of involuntary anesthetization persist into this century. In Frank Norris' *A Man's Woman* (1900), a woman nurse forcibly anesthetizes a child. In Norris' *Mc Teague* (1924), the quack dentist uses anesthesia to attempt to seduce a young female patient.

125. *Western Lancet* (1848), 7:365; B. Fordyce Barker, "On the Use of Anaesthetics in Midwifery," *Bulletin of the New York Academy of Medicine* (1862), 1:351, quoting a Dr. Watson; [Stanton] to Lucretia [Mott], October 22, 1852, reprinted in *Oven Birds*, p. 260.

126. Gregory, *Man-Midwifery*, pp. 43–44. For analysis of "domestic feminism," see note 74 above; Christopher Lasch, "The Woman Reformer's Rebuke," in *The World of Nations*, pp. 44–55.

Gregory also suspected that anesthesia was part of a plot by the profession to mystify midwifery so women could not understand or practice it, *Man-Midwifery*, p. 43.

127. Mann, *The Republic and The School*, p. 99; *Phil Med Ex*, (October 1847), n.s. 3:635.

128. Lyman, *Artificial Anaesthesia*, pp. 93–98; E. Hartshorne, *Remarks on the Case of Dr. B.* (1854); see also Moreton Stillé, *The Psychical Effects of Ether Inhalation*, bound with the above but separately paginated. See also Robert Druitt, *The Principles and Practice of Modern Surgery* (1860), p. 594; Samuel D. Gross, *A System of Surgery* (1866) 1:540. The *Philadelphia Medical Times* of 1877 drew the then-radical conclusion that, to protect physicians, more research was urgently needed on the subject of female eroticism, December 22, 1877, cited in Turnbull, *Artificial Anaesthesia*, pp. 283–84.

Most nineteenth-century texts urged male doctors never to anesthetize a woman without a female nurse or family member present. Yet truly bizarre sexual attacks on anesthetized patients still occur even today, *despite* the presence of witnesses. See Joan Vogel and Richard Delgado, "To Tell the Truth: Physicians' Duty to Disclose Medical Mistakes," *UCLA Law Review* (1980), 28:54, 78–79.

129. *Littell's Living Age* (June 12, 1847), 13:492; Hartshorne, *Remarks on the Case of Dr. B.*, p. 24.

130. *The Poems of Emily Dickinson*, edited by Thomas H. Johnson (1963), 1:181, manuscript c. 1861. Philadelphia *Presbyterian* (1847), 17:120, reprint from the London *Times*. See also William G. McLoughlin, ed., *The American Evangelicals, 1800–1900: An Anthology* (1968), p. 3; Ferguson, *Place of Suffering*, pp. 125–26. For a refutation, see Walter Kaufmann, "Suffering and the Bible," in *The Faith of a Heretic* (1961), pp. 137–69.

The classic formulation of this conflict later appeared in Aldous Huxley's *Brave New World:*

"But I don't want comfort. I want God, I want poetry, I want real danger, I want freedom, I want goodness, I want sin."
"In fact," said Mustapha Mond, "you're claiming the right to be unhappy."
"All right then," said the Savage defiantly, "I'm claiming the right to be unhappy."
"Not to mention the right to grow old and ugly and impotent; the right to have syphilis and cancer; the right to have too little to eat; the right to be lousy; the

right to live in constant apprehension of what may happen tomorrow; the right to catch typhoid; the right to be tortured by unspeakable pains of every kind." There was a long silence. "I claim them all," said the Savage at last.

Aldous Huxley, *Brave New World* (1960, 1932), p. 163.

131. *American Journal of Dental Science* (October 1848), quoted in W. Harry Archer, "The History of Anesthesia," in *The History of the Development of Anesthesia, Oral Surgery and Hospital Dental Service in the United States of America*, by Archer, Milton B. Asbell, and William B. Irby (1971), p. 390.

132. *Western Lancet* (1848), 7:364, emphasis in original; Thompson, "Anaesthesia," p. 7; Archer, "History of Anesthesia," p. 390.
Ramsbotham felt that the pain of uncertainty and decisionmaking would be worse for the patient than the pain of childbirth; see Ramsbotham to Simpson, January 23, 1852, Ramsbotham Papers. For additional opposition to anesthesia based on the profession's inability to monopolize it, see Flagg, *Ether and Chloroform*, p. 40.

133. Advertising was also blamed for inflating public expectations beyond what medicine felt it could accomplish and for encouraging patients to view ether as a cure-all for pain. For more on this subject, see ch. 5 below. For a typical attack on advertising, see the *Annalist* (January 1847), 1:167, and notes 149–50 below.

134. John Collins Warren, *Etherization; With Surgical Remarks* (1848), pp. 33–34; Bigelow, "Insensibility During Surgical Operations," p. 316; K. Bryn Thomas, "Chloroform or Ether—A Literary Question," *Anaesthesia* (1975), 30:88–89; Stephen Rogers, "Can Chloroform be Used to Facilitate Robbery?" *Papers Read Before the Medico-Legal Society of New York*, First Series, (1889), pp. 298–317.

135. Most of the sources on such activities were presented as arguments in favor of anesthetization and so are discussed in ch. 4 below. Plate 2 is from the collection of Buck Hill Associates, Johnsburg, N.Y., and is used with their permission; they assigned the date of 1845. For a discussion of the illustration used in the plate, see ch. 4 below.

136. For example, Bigelow, "Insensibility During Surgical Operations," p. 311; *Phil Med Ex* (January 1847), n.s. 3:19; Ramsbotham to Simpson, January 23, 1852, Ramsbotham Papers.

137. Joseph R. Gusfield, *Symbolic Crusade: Status Politics and the American Temperance Movement* (1963), ch. 2. For medical involvement, see Rush, "The Effects of Ardent Spirits Upon Man [1805]," in *Selected Writings*, pp. 334–41; and Rosenberg, *Cholera Years*.
Two new general accounts of alcoholism and prohibition in nineteenth-century America are unfortunately sketchy and sometimes unreliable on the role of medicine. W. J. Rorabaugh, *The Alcoholic Republic: An American Tradition* (1979) and Ian R. Tyrell, *Sobering Up: From Temperance to Prohibition in Antebellum America, 1800–1860* (1979).

138. *Annalist* (January 1847), 1:190.

139. T. L. Nichols, *The Curse Removed*, pp. 13–14.

140. *AJMS* (1849), 18:182; Clarke, "Anaesthesia in Surgery," p. 13; Duffy, "Obstetrical Anesthesia," pp. 34–35; Stillé, "Psychical Effects of Ether Inhalation."

141. Fülöp-Miller, *Triumph Over Pain*, p. 337; Charles E. Rosenberg, "The Bitter Fruit: Heredity, Disease, and Social Thought in Nineteenth-Century America," *Perspectives in American History* (1974), 8:191–93, for similar fears regarding alcohol.

142. *B Med Surg J* (1846), 35:435; Rhoda Truax, *The Doctors Warren of Boston* (1968), p. 198; Edward Warren, review of *Etherization in Childbirth*, p. 311. The problem was similar to the abuse of medicinal alcohol, though Edward Warren did not think it was nearly as serious.

143. *B Med Surg J* (1846), 35:435; (1847), 36:183; Rice, *Trials of a Public Benefactor*, p. 129, quoting the *Boston Post* of July 19, 1847. The holistic environmental medical science of the nineteenth century did not draw very sharp lines between health and morality—to take an unhealthy drug was sinful; conversely sinning was assumed to be bad for your health.

144. Turnbull, *Artificial Anaesthesia*, pp. 289–90.

145. *American Journal of Dental Science* 9 (October 1848), quoted in Archer, "History of Anesthesia," p. 390. For the most dramatic account of Wells' last days, see Fülöp-Miller, *Triumph Over Pain*, p. 181.

146. Morton's commercial activities have not been well studied. For brief glimpses, see Fülöp-Miller, *Triumph Over Pain*, pp. 131, 154; Rice, *Trials of a Public Benefactor;* Morton, *Letheon Circular.*

147. *Summary of the Transactions of the College of Physicians of Philadelphia* (1846–1849), 2:64–65; *NYJ Med* (January 1847), 8:122.

148. Quote from *Phil Med Ex* (December 1846), n.s. 2:719–20. For the Massachusetts Medical Society, see *B Med Surg J* (1846), 35:425. Ironically, unlike Letheon, most so-called "patent medicines" were never really patented, since the law required divulging the contents of a patented remedy and, after 1836, at least nominally required evidence of novelty. The truly secret patent nostrums were sold in patented-design bottles, or under registered trademarks, or with copyrighted labels instead. See James Harvey Young, *The Toadstool Millionaires: A Social History of Patent Medicines in America before Federal Regulation* (1961). Morton made the same point in his defense, *Letheon Circular*, pp. 23–25.

For other attacks on the patent as quackery, see Hodges, *Introduction of Ether*, p. 126; Eckenhoff, *Anesthesia from Colonial Times*, p. 26; *B Med Surg J* (1846), 35:356.

149. *American Journal of Dental Science* 9 (October 1848), quoted in Archer, "History of Anesthesia," p. 390, emphasis in original. Morton, *Letheon Circular*. For similar attacks on Simpson's self-promotional activities in the United Kingdom, see Youngson, *Scientific Revolution*, pp. 119–20.

150. The *Annalist* (January 1847), 1:167.

151. Van Ingen, *New York Academy of Medicine*, p. 32; Flagg, *Ether and Chloroform*, p. 32, emphasis in original. Greene, "Anesthesia and Surgery."

152. This controversy has been the major focus of most historical attention devoted to anesthesia and is generally available in any of the sources cited in ch. 1, note 2 above. Wells killed himself; Morton had a fatal seizure following a new charge by Jackson; Jackson's erratic behavior led to his institutionalization.

153. For the activities of the first AMA head in this regard, see Irwin Richman, *The Brightest Ornament: A Biography of Nathaniel Chapman, M.D.* (1967), ch. 12. For similar activities of Valentine Mott in New York, see Van Ingen, *New York Academy of Medicine*, pp. 50, 101—3. For the questionable role of Augustus A. Gould, treasurer of the Massachusetts Medical Society, in backing Morton's patent and advertising behind the scenes, see Bowditch, *History of Massachusetts General Hospital* (1851), pp. 300, 321. See also Young, *Toadstool Millionaires;* Stewart H. Holbrook, *The Golden Age of Quackery* (1959); David L. Dykstra, "The Medical Profession and Patent and Proprietary Medicines During the Nineteenth Century," *Bulletin of the History of Medicine* (September–October 1955), 29:401–19. Medical journals are still financially dependent on drug advertising.

Patents in general were highly controversial in Jacksonian America (like medical licenses in that regard). Patents, like licenses, were attacked as unfair government monopolies; patents, like licenses, were among the few available marks of personal distinction in a society that regarded individual distinction with intense ambivalence. For patents as "a peculiarly odious monopoly," see Bowditch, *History of Massachusetts General Hospital* (1851) p. 234. For the general views of Jacksonian William Leggett, see Marvin Meyers, *The Jacksonian Persuasion:*

Politics and Belief (1960, 1957), ch. 9; also ch. 3 for Tocqueville's concept of "venturous conservative." On patent law development, see A. Hunter Dupree, *Science in the Federal Government: A History of Policies and Activities to 1940* (1957), pp. 46–47.

154. Hooker, *Physician and Patient* ch. 10.

155. John Harvey Jr., "Ether, in Surgical Operations," unpublished M.D. thesis, University of Pennsylvania, 1851, p. 1, emphasis in original; Flagg, *Ether and Chloroform,* pp. 21, 54; *AJMS* (1850), 19:102. The superiority of empirical over theoretical knowledge of nature forms the contrast between Dr. Battius and the old Trapper in James Fenimore Cooper's, *The Prairie; A Tale* (1827). See also Shryock, *Development of Modern Medicine,* pp. 118–19.

156. *AJMS* (1850), 20:159–60, contains a good summary of the ideas of dental professionalizers. See also: Carl P. Lewis, Jr., "The Baltimore College of Dental Surgery and the Birth of Professional Dentistry, 1840," *Maryland Historical Magazine* (September 1964), 59:268–85; L. Laszlo Schwartz, "Historical Relations of American Dentistry and Medicine," *Bulletin of the History of Medicine* (November–December 1954), 28:542–49; Robert W. McCluggage, *A History of the American Dental Association* (1959); sketches of Bond and Baxley are in Kelly and Burrage, *American Medical Biographies.*

157. Edward Everett to Dr. Henry Holland, February 1, 1847, Everett Papers, vol. 80, reel 27, item 199. For a sample of dental opposition, see "T.E.B." [Bond] in *B Med Surg J* (1846), 35:445–48; J. F. Flagg in *B Med Surg J* (1846), 35:356, 407–8; (1847), 37:522.

158. Charles E. Rosenberg, "The American Medical Profession: Mid-Nineteenth Century," *Mid-America* (July 1962), 44:166.

159. John Collins Warren to W. T. G. Morton, December 1846, John C. Warren Papers, vol. 23, item 16.

160. *Phil Med Ex,* (December 1846), n.s. 2:719–20; *B Med Surg J* (1846), 35:445; *Annalist* (1846), 1:140, emphasis in original.

161. Fülöp-Miller, *Triumph Over Pain,* chs. 3–7.

162. Henry Burnell Shafer, *The American Medical Profession 1783–1850* (1936), p. 141; Paul F. Eve, "Mesmerism," *Southern Medical and Surgical Journal* (1845), n.s. 1:167–92.

163. Plates 3 and 4 courtesy New York Hospital Archives.

Davis' brew of 8 ounces of gum opium in 5 gallons of spirits probably worked reasonably well for the purpose. See Holbrook, *Golden Age of Quackery,* pp. 147–53, for the best account; also Young, *Toadstool Millionaires,* pp. 186–87. Ivan Illich, *Medical Nemesis: The Expropriation of Health* (1976), p. 151n, discusses Perry Davis but misinterprets him as a successor rather than a predecessor of anesthesia.

Davis' claim to originating the term "painkiller" was documented in an important early trademark infringement case, *Davis v. Kendall* 2 Durfee 566 (R.I.). See John J. Elwell, *A Medico-Legal Treatise on Malpractice and Medical Evidence,* (1871), pp. 196–97.

However, some locally made rivals undoubtedly developed the concept earlier. "Dalley's Magical Pain Extractor" boasted an 1839 founding date in its later advertising, see New York Hospital Archives. Other similar products circa 1850 included "A. E. Smith's Electric Oil," see flyer in Harvard School of Business, Business Archives, folder, drug misc—printed; "Hite's Pain Cure" of Staunton, Va., see bottle on display September 1979, Clements Library, University of Michigan, Ann Arbor; and "Aimar's Neurotic Oil," a South Carolina product, see Wm. Frost Mobley, *American Broadsides,* Catalog One (1980), item 47. "HAMLIN'S WIZARD OIL CURES ALL PAIN IN MAN OR BEAST," proclaimed the slogan on the rump of a circus elephant, portrayed swilling a bottle of wizard oil; see Ann Novotny and Carter Smith, *Images of Healing* (1980), p. 101. The *OED,* perhaps erroneously, gives an 1836 date for the first use of "painkiller" for a patent remedy.

164. *Patent Journal and Investor's Magazine,* January 23, 1847, pp. 578–80, re-

printed in *Milestones in Anesthesia: Readings in the Development of Surgical Anesthesia, 1665–1940*, [edited] by Frank Cole (1965), p. 43; see also "Painless Operations in Surgery," *Littell's Living Age* (June 1847), 13:481–96.

165. *New Orleans Medical and Surgical Journal* quoted in *B Med Surg J* (1846), 35:542; Jon Palfreman, "Mesmerism and the English Medical Profession: A Study of a Conflict," *Ethics in Science & Medicine* (1977), 4(1–2):51–66. For the ways in which mesmerism contributed to the acceptance of anesthesia, see ch. 4 below.

4. THE BENEFITS OF ANESTHESIA

1. Valentine Mott, *Pain and Anaesthetics: An Essay Introductory to a Series of Surgical and Medical Monographs* (1863), p. 8. For similar praise of anesthesia based on the "evil" of pain, see: Simpson, *Anaesthesia*, p. 232; Edward Warren, review of *Etherization in Childbirth*, p. 300; Harvey, "Ether, in Surgical Operations," p. 13; E. Jennie Chapin, "Chloroform," unpublished M.D. thesis, Female Medical College of Pennsylvania, February 1866, in Archives of the Medical College of Pennsylvania, Philadelphia, p. 28. I am indebted to Gina Morantz for helping me gain access to these Archives.

2. For anesthesia as a "moral" reform, see Edward Warren, *An Epitome of Practical Surgery for Field and Hospital* (Richmond: West and Johnson, 1863) quoted in Redding and Matthews, "Anesthesia During the American Civil War," p. 10. This Edward Warren was no relation to the Boston Warrens.

The essential evilness of pain had pre-anesthetic support in the theology of Augustine and Milton and the utilitarian philosophy of Bentham and Mill. See Daniel de Moulin, "A Historical-Phenomenological Study of Bodily Pain in Western Man," *Bulletin of the History of Medicine* (Winter, 1974), 48:540–70; see also the useful references in Maurice B. Strauss, ed., *Familiar Medical Quotations* (1968), pp. 353–354.

3. Mott, *Pain and Anaesthetics*, p. 5. For versions of the "boon to suffering humanity" quote, see Mott, "Remarks on the Importance of Anaesthesia from Chloroform in Surgical Operations, Illustrated by Two Cases," *Transactions of the New York Academy of Medicine* (1847–1857), 1:85; *AJMS* (1852), 23:192; Bowditch, *History of Massachusetts General Hospital* (1851), p. 218; *B Med Surg J* (1848), 38:255; (1847), 37:275, 346; Governor George N. Briggs to John Collins Warren, January 21, 1848, John C. Warren Papers, vol. 23, item 35; Harvey, "Ether, in Surgical Operations," p. 17; Clarke, "Anaesthesia in Surgery," p. 8; Eliza L. S. Thomas, "On the Propriety of Anaesthetic Agents in Surgical Operations," unpublished M.D. thesis, Female Medical College of Pennsylvania, February 1855, p. 1. And that is only a small sample.

For an introduction to the philosophical issues besetting a simple identification of pain with evil, see R. M. Hare, "Pain and Evil," *Proceedings of the Aristotelian Society* (1964), suppl. vol. 38:91–106; Abraham Edel, "Happiness and Pleasure," *Dictionary of the History of Ideas* (1973), 2:374–87; Roger Trigg, "The 'Evil' of Pain," in *Pain and Emotion* (1970), pp. 58–60; George Pitcher, "The Awfulness of Pain," *Journal of Philosophy* (July 23, 1970), 67:481–92. In an historical context, see Judith N. Shklar, "Putting Cruelty First," *Daedalus* (Summer, 1982), 111(3):17–27.

4. Thomas F. Harrington, *Harvard Medical School, A History*, (1905), 2:594; Bowditch, *History of Massachusetts General Hospital* (1851), p. 218; Enoch Hale to John Collins Warren, January 17, 1848, John C. Warren Papers, vol. 23, item 31; Thomas, "On the Propriety of Anaesthetic Agents," p. 2. See also Paul F. Eve, "Report of Operations performed under Anaesthetic Agents," *Southern Medical and Surgical Journal* (1849), n.s. 5:278.

5. Simpson to Ramsbotham, November 17, 1852, Ramsbotham Papers, emphasis

in original; for similar analogy between anesthesia and the abolition of lashing in the military, see Simpson to Ramsbotham, October 9, 1852, Ramsbotham Papers. Ramsbotham's reply was direct and to the point: "I really cannot see the least analogy between flogging female slaves and refusing to exhibit a poisonous gas. . . ." Ramsbotham to Simpson, November 29, 1852, Ramsbotham Papers.

Such advocates as Simpson portrayed anesthesia as a major feminist triumph and attacked critics as callous toward female suffering. For a typical American example, see I. R. Walker, "Anaesthesia and Anaesthetics," unpublished M.D. thesis, University of Michigan, 1862, p. 14.

Another popular analogy, at least on the level of metaphor, was between the use of anesthesia and the abolition of corporal punishments in the schools. See "The Use of Chloroform," *Punch*, February 5, 1848, quoted in R. M. Weller, *"Punch, On Anesthesia,"* *Anaesthesia* (1976), 31:1267–68; cartoon by "Cham" reprinted in the *Journal of the History of Medicine and Allied Sciences* (October 1946), 1:611.

For historians who have portrayed the introduction of anesthesia as linked to the humanitarian and benevolent spirit of the age, see Shryock, *Development of Modern Medicine,* p. 175; E. Douglas Branch, *The Sentimental Years, 1836–1860,* (1934, reprinted 1965), pp. 264–65; Kern, *Anatomy and Destiny,* p. 75; De Moulin, "Bodily Pain in Western Man"; James Turner, *Reckoning with the Beast: Animals, Pain, and Humanity in the Victorian Mind* (1980), ch. 5.

6. James Y. Simpson, *Answer to the Religious Objections Advanced Against the Employment of Anaesthetic Agents in Midwifery and Surgery* (1847).

7. Mary T. Seelye, "Relief of Pain as a Therapeutical Agent," unpublished M.D. thesis, Female Medical College of Pennsylvania, 1870. For similar arguments offered by non-believers, see Mordecai, "Effects of Chloroform," p. 17; Thompson, "Anaesthesia," p. 2. For the escapability of some pains through the use of reason, see Perry Miller, *The New England Mind: The Seventeenth Century* (1961, 1939), ch. 7; and *The New England Mind: From Colony to Province* (1961, 1953), ch. 21.

8. Thomas, "On the Propriety of Anaesthetic Agents," p. 14.

9. James Turner, "Anesthetics in Surgery and Parturition," unpublished M.D. thesis, University of Michigan, 1871, p. 26.

10. *Western Lancet* (1848), 8:247. See also: *AJMS* (1852), 23:163–64; Hooker, *Physician and Patient,* pp. 87–88.

11. Mott, "Remarks on the Importance of Anaesthesia," p. 86; Edward Warren, review of *Etherization in Childbirth,* p. 300. See also: *Ohio Medical and Surgical Journal* (1849), 2:72–79; "Report on Obstetrics and Diseases of Women," *Ninth Annual Meeting of the Illinois State Medical Society* (1859), p. 89. On the conflict between physicians and clergy, see Kett, *Formation of the American Medical Profession,* pp. 116–130.

12. Warren, *Etherization,* p. 68.

13. Shattuck, *Report,* pp. 293, 292. Shattuck was not as consistent in blaming the victims for their own pains as this quote implies. He also tells the parable of a virtuous country girl who moves to the city and is unable to fight off the vicious influences of her environment, pp. 267–68. Shattuck's report was as doctrinally eclectic as Mann's reports (which, interestingly, Shattuck quotes on pp. 293–94 in support of individual responsibility for pain).

14. Rosenberg, *Cholera Years,* chs. 7, 8, and 12. For a good discussion of the moral blindness of mechanical natural laws, see Francis Wayland, *The Elements of Moral Science,* edited by Joseph Blau (1963), pp. 100–21. "There is associated with natural laws no system of mercy; that dispensation is not revealed in Nature, [but] is contained in the Scriptures . . . ," explained Yale scientist Benjamin Silliman, quoted in Branch, *Sentimental Years,* p. 275.

15. Edward Warren, review of *Etherization in Childbirth,* p. 313. Austin Flint's review took a very similar approach, *Buffalo Medical Journal* (1848), 3:281. For an attack on Simpson as a zealous feminist, see Farr, "Opposition to Anaesthesia," p. 900. See also ch. 3 above for attacks on ether as philanthropy.

16. *Western Lancet* (1847), 6:56, emphasis in original; Warren, review of *Etherization in Childbirth,* pp. 301, 311. See also: "Report on Obstetrics and Diseases of Women," *Ninth Annual Meeting of the Illinois State Medical Society* (1859), p. 88; Henry, "Etherization, as a Surgical Remedy," p. 8; Friend, "Anaesthesia in Labour," p. 15; Mary T. Seelye, "Relief of Pain as a Therapeutical Agent." Not all pre-anesthetic physicians agreed; see Pascalis, "Theory of Pain," p. 31.

17. De Moulin, "Bodily Pain in Western Man," p. 559, traces the concept from the Greeks, through the Arab Avicenna, to modern times.

18. For the influence of anesthesia on the philosophical "mind-body problem," see the section on medical philosophy in ch. 11 below.

19. J. Mason Warren to W. H. Bissel, January 18, 1852, John C. Warren Papers, vol. 23, items 95, 97. For similar opinions, see: "Report of Medical Society of Virginia," p. 191; Joseph Pancoast, in Flagg, *Ether and Chloroform,* p. 147; Mott, "Remarks on the Importance of Anaesthesia," p. 86; William H. Van Buren, "Amputation at the Hip-Joint," *Transactions of the New York Academy of Medicine* (1847–1857), 1:130; Horner, "Anaesthetics," p. 24.

For transcripts of a major medical debate on whether anesthesia caused or prevented shock, see *Bulletin of the New York Academy of Medicine* (1864), 2:327–45. See also William M. Boling, "Remarks on the Use of Anaesthetic Agents, More Especially in Parturition," *New-Orleans Medical and Surgical Journal* (1851–52), 8:429–30; and also English, *Crile.*

20. Horner, "Anaesthetics," pp. 23–24; *Transactions of the College of Physicians of Philadelphia* (1846–1849), 7:404–7. See also Clarke, "Anaesthesia in Surgery," p. 7; Harvey, "Ether, in Surgical Operations," p. 13. For a pre-anesthetic view, see Samuel D. Gamble, "On the Influence of Pain in the Production of Death," *Southern Medical and Surgical Journal* (1838), 2:712.

21. Eve, "Report of Operations Performed Under Anaesthetic Agents," p. 278. For other claims that pain causes infection by lowering vital energy, see: Samuel D. Gross, "The Factors of Disease and Death After Injuries, Parturition, and Surgical Operations," *Reports and Papers, American Public Health Association* (1874–1875), 2:400–14, reprinted in *Medical America in the Nineteenth Century,* p. 191; "Painless Operations in Surgery," *Littell's Living Age* (June 1847), 13:492; Clarke, "Anaesthesia in Surgery," p. 7; Thomas, "On the Propriety of Anaesthetic Agents," p. 11.

Vitalist doctrines were used to marshall criticisms of anesthesia (see ch. 3, note 52) as well. The issue was whether pain *enhanced* or *depleted* vital energies.

22. Edward Warren, review of *Etherization in Childbirth,* p. 301. See also Mordecai, "Effects of Chloroform," pp. 22–24.

23. *B Med Surg J* (1866), 75:273–76, quoted in Wertz and Wertz, *Lying-In,* p. 118. H. R. Storer, leader of the medical crusade against abortion, agreed, Storer, *Eutokia: A Word to Physicians and to Women Upon the Employment of Anaesthetics in Childbirth* (1863), p. 6. Elimination of the pain of childbirth had other social benefits as well; it might make sex more enjoyable (or at least less traumatic) for Victorian ladies and thus help avoid race suicide, see Wertz and Wertz, *Lying-In,* p. 118. For a later period, see Lawrence G. Miller, "Pain, Parturition, and the Profession: Twilight Sleep in America," in *Health Care in America: Essays in Social History,* edited by Susan Reverby and David Rosner (1979), p. 28. On abortion in general, see James C. Mohr, *Abortion in America: The Origins and Evolution of National Policy* (1978).

24. Mott, "Remarks on the Importance of Anaesthesia," pp. 85, 86. See also John Collins Warren to George W. Norris, March 6, 1848, John C. Warren Papers, vol. 26.

25. Markwart Michler, "Medical Ethics in Hippocratic Bone Surgery," *Bulletin of the History of Medicine* (July–August 1968), 42:298.

26. Walt Whitman, "Song of Myself," and "The Wound-Dresser," in *Leaves of Grass,* (1958), pp. 79, 253; building on Whitman's imagery, T. S. Eliot portrayed Christ as a surgeon, "wounded" by his own "sharp compassion," T. S. Eliot, "East Coker," in "Four Quartets," *Complete Poems and Plays, 1909–1950* (1952), p. 127. I am indebted to Richard Selzer of Yale for this citation. See also Fredrickson, *Inner Civil War,* p. 93. A full discussion of surgical attitudes toward inflicted pain is presented in ch. 5 below.

27. William Lawrence to John Collins Warren, February 24, 1848, John C. Warren Papers, vol. 23, item 51; Jonathan Frederick May, "Cases of Amputation," *AJMS* (1851), 22:329.

28. Edward H. Horner, "Anaesthetics," unpublished M.D. thesis, University of Pennsylvania, February 1855, p. 1.

29. *AJMS* (1852), 23:449.

30. Robert Druitt, *Principles and Practice of Modern Surgery,* p. 592. Other quotes are from Thomas, "Propriety of Anaesthetic Agents," p. 9; Chapin, "Chloroform," p. 24; Henry, "Etherization as a Surgical Remedy," p. 8.

31. Peter Van Buren, "Anaesthesia," *Transactions of the Medical Society of the State of New York* (1858), pp. 70–77, provides one of the fuller lists of uses; Turnbull, *Artificial Anaesthesia,* pp. 135–44.

32. *American Journal of Insanity* (1865), 22:77, 59.

33. Druitt, *Principles and Practice of Modern Surgery,* p. 592; Gross, *System of Surgery,* p. 535; *AJMS* (1849), 18:514. For other specific examples of cases where anesthesia was useful to subdue patients, see Thomas, "On the Propriety of Anaesthetic Agents," pp. 8–10; Mordecai, "Effects of Chloroform," p. 24. The specific types of cases in which such control was believed especially important are discussed in ch. 8 below; my assessment of the frequency and significance of such cases in practice is in ch. 11 below.

The same *AJMS* article claimed that anesthesia was used "by way of experiment in ordinary cases, where there was no very definite object in view."

34. *The Semi-Centennial of Anaesthesia* (1897), p. 29.

35. Simpson to Ramsbotham, May 1, 1847, Ramsbotham Papers; see also Simpson, *Account of a New Anaesthetic Agent, as a Substitute for Sulphuric Ether in Surgery and Midwifery* (Edinburgh: Sutherland and Knox, 1847), reprinted in *Milestones in Anesthesia,* edited by Cole, p. 96. For an excellent discussion of this issue in a later period, see Judith Walzer Leavitt, "Birthing and Anesthesia: The Debate over Twilight Sleep," *Signs* (Autumn, 1980), 6:147–64.

36. Flagg, *Ether and Chloroform,* pp. 127–28; Mrs. Mann to Horace Mann, April 4, 1848, Mann Papers; Warren, *Etherization,* p. 76.

37. Jackson, *Manual,* pp. 7–8. Some critics of anesthesia regarded sensitivity to pain as an essential prerequisite for human freedom (see ch. 3 above). But others saw sensitivity as a source of slavery, because the capacity to suffer puts mankind at the mercy of those with the power to inflict suffering. For an example, see Hayman, "Economy of Pain." See also Flagg, *Ether and Chloroform,* p. x.

38. Warren, quoted in Raper, *Man Against Pain,* p. 94. Bigelow, "Insensibility During Surgical Operations," pp. 311–13; Harvey, "Ether in Surgical Operations," p. 18.

39. Bigelow, "Insensibility During Surgical Operations," pp. 311–13.

40. Henry Jacob Bigelow, "A History of the Discovery of Modern Anaesthesia," in *A Century of American Medicine, 1776–1876,* by Edward H. Clarke, et al. (1876), p. 87;

Hodges, *Introduction of Ether*, p. 23; Edward Warren, review of *Etherization in Childbirth*, p. 312. See also *B Med Surg J* (1846), 35:425; Bowditch, *History of Massachusetts General Hospital* (1851), p. 220; Frank K. Boland, *The First Anesthetic: The Story of Crawford Long* (1950), p. 46; J. Collins Warren, "Notes on the Discovery of Surgical Anesthesia," (1914), introduction to vol. 23 of John C. Warren Papers; Fülöp-Miller, *Triumph Over Pain*, pp. 94–110; Harvey, "Ether, in Surgical Operations," p. 4.

41. Flagg, *Ether and Chloroform*, pp. 19, 22. Interestingly enough, drug-experimenting students of the late 1960s and early 1970s revived this use of anesthetics. History is blended with recipes in Michael Shedlin and David Wallechinsky [The East Bay Chemical Philosophy Symposium] eds., *Laughing Gas: Nitrous Oxide* (1973). A more traditional account is Frederick B. Glaser, "Inhalation Psychosis and Related States," *Archives of General Psychiatry* (1966), 17:315–22. See also William U. Storms, "Chloroform Parties," *Journal of the American Medical Association* (July 9, 1973), 225:160.

42. Shedlin and Wallechinsky, *Laughing Gas*, chs. 7 and 9; Mostert, "States of Awareness During General Anesthesia," p. 75; Suzanne Hoover, "Coleridge, Humphry Davy, and Some Early Experiments with a Consciousness-altering Drug," *Bulletin of Research in the Humanities* (Spring, 1978), 81:9–27.

43. National Library of Medicine, Bethesda. Note the intertwined legs of the center figures. Robert Seymour (d. 1836) was a follower of noted illustrator George Cruikshank. Cruikshank may have drawn a version of this subject as well though I have not been able to locate a copy. I am grateful to Elizabeth E. Roth, Keeper of Prints, The New York Public Library, for the attribution and to Susan Badder for the information on Cruikshank. The original color print was signed by publisher T. McLean and dated "1/1/1830." See also Jürgen Thorwald, *The Century of the Surgeon* (1957), following p. 80.

44. February 6, 1847, quoted in Weller, "*Punch*, on Anaesthesia," p. 1268; in this case it was the *man* who used anesthetics to escape from his torment into hallucinogenic bliss.

45. December 18, 1847, quoted in Weller, "*Punch*, on Anaesthesia," p. 1271–72. In general, the British seem to have led in the development of such materials, the Americans copying or plagiarizing rather than innovating; but that was true of nineteenth-century humor magazines in general.

46. These included: heart, lung, and nerve diseases, plus wound infection, see ch. 3 above.

47. For specific attempts to refute each charge, see the notes to ch. 3 above.

48. *AJMS* (1850), 19:419, quoting the AMA Committee; *Western Lancet* (1847), 6:182; Lyman, *Artificial Anaesthesia*, p. 73. See also: "Report of a Committee of the Boston Society for Medical Improvement, on the Alleged Dangers Which Accompany the Inhalation of the Vapor of Sulphuric Ether," *B Med Surg J* (October 1861), 65:236, 241; *AJMS* (1850), 19:471; Thompson, "Anaesthesia," pp. 14–15; *AJMS* (1853), 25:519; Clarke, "Anaesthesia in Surgery," pp. 15, 28; Henry H. Smith, *The Principles and Practice of Surgery*, (1863), 1:170; Jona[than] Letterman, Circular Letter of October 30, 1862, in *Reports on the Operations of the Inspectors and Relief Agents of the Sanitary Commission, after the Battle of Fredericksburg . . .* , Sanitary Commission Document No. 57 (1862), pp. 6–8 (hereafter cited as Letterman, Circular Letter, for pp. 6–8, and as Sanitary Commission Document No. 57, for the entire document). I am indebted to Morris Vogel for calling my attention to this document.

49. For a good discussion of danger and professionalization, see Nicholas M. Greene, "A Consideration of Factors in the Discovery of Anesthesia and their Effects on its Development," *Anesthesiology* (1971), 35:521–22; Greene, *Anesthesiology and the University* (1975), p. 15.

50. *AJMS* (1850), 20:69, 149. See also John Bell, *A Treatise on Baths* (1859), p. 303. For the view that anesthetics *had* to be dangerous to work, see ch. 5 below.

51. Bigelow, "Insensibility During Surgical Operations," p. 316.

52. "Painless Operations in Surgery," *Littell's Living Age* (June 1847), 13:483–84; *B Med Surg J* (1846), 35:324.

53. George Rosen, "Mesmerism and Surgery: A Strange Chapter in the History of Anesthesia," *Journal of the History of Medicine and Allied Sciences* (October 1946), 1:527–50. The best study of the political implications and philosophic place of mesmerism in its initial phase is Robert Darnton, *Mesmerism and the End of the Enlightenment in France* (1968). See also: Jacques M. Quen, "Case Studies in Nineteenth Century Scientific Rejection: Mesmerism, Perkinsism, and Acupuncture," *Journal of the History of the Behavioral Sciences* (April 1975), 11:149–56; Fred Kaplan, "The Mesmeric Mania: The Early Victorians and Animal Magnetism," *Journal of the History of Ideas* (October–December 1974), 35:691–702.

54. This section draws together material presented in chs. 3 and 4. Only statements not previously documented here are footnoted, along with a few additional examples.

55. See also Ridings, "Anaesthetics," pp. 12, 27–28.

56. Contrast Giles, "Origin of Pain," pp. 2, 31, with Campbell, "Thesis on Anaesthesia," p. 26.

57. P. W. Allen, "On the Advantages of Anaesthesia and the Relative Value of Its Different Agents," *Eclectic Medical Journal* (October 1850), 2:434.

58. King, *Eclectic Obstetrics;* Hill, *Eclectic Surgery,* pp. 208–9.

59. Hill, *Eclectic Surgery,* pp. 208–9.

60. King, *Eclectic Obstetrics,* p. 656; [Walter Burnham,] "Chloroform: Its Advantages Over Ether As An Anaesthetic Agent," *Publications of the Massachusetts Eclectic Medical Society* (1860–1872), pp. 35–45.

61. Allen, "Advantages of Anaesthesia," p. 435; [Burnham,] "Chloroform."

62. Berman, "Neo-Thomsonianism," pp. 149–50.

63. See also ch. 5 below.

64. Medical concern over patient autonomy involved scientific, as well as social and professional, issues. Based on their environmentalist scientific theories, many nineteenth-century physicians considered the social and emotional aspects of the doctor-patient relationship to be a potent force in speeding or slowing recovery from disease. However, physicians could not agree whether medical paternalism or lay self-determination constituted the most health-promoting professional role. See Pernick, "Patient's Role."

65. Youngson, *Scientific Revolution,* and Farr, "Opposition to Anaesthesia," report no evidence of theological opposition in Britain.

5. ANESTHESIA AND THE ORIGINS OF UTILITARIAN PROFESSIONALISM

1. *AJMS* (1852), 23:455. Sargent's own position was somewhat more restrictive about the types of circumstances in which anesthesia was justified than were the views adopted by most physicians, but his statement about the nature of the choice accorded well with the majority view of the situation.

2. Mott, *Pain and Anaesthetics,* p. 8; see also J. C. Warren, "On the Use of Anaesthetics," *Trans AMA* (1850), 3:387. Porter, "Medical and Surgical Notes," *AJMS* (1852), 23:33. There were only a handful of surgeons who came close to denying that anesthesia had *any* valid drawbacks; one was Harvey, "Ether, in Surgical Operations," pp. 7–8, 9. See also ch. 6, notes 29–32 below.

3. Porter, "Medical and Surgical Notes," *AJMS* (1852), 23:33; *Trans AMA* (1848), 1:176. For identical sentiments, see Horner, "Anaesthetics," p. 29.

4. "Suffering" refers to the *emotional* effects of pain, as distinguished from its

physical effect on the body. Whereas most nineteenth-century physicians separated these two aspects of pain, many were imprecise in their language, and others rejected the mind-body duality that this distinction implies. Thus, while I have tried to keep the terms separate whenever appropriate, it is not always possible to distinguish the physical from the emotional aspects of "pain" as used by nineteenth-century physicians.

5. *Trans AMA* (1849), 2:246; *NYJ Med* (March 1848), 10:243; Gregory, *Man-Midwifery*, p. 43; see also ch. 4, notes 16–24 above.

6. For present-day problems that raise similar issues, see note 134 this chapter, below.

7. See ch. 2 above.

8. William Potts Dewees, *An Essay on the Means of Lessening Pain, and Facilitating Certain Cases of Difficult Parturition* (1806), p. 43; Dewees, "Examination of Dr. Osburn's Opinion," p. 278.

However, one pre-anesthetic heroic practitioner denied that pain was a disease, Pascalis, "Theory of Pain," p. 31.

9. Shafer, *American Medical Profession*, pp. 140–41. For the classical observation that one pain can block perception of another, see Hippocrates, *Aphorisms*, 2:46, in *Hippocrates*, W. H. S. Jones, trans. (1931), 4:119.

10. Dewees, *Lessening Pain and Facilitating Parturition;* Dewees, "Examination of the Physical Necessity of Pain." Dewees was uncertain whether the pain itself was a disease, whether it was caused by a disease of the nerves, or whether it was caused by a disease of the uterus; see "Examination of Dr. Osburn's Opinion," pp. 272, 280; A. Clair Siddall, "Bloodletting in American Obstetric Practice, 1800–1945," *Bulletin of the History of Medicine* (Spring, 1980), 54:101–110.

11. Edward Warren, review of *Etherization in Childbirth*, p. 314; "Report on Obstetrics and Diseases of Women," Illinois State Medical Society, p. 96; see also *AJMS* (1852), 23:193, 280; *AJMS* (1851), 22:112; Thompson, "Anaesthesia," p. 24. Dickson, "Introductory Lecture on Pain and Death," p. 56; *Dental Cosmos* (1869), 11:48.

See also Catherine M. Scholten, " 'On the Importance of the Obstetrick Art': Changing Customs of Childbirth in America, 1760–1825," *William and Mary Quarterly*, (July 1977), 3d ser. 34:439–40.

12. Boling, "Remarks on Anaesthetic Agents," p. 287.

13. H. R. Storer, "As to the Practically Absolute Safety of Profoundly Induced Anaesthesia in Childbirth as Compared with its Employment in General Surgery," *Edinburgh Medical Journal* (1877), 22:741–43. Barker, "Anaesthetics in Midwifery," *Transactions of the New York Academy of Medicine* (1857), 2:255.

14. King, *Eclectic Obstetrics*, p. 506; see ch. 4 above.

15. "Report of the Medical Society of Virginia," p. 182.

16. William E. Horner to John Collins Warren, January 18, 1848, John C. Warren Papers, vol. 23, item 33. See also Robley Dunglison to John Collins Warren, January 29, 1848, John C. Warren Papers, vol. 23, item 40; Morton, *Letheon Circular*, pp. 42–47; Thompson, "Anaesthesia," p. 15; Kidd, *Manual*, p. 193.

17. [Samuel Gridley Howe], *Report of a Minority of the Special Committee of the Boston Prison Discipline Society, Appointed at the Annual Meeting, May 27, 1845* (1846), p. 43. Howe was speaking of penology, using the metaphorical comparison with medicine and contrasting the "curative" with the punitive functions of punishment. I have not been able to ascertain Howe's opinions on the use of anesthesia; he was no longer actively practicing medicine at this time. For Howe's hydropathy, see Schwartz, *Howe*, p. 93. Gastineau, "Sick and Suffering Sisterhood."

18. Reprinted in *Buffalo Medical Journal* (1848), 3:677. See also the homeopathic

endorsement in McClelland, "Dissertation on Anaesthesia in Labor," p. 7. Duns, *Simpson*, p. 222.

19. John Upton Riggs, "Anaesthetics," unpublished M.D. thesis, University of Michigan, 1868, pp. 8–9. See also notes 132–34 this chapter.

20. James Jackson to John Collins Warren, February 12, 1849, in John C. Warren Papers, vol. 23, item 72; *Ohio Medical and Surgical Journal* (1848), 1:200; *AJMS* (1867), 53:181; Thomas Bryant, *The Practice of Surgery* (1873), p. 927.

21. Flint, "Conservative Medicine," in *Medical America*, p. 138; Duns, *Simpson*, p. 256.

22. T. Gaillard Thomas, *Introductory Address Delivered at the College of Physicians and Surgeons, New York, October 17th, 1864* (New York: Trafton, 1864), p. 31, as quoted in Rosenberg, "Therapeutic Revolution," p. 498. For many similar examples, see Warner, "Nature-Trusting Heresy," e.g., p. 317.

23. *AJMS* (1851), 21:493.

24. *Phil Med Ex* (June 1847), n.s. 3:380. See also "Report of the Standing Committee for the Year 1849," *Transactions of the Medical Society of New Jersey* (1766–1858), 1:455.

25. *Edinburgh Review* (1850), 92:12, quoted in Richard H. Shryock, "The History of Quantification in Medical Science," *Isis* (June 1961), 52:233.

26. *AJMS* (1852), 23:156; Hooker, *Physician and Patient*, pp. 53, 54–55, 57.

27. Mott, *Pain and Anaesthetics*, p. 8. See also Mott, "Remarks on the Importance of Anaesthesia," p. 86; Harvey, "Ether, in Surgical Operations," p. 9.

28. Friend, "Anaesthesia in Labour," p. 14; *Western Lancet* (1848), 7:362; *NYJ Med* (March 1848), 10:243; Daniel Henry Muir, "Anaesthesia," unpublished M.D. thesis, University of Michigan, 1871, pp. 22–23. See also Horner, "Anaesthetics," p. 23; Mordecai, "Effects of Chloroform," p. 19.

29. *Western Lancet* (1847), 6:55–56, emphasis in original.

30. Henry, "Etherization, as a Surgical Remedy," pp. 8–9. See also *AJMS* (1852), 23:449; "Report of the Medical Society of Virginia," p. 181. Emphasis in original.

31. Shryock, "History of Quantification," p. 233.

32. For a few examples see *AJMS* (1851), 21:178–83; (1852), 23:450–55; (1854), 28:13–20; *Trans AMA* (1848), 1:214–21; George W. Norris, "Statistical Account of the Cases of Amputation Performed at the Pennsylvania Hospital From January 1, 1850, to January 1, 1860 . . . ," *Pennsylvania Hospital Reports* (1868), 1:149–64.

The errors, discussed in my assessment of the data in ch. 11 below, consisted primarily of failure to print the cases in which anesthesia had not been used, failure to control for other variables in a time series, and inaccuracies in recording the actual administration of anesthetics to specific patients. The concept of statistical controls was still extremely new and had not been widely disseminated. For one example, see "Report of the Medical Society of Virginia," p. 182.

33. Flint, "Conservative Medicine," p. 135; Bowditch, in Kaufman, *Homeopathy*, p. 112. For similar emphasis on synthesis and anti-extremism as the key to conservative medical ideology, see Bigelow, *Brief Expositions*, esp. pp. 16–17; Austin Flint, "Remarks on the Numerical System of Louis," *New York Journal of Medicine and Surgery* (1841), 4:283–303.

34. In *Illness as Metaphor*, Susan Sontag argues that the metaphorical use of disease and medicine obscures our understanding of these vital matters (1978). For my criticism of this view, see *Journal of the History of Medicine and Allied Sciences* (1980), 35:346–48; see also Owsei Temkin, "Metaphors of Human Biology," in *Double Face of Janus*.

Aileen S. Kraditor, *Means and Ends in American Abolitionism: Garrison and His*

Critics on Strategy and Tactics, 1834–1850 (1969, 1967), esp. chs. 2 and 4; John Demos, "The Anti-slavery Movement and the Problem of Violent 'Means,' " *New England Quarterly* (December 1964), 37:501–26.

35. Howard Mumford Jones, ed., *Emerson on Education*, (1966), p. 224. Emerson declared the difference between use of "this drug, and the . . . following of nature," to be "precisely analogous to the difference between the use of corporal punishment and the methods of love." Emerson denounced the use of force as "this quack practice," and advised instead to "adopt the pace of Nature."

36.

Nor is severe punishment to be regarded as the "last resort." When it may be inflicted at all, it is the first resort, and the true remedy. Allow me to illustrate: A skilful physician is called to prescribe for a patient. . . . If the doctor resorts to herb drinks and tonics in the case supposed, he is a quack, and his patient will die while the tender hearted simpleton is experimenting upon him. But the *"calomel"* is given and the patient recovers. So with punishment. . . . [I]f the case is one that requires great severity, that kind of punishment must be inflicted promptly and faithfully,

Hiram Orcutt, *The Discipline of the School* (1881, 1871), p. 8. Note that the issue here is not just pain vs. painlessness but Art vs. Nature. For other approving comparisons between the art of the heroic physician and the art of the flagellating schoolmaster, see: *New York Teacher* (1852–1853), 1:301; *Teachers' Advocate* (1845), 1:55; *Massachusetts Teacher* (1848), 1:274; (1849), 2:9.

Horace Mann humorously compared the total abolition of corporal punishment with the medical doctrines of Sylvester Graham, see Massachusetts *Common School Journal* (May 1841), 3:154.

37. *New York Tribune,* May 29, 1862, as quoted by Robert F. Durden, "Ambiguities in the Antislavery Crusade of the Republican Party," in *The Antislavery Vanguard,* p. 384.

John Brown was not the only advocate of violent means to combine medical and religious metaphors in support of bloodletting. For lesser known uses of the medical metaphor, see Daniel Aaron, *The Unwritten War: American Writers and the Civil War* (1975, 1973), pp. 19, 118, 174; Wilson, *Patriotic Gore,* p. 347.

38. Hydropathist Mary Gove Nichols compared "the lancet, and poison, and operative surgery," to the "hangman, general, or jailor," in "Woman the Physician," *Water-Cure Journal* (October 1851), 12:3. For the links between nonresistance and vegetarianism, see William S. Tyler to Edward Tyler, October 10, 1833, reprinted as "Grahamites and Garrisonites," [edited] by Thomas H. Le Duc, *New York History* (April 1939), 20:189–91. For the areas of ideological overlap in general, see Walters, *Antislavery Appeal.* Thomas James Mumford, *Memoir of Samuel Joseph May* (1873), pp. 174, 186, 259, contains a few additional glimpses. See also Robert S. Fletcher, "Bread and Doctrine at Oberlin," *Ohio State Archeological and Historical Quarterly* (January 1940), 49:58. I am indebted to Gina Morantz for this last citation.

39. Hawthorne thus advocated only a limited war for the border states and compared the process to the way a conservative surgeon would conduct an amputation. See Aaron, *Unwritten War,* p. 47.

Horace Mann was extremely fond of using the conservative physician's calculus of suffering as a model to explain his self-professedly moderate stand on corporal punishment.

We do not then inflict punishment wholly because it is deserved; but we inflict it that we may ward off a greater evil by a less one,—a permanent evil by a temporary one. We administer it, only as a physician sometimes administers poison to a sick man,—not because poison is congenial to the healthy system, nor, indeed because poison is congenial to the diseased system;

but because it promises to arrest a fatal malady . . . . [T]he evil of punishment should always be compared with the evil proposed to be removed by it; and, in those cases only, where the evil removed preponderates over the evil caused, is punishment to be tolerated,

Horace Mann, *Lectures on Education* (1855), p. 304. See also *Annual Reports of the Secretary of the Board of Education of Massachusetts; Fourth Annual Report, for 1840,* in *The Life and Works of Horace Mann* (1891), 3:66; *Ninth Annual Report, for 1845,* in *Life and Works,* 4:40; Louis Filler, ed., *Horace Mann On the Crisis in Education,* (1965), pp. 148–49, 190–91.

But Mann hoped that with the gradual perfection of humanity, eventually both dangerous drugs and physical punishments might *almost* be eliminated. "When the arts of health and of education are understood, neither poison nor punishment will need to be used, unless in most extraordinary cases," *Fourth Annual Report, for 1840,* in *Life and Works,* 3:66.

For a similar use of the conservative calculus to justify a cost-benefit approach to school punishments, see *Massachusetts Teacher* (1848), 1:253. See also Kraditor, *Means and Ends,* pp. 28, 179–89.

On physical punishments, see Myra Glenn, *Campaigns Against Corporal Punishment* (forthcoming); Carl F. Kaestle, "Social Change, Discipline, and the Common School in Early Nineteenth-Century America," *Journal of Interdisciplinary History* (Summer, 1978), 9:1–17.

40. For Whitman's identification with the language of conservative medicine, see notes 109–12 this chapter, below. Interestingly, while most metaphors for the war involved the *inflicted* pains of amputation, bloodletting, etc., Whitman chose to see the war in terms of *natural* pain, "the parturition years" of the new Union, quoted in Aaron, *The Unwritten War,* pp. 56–57.

41. For various uses of the heroic *metaphor* by opponents of heroic medical *practice,* see Aaron, *The Unwritten War,* p. 28, quoting Dr. Oliver Wendell Holmes; Schwartz, *Samuel Gridley Howe,* pp. 201–22 for Howe's support of John Brown's efforts to purge the land with blood; for a general account of the conversion of pre–war pacifists to the use of force, see Fredrickson, *Inner Civil War,* esp. p. 61. A well-known example is Horace Bushnell, "Our Obligations to the Dead," (1865), reprinted in *The American Evangelicals, 1800–1900: An Anthology,* edited by William G. McLoughlin (1968), p. 155.

42. James Y. Simpson, "Account of a New Anaesthetic," reprinted in *Milestones in Anesthesia,* edited by Cole, p. 97. For a current example, see *New England Journal of Medicine* (June 7, 1979), 300:1330.

43. For an extended discussion of professionalism, its definition, functions, and historical evolution, see the afterword, below.

44. Quoted in James Crewdson Turner, "The Emergence of a Modern Sensibility: Love for Animals and the Anglo-American Mind," a longer unpublished draft version of his *Reckoning with the Beast* (1977).

45. T. S. Eliot, "East Coker," in "Four Quartets," *Complete Poems and Plays, 1909–1950* (1952), p. 127.

46. Rice, *Trials of a Public Benefactor,* p. 42. For similar descriptions, see *New York Herald,* July 21, 1841; Youngson, *Scientific Revolution,* pp. 24–39.

47. Michler, "Medical Ethics," pp. 298–300. On this question, however, ancient medicine was far from unanimous; see below.

48. Michler, "Medical Ethics," p. 301. Hippocratic doctrine permitted the use of anodynes but only if they were deemed completely safe; see Seeman, *Man Against Pain,* pp. 57–58.

49. Celsus, *De Medicina,* translated by W. G. Spencer, Loeb Classical Library (3 vols, Cambridge, Mass.: Harvard University Press, 1935–38), 3:297; quoted in Guido Majno, *The Healing Hand: Man and Wound in the Ancient World* (1975), p. 355. See also de Moulin, "Pain in Western Man," p. 561; Robinson, *Victory Over Pain,* pp. 12, 21.

50. Stephen W. Williams, *American Medical Biography* (1967 reprint of 1845 edition), pp. 445–46.

51. Sykes, *Hundred Years of Anesthesia,* 2:169, quoting the *Lancet,* June 30, 1877, p. 934; Dickinson Crompton, "Reminiscences of Provincial Surgery," *Guy's Hospital Reports* (1887), 29:144. For a similar American account, see Stephen Smith's description of his first operation experience—the 1847 nonanesthetized reduction of a strangulated hernia in a laborer, "Reminiscences of Two Epochs: Anaesthesia and Asepsis," *Bulletin of the John Hopkins Hospital* (1919), 30:273–78.

52. Samuel Cooper, *A Dictionary of Practical Surgery,* (1822), 2:443. For an American example, see the biography of Joseph Parrish in Williams, *American Medical Biography,* p. 435. For Darwin, see Donald Fleming, "Charles Darwin, the Anaesthetic Man," *Victorian Studies* (March 1961), 4:219–36; Youngson, *Scientific Revolution,* p. 26.

Of course, the discovery of anesthesia did not wholly eliminate the need for professional socialization as a defense against pain, as Merton, Becker, and others have shown. One of the more sensitive recent sociological studies is Wendy Carlton, *"In Our Professional Opinion": The Primacy of Clinical Judgement Over Moral Choice* (1978).

53. Samuel Rezneck, "A Course of Medical Education in New York City in 1828–29: The Journal of Asa Fitch," *Bulletin of the History of Medicine* (November–December 1968), 42:560, 561.

54. J. Collins Warren, *Influence of Anaesthesia on the Surgery of the Nineteenth Century* (1906), p. 4. See also Smith, *Principles and Practice of Surgery,* 1:175–76.

55. Berlant, *Profession and Monopoly,* p. 86.

56. *AJMS* (1852), 23:453. See also Rothstein, *American Physicians,* p. 252.

57. John Pearson, *Principles of Surgery* (1832), p. vii. This was the American edition of a 1788 London publication. Before the discovery of ether, only 15 percent of those admitted to the *surgical* wards of the Massachusetts General Hospital ever received any *operative* surgical treatment. Massachusetts General Hospital, Surgical Casebooks.

58. See ch. 3, note 57 above.

59. Benjamin Rush, *Sixteen Introductory Lectures to Courses of Lectures Upon the Institutes and Practice of Medicine* (1811), p. 213; Coulter, *Science and Ethics,* p. 56.

60. For testimony on the physical painfulness of heroic bloodletting, see Blackwell, *Pioneer Work,* pp. 41, 206. For examples of Rush's nationalistic propaganda, see Rush to John Coakley Lettsom, May 13, 1804, in *Letters of Benjamin Rush,* 2:881–82. See also Coulter, *Science and Ethics,* pp. 56–57.

61. Anthony A. Benezet, *The Family Physician* (Cincinnati: W. H. Woodward, 1826), quoted in John B. Blake, "From Buchan to Fishbein: The Literature of Domestic Medicine," in *Medicine Without Doctors,* edited by Guenter B. Risse, Ronald L. Numbers, and Judith Walzer Leavitt (1977), p. 16.

". . . it is better to urge the expulsion of the cause of disease even by the increase of irritation and pain . . . ," agreed one young frontier practitioner in 1850, Samuel Willard to Dear Father, July 4, 1850, Samuel Willard Papers, Illinois State Historical Society Library, Springfield, also quoted in Jack Northrup, "Letters of a Frontier Doctor," *Bulletin of the History of Medicine* (January–February 1973), 47:89. For more on American nationalism and painful medicine, see Kaufman, *Homeopathy,* pp. 9–11; and Ronald L. Numbers and John Harley Warner, "The Maturation of American Medical Science," in *Scientific Colonialism, 1800–1930: A Cross-Cultural Comparison,* edited by Nathan Reingold and Marc Rothenberg (forthcoming).

62. Rothstein, *American Physicians,* p. 221; see ch. 3 above.

63. Williams, *American Medical Biography,* p. 537. Though they portrayed themselves as frontiersmen and did spend varying amounts of time in isolated rural areas while perfecting their innovations, all these men were highly trained, relatively well traveled and basi-

cally cosmopolitan in outlook. See also sketch of John Hart, in Williams, p. 231; Flexner, *Doctors on Horseback*.

James Eckman, "Anglo-American Hostility in American Medical Literature of the Nineteenth Century," *Bulletin of the History of Medicine* (January 1941), 9:31–71; Allen O. Whipple, *The Evolution of Surgery in the United States* (1963), pp. 5, 16; *Trans AMA* (1848), 1:287.

64. William Gibson, *The Institutes and Practice of Surgery*, (1827), 1:123.

65. Thompson, "Anaesthesia," p. 10. For suffering as "trivial," see Clarke, "Anaesthesia in Surgery," pp. 4–5, paraphrasing Magendie; the original is quoted by S. W. Barker, "Anesthesia," p. 457.

66. *AJMS* (1852), 23:193, emphasis in original.

67. *B Med Surg J* (1870), n.s. 5:147; *Ohio Medical and Surgical Journal* (1857), 9:333. For similar sentiments, see *NYJ Med* (1848), 10:243; *Ohio Medical and Surgical Journal* (1850), 2:203.

68. Horner, "Anaesthetics," pp. 29–31; *Trans AMA* (1849), 2:246; *NYJ Med* (March 1848), 10:243; Gregory, *Man-Midwifery*, p. 43. See also: *Western Lancet* (1847), 6:56; *American Journal and Library of Dental Science*, quoted in Rice, *Trials of a Public Benefactor*, p. 117; *B Med Surg J* (1846), 35:447; Mohr, *Abortion*, p. 34.

69. Mott, *Pain and Anaesthetics*, p. 8; John Erichsen, *The Science and Art of Surgery*, edited by John H. Brinton (1854), p. 29; C. R. Gilman, quoted in the *AJMS* (1852), 23:192, emphasis in original. See also *British Medical Journal* quoted in *B Med Surg J* (1870), n.s. 5:145; Thomas, "On the Propriety of Anaesthetic Agents," pp. 13–14, emphasis in original. *Dental Cosmos* (1866), 7:634.

70. Dickson, "Pain and Death," p. 61. By the 1870s in Britain, a few physicians and others were publicly urging mercy killing; the agent suggested from the very first was chloroform, W. Bruce Fye, "Active Euthanasia: An Historical Survey of Its Conceptual Origins and Introduction to Medical Thought," *Bulletin of the History of Medicine* (1979), 52:492–502, esp. 498. By 1905, Dr. William Osler lightheartedly suggested chloroforming everyone at age sixty. He got the idea from Anthony Trollope's midcentury story, "The Fixed Period," see Osler, *Aequanimitas; With Other Addresses*, (1906), pp. 391–411. According to Arthur Schlesinger Jr., President William Howard Taft endorsed Osler's idea as a way of disposing of ex-presidents, *Parade Magazine*, June 21, 1981, p. 6.

71. G. W. Peck, "On the Use of Chloroform in Hanging," *American Whig Review* (September 1848), 8:283–96; Henry J. Bigelow, "Execution by Hanging," in *Surgical Anaesthesia: Addresses and Other Papers* (1900) pp. 376–78. For one of the earliest reports of such an execution, see the *Brooklyn Daily Eagle*, May 3, 1847, p. 2, col. 3.

72. Warren, *Etherization*, p. 70. See also Jackson, *Manual*, pp. 101–4; Jackson reprints many of Warren's cases and adds a few of his own. Turnbull, *Artificial Anaesthesia*, pp. 59–61, and p. 262 for anesthetics and active euthanasia of animals by the SPCA.

For the wary reaction of American Catholics to anesthetic euthanasia, see "The Moral Limit in the Use of Anaesthetics," *American Ecclesiastical Review* (1890), 3:198–204.

73. John Duffy, "Science and Medicine," in *Science and Society in the United States*, edited by David D. Van Tassel and Michael G. Hall (1966), p. 122; Austin Flint, "Conservative Medicine," in *Medical America*, edited by Brieger, p. 141; *AJMS* (1852), 23:394; Fülöp-Miller, *Triumph Over Pain*, p. 72; Rothstein, *American Physicians*, pp. 190–94; Warner, "Physiologic Theory"; David T. Courtwright, *Dark Paradise: Opiate Addiction in America before 1940* (1982), pp. 42–54; H. Wayne Morgan, *Drugs in America: A Social History 1800–1980* (1981). An 1884 survey found morphine to be the second most commonly prescribed drug in Boston, Coulter, *Science and Ethics*, p. 377.

74. J. Mason Warren to Isaac Parrish, March 28, 1848; John Collins Warren to

Isaac Parrish, April 30, 1848, both in Warren Family Papers, vol. 26. Manuscript notes of lecture by Henry H. Smith, taken by John Hainson Rodgers, n.d., in the margins of Henry H. Smith, *Syllabus of the Lectures on the Principles and Practice of Surgery, Delivered in the University of Pennsylvania* (Philadelphia: T. K. and P. G. Collins, Printers, 1855), p. 35, located in the Special Collections, George Harrell Library, Penn State University College of Medicine, Hershey, Pa. See the full debate on this issue in *Trans AMA* (1850), 3:331–38, esp. 333.

75. S. W. Mitchell, *Injuries of Nerves and Their Consequences* (1872); Ronald Melzack, *The Puzzle of Pain* (1973), p. 61. Charles W. Parsons of Rhode Island actually had begun such experiments as early as 1850, see *AJMS* (1851), 21:306–19.

76. For a popular-history account, see Fülöp-Miller, *Triumph Over Pain*, chs. 3–7.

77. Darrel Amundsen, "The Physician's Obligation to Prolong Life: A Medical Duty without Classical Roots," *The Hastings Center Report* (August 1978), p. 27.

78. De Moulin, "Bodily Pain," p. 562. However, Galen "abhor[red] more than anyone" the use of soporific drugs, presumably including most narcotics, Robinson, *Victory Over Pain*, pp. 12, 21.

79. For other examples, see Robinson, *Victory Over Pain;* Strauss, *Familiar Medical Quotations*, p. 410.

The barber-surgeon, Bailly of Troyes, was prosecuted at the instigation of Guy Patin, the leader of the Paris physicians, see Fülöp-Miller, *Triumph Over Pain*, pp. 21–23. Patin sought to prevent *any* use of internal medicines by barber-surgeons, but he was particularly opposed to the danger of their giving narcotics. See Francis R. Packard, *Guy Patin and the Medical Profession in Paris in the Seventeenth Century* (1925), p. 239, on this specific antipathy. See also Toby Gelfand, *Professionalizing Modern Medicine: Paris Surgeons and Medical Science and Institutions in the Eighteenth Century* (1980); Robinson, *Victory Over Pain*, p. 40.

80. De Moulin, "Pain in Western Man," p. 554. For nineteenth-century reference to Bacon's precedent, see *Westminster Review* (1859), 71:70.

81. John Gregory, *Lectures on the Duties and Qualifications of a Physician* (London: W. Strahan, 1772), p. 37, quoted in Laurence B. McCullough, "Historical Perspectives on the Ethical Dimensions of the Patient-Physician Relationship: The Medical Ethics of Dr. John Gregory," *Ethics in Science and Medicine*, (1978), 5(1):52, and 49 for the influence of Hume and Bacon.

82. Percival, *Medical Ethics*, pp. 71, 98, 221, for both codes. Relieving pain was not the only duty that Percival held might outweigh the duty to preserve life; Percival also believed a doctor's obligations to the state could require medical participation in criminal trials, whippings, and executions, e.g., pp. 161–65. See also Dickson, "Pain and Death," p. 55.

83. *Christian Examiner* (May 1842), 32:268. The Unitarian *Examiner*, however, doubted whether homeopathy could be proved to work. They took a skeptical attitude toward the claims of all curative systems, including homeopathy.

84. Blackwell, *Pioneer Work*, p. 41; *B Med Surg J* (1847), 36:128; Coulter, *Science and Ethics*, pp. 114–18.

85. Coulter, *Science and Ethics*, p. 162.

86. Campbell, "Thesis on Anaesthesia," p. 32.

87. Oliver Wendell Holmes, *Medical Essays, 1842–1882* (1892), p. 365.

88. Coulter, *Science and Ethics*, pp. 371–73. For orthodox attacks on the stoicism required by homeopathy, see Bigelow, *Rational Medicine*, p. 43; *Western Lancet* (1848), 8:312.

89. *Transactions of the Homeopathic Medical Society of the State of New York*, (1865), pp. 121–28.

90. *Philadelphia Bulletin*, "Female Physicians," reprinted in *The Water-Cure Journal* (January 1860), 29:3–4.

91. Herman Melville, *White-Jacket*, edited by Hennig Cohen (1967, 1850), p. 249.

92. Melville, *White-Jacket*, p. 250.

93. Bigelow, "Inaugural Lecture," in *Surgical Anaesthesia*, p. 226; Hooker, *Physician and Patient*, pp. 385–89, and quotation in *AJMS* (1852), 23:158; Stevens quote in *Trans AMA* (1848), 1:30, quoted by Barbara Rosenkrantz, "The Search for Professional Order," p. 113. See also Kidd, *Manual*, p. 193.

94. *B Med Surg J* (1849), 40:370; Rosenberg, *Cholera Years*, p. 156. Rothstein, *American Physicians*, p. 221.

95. Duffy, *Public Health in New York*, p. 466; Rothstein, *American Physicians*, p. 221.

96. Thompson, "Anaesthesia," pp. 8–9.

97. Hooker, *Physician and Patient*, pp. 385–89, emphasis in original. See also *AJMS* (1852), 23:175; *Western Lancet* (1848), 8:128. Compare these nineteenth-century views with Osler's *Aequanimitas* of 1889.

98. Bigelow, *Rational Medicine*, pp. 52–53. See also Charles H. Sackrider, "Ether and Chloroform," unpublished M.D. thesis, University of Michigan, 1856, pp. 29–30; Blackwell, *Pioneer Work*, p. 56; Thomas, "On the Propriety of Anaesthetic Agents," pp. 2, 13.

99. Lamentations 3:64–65 (Revised Standard Version). The King James Version reads "sorrow of heart" rather than "hardness"; "hardness" is clearly the correct translation, but the Revised Standard Version was not published until 1881. For Sigourney, see *Oven Birds*, pp. 57–72.

There are many excellent studies of this literature. I have found the most useful to be: Barbara Welter, "The Cult of True Womanhood," *American Quarterly* (Summer, 1966), 18:151–74; and Christopher Lasch, "The Woman Reformer's Rebuke," in *The World of Nations* (1974).

100. See ch. 3, note 107 above, and Alexis de Tocqueville, *Democracy in America* (1945), 2:222–23. James H. Averill, *Wordsworth and the Poetry of Human Suffering* (1980).

101. John William Ward, *Andrew Jackson, Symbol for an Age* (1955). Ward does not mention this aspect of Jackson's appeal, however. Hickory is a tough wood, second only to birch as a favorite switch of schoolmasters. Richard Slotkin, *Regeneration Through Violence: The Mythology of the American Frontier, 1600–1860* (1973); W. Eugene Hollon, *Frontier Violence* (1974); F. O. Matthiessen, *American Renaissance* (1941), pp. 641–45; Wilson, *Patriotic Gore*, pp. 507–18. See also Nicholas M. Greene, "A Consideration of Factors in the Discovery of Anesthesia and their Effects on Its Development," *Anesthesiology* (1971), 35:517.

102. Lewis O. Saum, "Death in the Popular Mind of Pre-Civil War America," *American Quarterly* (December 1974), 26:483–84; Daniel J. Boorstin, *The Americans: The National Experience* (1967, 1965), pp. 101–104; Peter G. Filene, *Him/Her/Self: Sex Roles in Modern America* (1975). However, one must be wary of reading back the Social Darwinism and Taylorism of the turn of the century into the earlier period, especially by lumping them all together as "modernization."

103. Nancy F. Cott, *The Bonds of Womanhood: "Woman's Sphere" in New England, 1780–1835* (1977), offers perceptive comments on this dichotomy and traces its roots to before the Victorian era.

104. See also Fleming, "Charles Darwin."

105. Walt Whitman, "Song of Myself," in *Leaves of Grass* (1958), p. 68.

106. Whitman, "Song of Myself," p. 78.

107. Whitman, "Song of Myself," p. 79.

108. Whitman, "A Song of Joys," in *Leaves of Grass*, pp. 162, 163.

109. Harold Aspiz, *Walt Whitman and the Body Beautiful*, (1980), p. 37; see also p. 97.

110. Whitman, "Song of Myself," p. 94.

111. Whitman, "The Wound-Dresser," in *Leaves of Grass*, pp. 253, 254. See also "Hospital Scenes and Persons," in *Specimen Days*, in *The Portable Walt Whitman*, edited by Mark Van Doren (1945), p. 508.

112. Whitman, "A Woman Waits for Me," in *Leaves of Grass*, p. 106. In poems like "I Sit and Look Out," and "To a Foil'd European Revolutionaire," Whitman expresses a passive acceptance of suffering. But this passivity is only half of Whitman's response to pain. Its antithesis comes in the active relief provided by the "Wound Dresser." The flaw in Whitman's synthesis is not simply that he accepts suffering as "necessary" but that he varies what is "necessary" according to his perceptions of individual need—a flaw he shared with conservative medicine; see chs. 6 and 11 below.

For Whitman's basically conservative response to anesthetics, see *Brooklyn Daily Eagle*, October 14, 1847, p. 2, col. 3.

113. For versions of varying sophistication, see Kaufman, *Homeopathy;* Rothstein, *American Physicians*, pp. 125–73, 217–43.

114. James, "Essay on Surgery," p. 27, (1857).

115. Campbell, "Thesis on Anaesthesia," pp. 28, 31, (1866); McClelland, "Dissertation on Anaesthesia in Labor," pp. 12, 15, (1867); Ridings, "Essay on Anaesthetics," pp. 27–29, (1868).

116. *Hahnemannian Monthly* (1868–69), 4:180.

117. John M. Criley, "Anaesthesia in Labor," unpublished M.D. thesis, Homoeopathic Medical College of Pennsylvania, 1869, p. 19, see also p. 9; in Hahnemann University Archives, Philadelphia.

118. Gilchrist, *Syllabus*, pp. 20–22.

119. John K. Wade, "Dissertation on Anaesthetics in Labor," unpublished M.D. thesis, Hahnemann Medical College, 1882, pp. 2–3, 8–9, Hahnemann University Archives, Philadelphia.

120. *Transactions of the Homoeopathic Medical Society of the State of New York* (1865), p. 67; Gilchrist, *Syllabus*, p. 20.

121. Bullard, "Thoughts About Doctors," pp. 354, 355.

122. Miller, "Pain, Parturition, and the Profession," pp. 31–32.

123. Gastineau, "Sick and Suffering Sisterhood"; Schwarz, *Kellogg*, pp. 55–56, 112; Gaustad, *Rise of Adventism*. In 1873, Russell T. Trall allowed that anesthesia might be used in "exceedingly dangerous, painful, or protracted" operations, though he "always" preferred "magnetism" in susceptible individuals; *The Hydropathic Encyclopedia* (1873), 2:331.

124. This consideration of pain, suffering, and danger by no means exhausts the list of advantages and disadvantages that had to be weighed in anesthetic decisionmaking. For example, many physicians saw anesthesia as posing a conflict between their own medical judgment and the desires of their patients. These doctors had to choose between paternalism and autonomy as the proper form of professional-client relationship. Since midcentury environmental medicine insisted that both too much and too little freedom could directly cause disease, the question of how much choice to allow patients in therapy involved both technical and ethical considerations; see Pernick, "Patient's Role."

While some physicians insisted on absolute paternalism, and others lauded patient choice (see chs. 3 and 4 above), most adopted an intermediate approach. Following such models as Worthington Hooker, and Thomas Percival's widely cited injunction to unite "authority" with "condescension," *Medical Ethics*, p. 71, conservative surgeons like Frank Hamilton and Alfred C. Post allowed patients to have their own way in the use of anesthetics, but only when they absolutely demanded it, *Bulletin of the New York Academy of Medicine* (1864), 2:333; Hamilton, *Military Surgery*, pp. 622–23; Raper, *Man Against Pain*, pp. 105–6. However, in practice, most physicians seem to have been more flexible; for my assessment of actual practice see ch. 11 below.

125. Versions of the hedonistic calculus were, however, discussed by Enlightenment American intellectuals; see Garry Wills, *Inventing America: Jefferson's Declaration of Independence* (1978), chs. 10, 18, 20, and 23; see also Howard Mumford Jones, *The Pursuit of Happiness* (1966, 1953). For the influence on Edwards and Hopkins, see McLoughlin, *American Evangelicals,* p. 7; for the nineteenth century see Wayland, *Elements of Moral Science,* pp. 89–93. See also Paul A. Palmer, "Benthamism in England and America," *American Political Science Review* (October 1941), 35:855–71.

For American ambivalence toward utilitarian calculation in general, see Patricia C. Cohen, "A Calculating People: The Origins of a Quantitative Mentality in America," unpublished Ph. D. dissertation, University of California, Berkeley, 1977; Ralph Lerner, "Commerce and Character: The Anglo-American as New-Model Man," *William and Mary Quarterly* (January 1979), 3d ser. 36:3–26; and especially, Perry Miller, "The Romantic Dilemma in American Nationalism," in *Nature's Nation,* pp. 199–201. For the slowness of both the utilitarian calculus and the probability calculus to influence American medicine, see Shryock, "Quantification in Medical Science," pp. 224–25, 233; Estes, *Hall Jackson.* For the development of medical statistics and controlled studies before Louis, see Abraham Lilienfeld, "*Ceteris Paribus:* The Evolution of the Clinical Trial," *Bulletin of the History of Medicine* (Spring, 1982), 56:1–18.

126. Kidd, *Manual,* unpaginated front leaf.

127. Charles D. Meigs, *Females and Their Diseases* (1848), pp. 311–13; see also Rosenberg, "Therapeutic Revolution," p. 503.

128. See, for example, the furor provoked among conservatives by Surgeon General Hammond's attempt to completely ban calomel; Gert Brieger, "Therapeutic Conflicts and the American Medical Profession in the 1860s," *Bulletin of the History of Medicine* (May—June 1967), 41:215–22. For the belief that conservatism would legitimate the moderate continuation of nonanesthetic surgery, see *Buffalo Medical Journal* (1848), 3:70; for conservatism as sanctioning the moderate use of unpopular anesthetics, see Frederick D. Lente, "Anesthesia in Surgery. How its Dangers are to be Avoided," *NYJ Med* (1855), n.s. 15:196. See also Austin Flint, quoted in Warner, "Nature-Trusting," p. 316.

129. Rosenberg, "Therapeutic Revolution," pp. 503–504.

130. Warner, "Nature-Trusting"; Bryan, "Bloodletting."

131. Druitt, *Principles and Practice of Surgery,* p. 594. See also James Jackson to John Collins Warren, February 12, 1849, in Warren Papers, vol. 23, item 72.

132. Kidd, *Manual,* p. 90.

133. Bryant, *Practice of Surgery,* p. 927; *Ohio Medical and Surgical Journal* (1848), 1:200; McClelland, "Dissertation on Anaesthesia in Labor," p. 8; see also Boling, "Remarks on Anaesthetic Agents," pp. 431, 433.

134. *AJMS* (1867), 53:181. Youngson, *Scientific Revolution,* pp. 87–88, understands that anesthetic use involved a risk-benefit calculation, but he overlooks the ethical and professional dimensions of such decisions. Thus, he erroneously concludes that, by 1850, it had been proved that chloroform was safe and should have been used, p. 214.

For present-day ethical and scientific issues in medical utilitarianism, see The Hastings Center, "Values, Ethics, and C.B.A. in Health Care," *The Implications of Cost-Effectiveness Analysis of Medical Technology* (1980), pp. 168–82; Gina Bari Kolata, "Clinical Trials: Methods and Ethics are Debated," *Science* (1977), 198:1127–31; William W. Lowrance, *Of Acceptable Risk: Science and the Determination of Safety* (1976); Renée C. Fox, "The Evolution of Medical Uncertainty," *Milbank Memorial Fund Quarterly* (Winter, 1980), 58:1–49.

135. For the present/future issue, see *AJMS* (1852), 23:394.

136. The problem of applying the universal laws of biology to the individualized art of patient care has interesting parallels with the question of "rule" utilitarianism. See John Rawls, "Two Concepts of Rules," J. J. C. Smart, "Extreme and Restricted Utilitarianism,"

and H. J. McCloskey, "An Examination of Restricted Utilitarianism," all in *John Stuart Mill, Utilitarianism,* edited by Samuel Gorovitz (1971), pp. 175–216.

6. FROM THE UNIVERSAL TO THE PARTICULAR

1. Walter Lowenfels, *Walt Whitman's Civil War* (1961), p. 113.

2. Talcott Parsons regarded universalism as a basic value orientation of professionalism; Merton, Berlant, and others since have pointed out the professional tension between universalism and particularism; see afterword, notes 11–12, below.

3. Some of the following statements applied only to chloroform and are noted as such; others applied to all anesthetics; a few applied only to ether. Today, chloroform is thought to be much more variable in effect from individual to individual than ether is.

4. *AJMS* (1852), 22:497. This article, reprinted from a Dublin journal, used the words "chloroform" and "anaesthesia" interchangeably. The article was strongly endorsed by the editor of the *AJMS,* but it is not clear whether the endorsement was meant to apply to both anesthetics or to chloroform alone. At this time, many British hospitals used only chloroform, but most American hospitals used both agents, see ch. 10 below.

5. Alfred Hunter Voorhies, "Chloroformum," unpublished M.D. thesis, University of Pennsylvania, February 1860, p. 18.

6. Chapin, "Chloroform," pp. 12–13.

7. Lyman, *Artificial Anaesthesia,* pp. 48, 49–50. Lyman regarded his strictures as applying "principally" to chloroform, but even with ether, he felt that the dangers existed and varied significantly from person to person. "No anaesthetic agent can be used without incurring the risk of a certain amount of danger—. . . . Every patient should, therefore, be made an object of careful study before the act of inhalation is commenced, and all possible contraindications should be scrupulously noted," p. 50.

8. *Trans AMA* (1848), 1:183–84.

9. *AJMS* (1850), 19:100.

10. F[itz]W[illiam] Sargent, *On Bandaging and Other Operations of Minor Surgery* (1856), p. 360.

11. *B Med Surg J* (August 1847), 37:32, emphasis in original.

12. Thompson, "Anaesthesia," p. 11. See also *AJMS* (1852), 23:255; Henry, "Etherization, as a Surgical Remedy," p. 10.

13. One possible exception is Hosack, who thought the variability of anesthetics would prove to be "a rare exception comparatively," *B Med Surg J* (August 1847), 37:32.

14. *Trans AMA* (1848), 1:227, 183; see also "Report of the Medical Society of Virginia," p. 198.

15. Flagg, *Ether and Chloroform,* p. 31, emphasis in original; p. 40, emphasis added.

16. *Western Lancet* (1848), 7:362.

17. *Western Lancet* (1848), 7:363, emphasis in original.

18. Friend, "Anaesthesia in Labour," p. 14.

19. *St. Louis Medical and Surgical Journal* (1850), 7:315. The author was afraid ether would be used as indiscriminately as opiates were.

20. Thompson, "Anaesthesia," pp. 7, 11. See also Greene, "Factors in the Discovery of Anesthesia and Its Development," pp. 521–22; Greene, *Anesthesiology and the University,* pp. 15, 42, 148. For a somewhat different assessment of the connection between anesthetic variability and professionalism, see L. D. Vandam, "Early American Anesthetists: The Origins of Professionalism in Anesthesia," *Anesthesiology* (1973), 38:264–74. Vandam does

not take into account the difference between nineteenth- and twentieth-century concepts of professionalism and so concludes that there was no professionalism in anesthesia administration before this century.

21. Thompson, "Anaesthesia," p. 2. Pioneer ether manufacturer Dr. Edward R. Squibb ranked the search for a "universally applicable anaesthetic" among the leading professional "heresies," *New York Medical Journal* (April 1871), 13:385.

22. Illich, *Medical Nemesis,* ch. 3. My disagreement here is not with Illich's point that people today are dependent on medical painkillers but with his historical analysis of how that dependency came about. Illich sees the dependency as caused by the profession; I see it as originating with patient demands. Thus, he feels the problem could be solved by deprofessionalization; I do not.

The only one of John Collins Warren's correspondents who regarded anesthesia as a "panacea" was a lay person, H. A. S. Dearborn to John Collins Warren, January 25, 1848, John C. Warren Papers, vol. 23, item 37. The letter goes on to praise the "certainty" of surgery compared with medicine. Henry Alexander Scammell Dearborn was a Whig politician and son of General Henry Dearborn.

23. See above, ch. 3, note 163, emphasis added.

24. *Western Lancet* (1847), 6:182.

25. *AJMS* (1850), 19:419. See also *AJMS* (1852), 23:255.

26. "Report of the Medical Society of Virginia," p. 198. See also Ramsbotham to Simpson, August 10, 1853, Ramsbotham Papers, for the view that patients' "different constitutions" required a professional to "calculate the exact dose."

27. Smith, *Principles and Practice of Surgery,* 1:170–71. See also ch. 4, notes 48–49 above. Here, it is not simply the presence of danger but its individual variability that necessitates professional control.

28. Greene, "Factors in the Discovery of Anesthesia and its Development," pp. 521–22.

29. Simpson to Ramsbotham, May 1, 1847, Ramsbotham Papers, emphasis in original; Mayo G. Smith, *A Treatise on the Inhalation of Ether for the Prevention of Pain* (1848), bound with Smith, *A Popular Treatise on the Teeth,* pp. 47, 22; for the Poor House, see *AJMS* (1850), 20:341; J. T. Metcalfe, "On the Purity and Use of Chloroform," *Transactions of the New York Academy of Medicine* (1847–1857), 1:149; Chisholm, *Manual,* p. 434, emphasis in original; Bigelow, *Surgical Anaesthesia,* p. 131.

30. Harvey, "Ether, in Surgical Operations," pp. 7–9.

31. Quoted by Eve, "Report of Operations Under Anaesthetic Agents," p. 281. Eve himself, however, cited a few conditions in which he never used anesthetics, other conditions in which he used them only "in some cases," and others for which he used them "in some instances producing only a partial state of insensibility, in all exercising great caution," pp. 279–81.

32. Ramsbotham to Simpson, August 10, 1853, emphasis in original; Simpson to Ramsbotham, August 15, 1853, Ramsbotham Papers.

33. For my assessment of the actual impact of anesthesia on professional power, see ch. 11 below.

34. Simpson, *Anaesthesia,* pp. 246–47. Titles and degrees are as listed on the title page of the Philadelphia edition. See also pp. 234–35. For the role of class and race in pain perception, see ch. 7 below; for the influence of class and race on anesthetization, see chs. 8 and 9 below.

35. In other words, to assess the degree of individualization in any biological theory, it is necessary to specify *both* the amount of variation possible in any one characteristic and the number of characteristics felt to be important.

36. These basic four types, or "temperaments," were expanded by later scholastics to as many as forty different categories, Erwin H. Ackerknecht, "Diathesis: The Word and the Concept in Medical History," *Bulletin of the History of Medicine* (Fall, 1982), 56:319.

37. The discussion above is based on Temkin, *Galenism;* and Rudolph E. Siegel, *Galen's System of Physiology and Medicine* (1968).

38. Rush, "The Progress of Medicine," in *Selected Writings,* pp. 235–36; Charles Caldwell, *Autobiography,* edited by Harriot W. Warner (1968, reprint of 1855 edition), p. 153. See also ch. 2 above.

39. Rush, "The Progress of Medicine," in *Selected Writings,* p. 231; Coulter, *Science and Ethics,* pp. 37–39.

40. Caldwell, *Autobiography,* pp. 185–86.

41. Rush, "The Progress of Medicine," in *Selected Writings,* p. 236.

42. Pernick, "Politics, Parties, and Pestilence," p. 575; Rush, "The Progress of Medicine," in *Selected Writings,* pp. 236–37.

43. Rush, "The Progress of Medicine," in *Selected Writings,* p. 238.

44. See also Berlant, *Profession and Monopoly,* p. 88.

45. Rush, "Observations and Reasoning in Medicine: A Lecture," (1791), in *Selected Writings,* pp. 245–53; Caldwell, *Autobiography,* p. 125.

46. Rush, "The Progress of Medicine," in *Selected Writings,* p. 236.

47. Thatcher, *American Medical Biography* (1967, reprint of 1828 edition), 2:54.

48. Rush to John Coakley Lettsom, May 13, 1804; Rush to John Syng Dorsey, May 23, 1804, in *Letters of Benjamin Rush,* edited by Lyman H. Butterfield (1951), 2:881, 882. See also Rush, "Observations and Reasoning," in *Selected Writings,* pp. 245–53; Rosenberg, "Therapeutic Revolution," p. 494, quoting Elihu Hubbard Smith, *Diary of Elihu Hubbard Smith* (Philadelphia: American Philosophical Society, 1973), September 18, 1795, p. 59. Rosenberg's extremely valuable article does not clearly differentiate between the individualization of *therapeutic modalities* and the individualization of *doses* within a uniform routine therapeutic mode.

49. Benjamin Rush, *An Enquiry into the Effects of Public Punishments Upon Criminals and Upon Society* (1787), reprinted in *A Plan for the Punishment of Crime: Two Essays,* edited by Negley K. Teeters (1954), pp. 11–12. See also Jeremy Bentham, *An Introduction to the Principles of Morals and Legislation,* ch. 14, part 14, rule 6:

> *Attend to circumstances influencing sensibility.* It is further to be observed, that owing to the different manners and degrees in which persons under different circumstances are affected by the same exciting cause, a punishment which is the same in name will not always either really produce, or even so much as appear to others to produce, in two different persons the same degree of pain: therefore
> *That the quantity actually inflicted on each individual offender may correspond to the quantity intended for similar offenders in general, the several circumstances as influencing sensibility ought always to be taken into account,*

in *Philosophical Perspectives on Punishment,* edited by Ezorsky, p. 59, emphasis in original.

50. Rush, *A Plan for the Punishment of Crime,* p. 12; Rush to Jeremy Belknap, June 6, 1791, *Letters of Benjamin Rush,* 1:583.

51. Thomson eventually expanded his list of medicines to six; his followers, however, in an attempt to mystify and professionalize his antiprofessional system, soon added a whole pharmacopoeia of "Thomsonian" medicines. See ch. 2 above, and Rosenberg, *Cholera Years,* p. 71.

52. Coulter, *Science and Ethics,* pp. 41–46.

53. Pernick, "Politics, Parties, and Pestilence," pp. 574, 576.

54. For a similar conflict within English medicine, see Niebyl, "The English Bloodletting Revolution."

55. Williams, *American Medical Biography*, p. 210. Goodhue lived from 1759–1829. In both England and America, such variation of therapy according to social class appealed to many elitists. But, despite Rush's attempts to brand his medical opponents as *all* monarchists, the advocates of class-based distinctions in therapy included many radical democrats as well.

56. Hooker, *Physician and Patient*, p. 56, emphasis added. Hooker still regarded dosage as more variable than the therapeutic modality.

57. Hooker, *Physician and Patient*, p. 57.

58. Flint, "Conservative Medicine," in *Medical America in the Nineteenth Century*, p. 138, emphasis in original.

59. Edward H. Dixon, *Woman and Her Diseases, from the Cradle to the Grave: Adapted Exclusively to Her Instruction in the Physiology of Her System . . .* (1859), p. 49.

60. Flint, "Conservative Medicine," in *Medical America in the Nineteenth Century*, pp. 140–41.

61. Williams, *American Medical Biography*, p. 210, emphasis in original. See also Frank H. Hamilton, "Abuse of Drugs," Address at Buffalo, New York, 1877, clipping in Hamilton Case Book, vol. 12 back end flap.

62. Flint, "Conservative Medicine," in *Medical America in the Nineteenth Century*, p. 141; Hooker, *Physician and Patient*, p. 57; Rothstein, *American Physicians*, pp. 186–96; Smith, "Quinine and Fever."

63. *AJMS* (1850), 19:472.

64. Smith, "Quinine and Fever"; John B. Blake, *Safeguarding the Public: Historical Aspects of Medicinal Drug Control* (1970). It was only after the doctrines of conservative medicine led physicians to concern themselves with quantifying individual differences in dosage that the medical profession really began to take an interest in drug adulteration; before the mid-nineteenth century, physicians simply kept administering a drug until it "worked," without paying much attention to the dosage. Adulteration might defraud the patient, but it was not seen as being a *health*-threatening crime (unless the adulterant was poisonous of course). For the early involvement of conservative physicians with drug purity laws, see *Trans AMA* (1848), 1:311–32.

65. Flint, "Conservative Medicine," in *Medical America in the Nineteenth Century*, pp. 135–36. Professional ideology was part of the paradigm that shaped the physician's concept of what was and what was not medical "knowledge."

66. Quoted in Rosenberg, *Cholera Years*, p. 158, emphasis in original. See Rosenberg, "American Medical Profession: Mid Nineteenth Century," p. 166; *AJMS* (1850), 19:471; Hamilton, "Abuse of Drugs," Case Book 12.

67. For the economics of medical sectarian competition, see Rothstein, *American Physicians;* Paul Starr, "Medicine, Economy and Society in Nineteenth-Century America," *Journal of Social History* (June 1977), 10:588–607; George Rosen, *Fees and Fee Bills: Some Economic Aspects of Medical Practice in Nineteenth Century America, Bulletin of the History of Medicine,* Supplement No. 6 (1946).

68. See notes 59–62 above.

69. For a good analysis of this conflict during the Civil War, see Brieger, "Therapeutic Conflicts." One conservative who did support such a complete ban was New Yorker Stephen Smith.

70. "Routine Practice," *B Med Surg J* (January 11, 1883), 108:42–43; Rosenberg, "Therapeutic Revolution," p. 503.

71. Flint, "Conservative Medicine," in *Medical America in the Nineteenth Century*, p. 138.

72. "Routine Practice," p. 43.

73. *AJMS* (1853), 15:202, emphasis in original.

74. Conservative physicians often concluded that the hard work and frugal life of the industrious poor made them far healthier than the idle, dissipated rich. For the application of such beliefs to class differences in pain sensitivity, see ch. 7 below. For their application to anesthetic use, see chs. 8 and 9 below.

75. Martial Dupierris, "Reduction of a Femoral Dislocation, of Six Months' Standing, by Manipulation," *North American Medico-Chirurgical Review* (Philadelphia) (1857), 1:294. For the converse, a case in which anesthesia was given explicitly to reward a cooperative, noncomplaining patient, see *AJMS* (1851), 22:271.

76. For other examples of racial variations in the prescription of specific medical remedies and their dosages, see: John Stainbach Wilson, "The Negro—His Peculiarities as to Disease," *American Cotton Planter and the Soil of the South* (1859), n.s. 3:229, cited with many other examples in Todd Savitt, *Medicine and Slavery: The Diseases and Health Care of Blacks in Antebellum Virginia* (1978), p. 14. Other racial variations in therapy are prescribed in A. P. Merrill, "An Essay on Some of the Distinctive Peculiarities of the Negro Race," *Memphis Medical Recorder* (1855), 4:15, 136, 138, 326; John S. Haller, "The Negro and the Southern Physician: A Study of Medical and Racial Attitudes, 1800–1860," *Medical History* (July 1972), 16:245, 246, 248, 250, 252. For an interesting example from a British opponent of universal depletion, see Thomas Trotter, *A View of the Nervous Temperament; Being a Practical Inquiry Into the Increasing Prevalence, Prevention, and Treatment of Those Diseases Commonly Called Nervous, Bilious, Stomach & Liver Complaints . . .* (1808), pp. 111, 123, 126, 142, 219. I am deeply in debt to Kurt Zimansky for first mentioning this very useful work to me.

For general accounts of Cartwright and Nott, see William Stanton, *The Leopard's Spots: Scientific Attitudes Toward Race in America, 1815–59* (1960); George M. Fredrickson, *The Black Image in the White Mind: The Debate on Afro-American Character and Destiny, 1817–1914* (1971), ch. 3.

77. *New York Teacher* (1852–1853), 1:70. Identical sentiments, including the medical analogy, are in the *Massachusetts Teacher* (1851), 4:38. See also Michael Katz, *The Irony of Early School Reform: Educational Innovation in Mid-Nineteenth Century Massachusetts* (1968), p. 169.

78. Charles Grandison Finney, *Lectures on Revivals of Religion*, edited by William G. McLoughlin (1960 reprint of 1835 edition) pp. 199, 201. Finney's example too included a medical analogy, p. 199.

79. The relation between changes in professionalism and the discovery of individual variations was noted briefly by Willard Gaylin, *Partial Justice: A Study of Bias in Sentencing* (1975, 1974), pp. 195–96. For a recent assessment of the general problem, see John Higham, "Hanging Together: Divergent Unities in American History," *Journal of American History* (June 1974), 61:5–28; see also Higham, *From Boundlessness to Consolidation: The Transformation of American Culture 1848–1860* (1969); Yehoshua Arieli, *Individualism and Nationalism in American Ideology* (1964). Among the many other works dealing with general aspects of this vast issue are Boorstin, *The Americans: The National Experience;* Rush Welter, *The Mind of America, 1820–1860* (1975); Russel Blaine Nye, *Society and Culture in America, 1830–1860,* (1974). Robert Wiebe, *The Segmented Society: An Historical Preface to the Meaning of America* (1975), does the best job of relating this tension to professionalism. See also Arthur Mann, *The One and the Many: Reflections on American Identity* (1979); and J. R. Pole, *American Individualism and the Promise of Progress* (1980).

80. Quoted in Lowenfels, *Walt Whitman's Civil War*, p. 113. For identical sentiments in an explicitly medical context, see Whitman, *Memoranda During the War*, p. 31.

81. Whitman, "Salut au Monde!" in *Leaves of Grass*, pp. 127–36. Quote is from "Song of Myself," in *Leaves of Grass*, p. 79.

82. For bathing, see *AJMS* (1850), 20:149.

83. *Trans AMA* (1848), 1:183–84.

84. *Trans AMA* (1848), 1:227. An editorially endorsed article in the *AJMS* illustrates the combination of individual variation with particularized rules. While declaring that a physician "cannot be too particular" in "consider[ing] the actual condition of the patient" before using anesthetics, the article also said that individual variations could be codified into "certain rules . . . which should be observed . . . rigidly," *AJMS* (1851), 22:491, 490.

85. The contents of these indications and contraindications are the topic of ch. 8 below.

86. Mott, *Pain and Anaesthetics.*

87. See, for example, Pennsylvania Hospital Fracture Book for 1852, list of rules for keeping of records. See Vogel, "Patrons, Practitioners, and Patients," for the general conflict between managers and physicians.

88. Greene, "Factors in the Discovery of Anesthesia and its Development," pp. 521–22.

89. *British Medical Journal,* quoted in *B Med Surg J* (February 1870), n.s. 5:145; comment, apparently by Jacob Bigelow, in the page proofs of the article. The page proofs are in a collection of uncatalogued "Ether Material," now in the Countway Library of Medicine, Boston, originally donated by William Sturgis Bigelow to the Treadwell Library (and from there donated to the Massachusetts General Hospital).

90. Greene, "Factors in the Discovery of Anesthesia and its Development," pp. 521–22. Interestingly, whereas mesmerism-anesthesia fit the professional requirement for wide individual variations, these variations could not be reduced to rules, no matter how particularized; while uncertainty was good within limits, mesmerism was rejected in part because it exceeded all such limits.

91. Bacon, *Essays,* ed. by Henry Morley (n.d.), no. 30, p. 171. I am indebted to Carol Pollard for this citation.

92. For a general survey of these developments, see Coulter, *Science and Ethics,* pp. 41–46, and ch. 4. In addition to the racial variations cited in note 76 above, see Shafer, *American Medical Profession,* pp. 99, 100, 140; Bryan, "Bloodletting in American Medicine," esp. pp. 518, 526; *AJMS* (1853), 25:30, 202, for an assortment of examples.

93. For a good discussion of Bowditch, see Rosenkrantz, *Public Health and the State,* pp. 57–71. Bowditch, son of a well-known mathematician, believed that therapeutics could truly become a calculus, but he was not as extreme in that regard as some others, notably Edward Jarvis; see Rosenkrantz, p. 47n.

The concept that therapeutic rules could be formulated at some point in between Rush's universalistic rules and the romantic individualism of treating every case as unique was directly linked to the contemporary development of the "specific disease" concept—the idea that there were a large but finite number of specific diseases, rather than Rush's monolithic "fever," or the assertion that every individual's disease was unique; see Rosenberg, "Therapeutic Revolution."

94. For a closely related point, the connection between vital statistics registration and social control, see Jarvis' comments in *AJMS* (1852), 24:150. For beef soup, see Rosenberg, "And Heal the Sick: The Hospital and the Patient," p. 432.

95. Morris Vogel, "The Civil War and the Hospital," unpublished graduate seminar paper, University of Chicago, 1969; Fredrickson, *Inner Civil War,* ch. 7; Letterman, "Circular Letter," in *Sanitary Commission Document No. 57;* Mott, *Pain and Anaesthetics.*

96. Meigs, *Females and their Diseases,* pp. 21–23.

97. T. Childs, *Rational Medicine: Its Past and Present . . .* (New York: Baker & Godwin, 1863), pp. 17, 18, as quoted in Shryock, "The History of Quantification in Medical Science," p. 222.

98. Meigs, *Females and their Diseases,* pp. 311–13.

99. "Routine Practice," p. 43.

100. "Routine Practice," p. 43. See also the comments of Arthur John Brock, M.D., "Introduction," in *Galen On the Natural Faculties* (1963, 1916), p. xxxix:

What Galen combated was the tendency, familiar enough in our own day, to reduce medicine to the science of finding a label for each patient, and then treating not the patient, but the label. (This tendency, we may remark in parenthesis, is one which is obviously well suited for the *standardising* purposes of a State medical service. . . .)

I am indebted to my colleague Jay Gold for this reference, emphasis in original.

101. See note 90 above.

102. *AJMS* (1850), 19:471.

103. Meigs, *Females and their Diseases.*

104. James McNaughton, *Address on the Homoeopathic System of Medicine, February 6, 1838* (Albany: n.p., 1838), p. 26, as quoted in Harris Coulter, "Orthodox and Sectarian Medicine in the United States: The Struggle of the American Medical Association with the Homoeopathic and Eclectic Physicians," a longer typescript version of his *Science and Ethics,* p. 252. This quote is edited to remove the reference to Jews in the published version, p. 168. This attack was against the formularies of homeopathy, but the basic idea applied to orthodox formularies as well, see also Coulter, *Science and Ethics,* p. 169.

Opposition to Morton interestingly included the rumor that he had married a Jew and been circumcised!; see Edward N. Bates to Albert Blodgett, October 17, 1906, Albert Blodgett Papers, Countway Library of Medicine, Boston.

Ironically, it was this same insistence that medicine not be reduced to a formula that, while barring "undesirable" men from the profession, provided an opening for the entry of middle-class native *women.* See Morantz, " 'Connecting Link.' " By the late nineteenth century, the American feminist movement was seriously split between those who saw rights for women as part of a larger movement on behalf of all oppressed groups and those who saw rights for middle-class native white women as a counterbalance to the influence of immigrants and blacks. The story was first outlined by Eleanor Flexner, *Century of Struggle: The Woman's Rights Movement in the United States* (1970, 1959), pp. 142–46, 216–20. See also Jill Ker Conway, "Women Reformers and American Culture, 1870–1930," *Journal of Social History* (1971–1972), 5:164–77; and Lasch, "Woman Reformer's Rebuke," in *World of Nations.*

105. For "niggerology," see Fredrickson, *Black Image,* p. 78.

106. Hooker, *Physician and Patient,* p. 58.

107. Quoted in Lowenfels, *Walt Whitman's Civil War,* p. 113.

108. For "clock-work" see *New York Teacher* (1853–1854), 3:352. For similar use of machine metaphors to praise classroom efficiency, see *Teachers' Advocate* (1845), 1:667; *Massachusetts Teacher* (1851), 4:366–67; and Selwyn K. Troen, *The Public and the Schools: Shaping the St. Louis System, 1838–1920* (1975), pp. 149, 150–51.

For "teaching machine" and "teaching-jenny," as well as "formularies," see *Teachers' Advocate* (1845), 1:179. This volume was misnumbered in places; this page is the *second* of two page 179s. For similar examples of opposition to standarized teaching as machine-like, see *New York Teacher* (1856–1857), 6:165; *Teachers' Advocate* (1845), 1:195, 385, 500, 506.

The *Teachers' Advocate* was the predecessor of the *New York Teacher* as the organ of the New York State Teachers' Association; the *Massachusetts Teacher* was the organ of the Massachusetts Teachers' Association.

109. *New York Teacher* (1853–1854), 2:260, 207–9.

110. See the extremely perceptive comment by David Rothman, *Journal of Interdisciplinary History* (Autumn, 1971), 2:377, in reviewing *Children and Youth in America: A Documentary History,* edited by Robert H. Bremner et al.

111. Katz, *Irony of Early School Reform.*

112. There are interesting similarities and dissimilarities with the process of legal codification, especially in the area of judicial discretion vs. determinate sentencing in criminal cases. For an analytic framework that would have allowed for such comparisons and contrasts, see Miller, *Life of the Mind in America,* Book Two. Legal historians whose works have stressed the nineteenth-century conflict between formal laws and individual judicial discretion include Morton J. Horwitz, Morton White, William Nelson, and Jamil S. Zainaldin. See also Haskell, *Emergence of Social Science.*

Modern social history bears a striking resemblance to nineteenth-century conservative medicine in its attempt to reconcile generalizations with individuality through quantification. But, as with conservative medicine, quantitative history must beware of mistaking particularism for individualism, of assuming that adding more variables to an equation captures the essence of individual variation. Of course, the parallel can be stretched too far, but I believe it is worth serious consideration.

7. "THEY DON'T FEEL IT LIKE WE DO"

1. "Sensitivity" or "sensitiveness" was an everyday word, defined by Francis Wayland as meaning the capacity to be pleased or pained, Wayland, *Elements of Moral Science,* p. 89. "Sensibility" had both a narrow medical and a diffuse general meaning. Medically, as defined by Haller in 1762, "sensibility" referred to the reactiveness of sensory nerves; as contrasted with "irritability," which referred to the reactiveness of muscles. A related term was "excitability," used by vitalists and especially Brounonians to refer to the amount of nerve force. Even in the medical literature, however, both "irritability" and "excitability" were sometimes confused with "sensibility," and used to refer to variations in nerve response. See Albrecht von Haller, "A Dissertation on the Sensible and Irritable Parts of Animals," translated by Owsei Temkin, *Bulletin of the History of Medicine* (October 1936), 4:651–99; Fielding H. Garrison, *Garrison's History of Neurology,* revised by Lawrence C. McHenry, Jr. (1969), pp. 75, 109. But "sensibility" also had a broader, nonmedical meaning in the terminology of Victorian Romanticism, meaning roughly "aliveness and receptivity to sensation and emotion, to the sublime and the pathetic," paraphrasing *OED,* 9:461. All these terms, however, included the concept of "capacity to feel physical pain." The difference between "sensitivity" and "endurance" is discussed at length below. For nineteenth-century American definitions, see John Harrison, "Sensation," *New-Orleans Medical and Surgical Journal* (1849–50), 6:427–28.

For a brief note on the pervasiveness of the assumption that people differed in pain sensitivity, see Charles E. Rosenberg, "Science and American Social Thought," in *Science and Society in the United States,* edited by David D. Van Tassel and Michael G. Hall (1966), p. 137. For a brief provocative explanatory scheme that encompasses such variations, see Wiebe, *Segmented Society,* pp. 87–88. For some already cited nineteenth-century statements of variations in pain sensitivity, see ch. 6, notes 10 and 20 above; Chapin, "Chloroform," pp. 12–13.

2. F[rançois] Magendie, *An Elementary Compendium of Physiology,* translated by E. Milligan (1824), p. 98; see also pp. 99, 115.

3. Ronald Melzack, *The Puzzle of Pain* (1973), chs. 1, 2. For early twentieth-century examples, see note 40 below. For current examples, see note 60 below.

4. Siegel, *Galen's System of Physiology,* p. 209; Temkin, *Galenism,* p. 103. For nineteenth-century survival of temperament as a guide to sensitivity, see P. M. Roget, *Outlines of Physiology* (1839), p. 360; *Dental Cosmos* (1869), 11:230.

5. For important eighteenth-century precedents in France and Scotland, see Martin S. Staum, *Cabanis: Enlightenment and Medical Philosophy in the French Revolution* (1980),

especially pp. 212–31, 257, 311; Christopher Lawrence, "The Nervous System and Society in the Scottish Enlightenment," *Natural Order: Historical Studies of Scientific Culture,* edited by Barry Barnes and Steven Shapin (1979), pp. 19–40.

6. The story of the "Princess on the Pea," for example, first collected by the Grimms, has been traced back to classical India. Stith Thompson, *Motif-Index of Folk-Literature* (1966), 3:375. I am indebted to David Hufford for helping me find my way through the folklore indexes. For more on this story in Victorian society, see note 18 below.

7. Stephen Tracy, *The Mother and Her Offspring* (New York, 1860), p. xv, quoted in Carroll Smith-Rosenberg and Charles Rosenberg, "The Female Animal: Medical and Biological Views of Woman and Her Role in Nineteenth-Century America," *Journal of American History* (September 1973), 60:334; Robley Dunglison, *Human Physiology* (1832), 2:453; Dunglison retained the same passage through many successive editions; see *Human Physiology,* 7th ed. (1850), 2:657; Meigs, *Females and their Diseases,* p. 50; Holmes, *Elsie Venner,* p. 69; *Preamble and Resolution of the Philadelphia County Medical Society upon the Status of Women Physicians, with A Reply by a Woman* (1867) reprinted in *The Female Experience: An American Documentary,* edited by Lerner, p. 409; Morrill Wyman, *Progress in School Discipline: Remarks of Dr. Morrill Wyman, of Cambridge, in Support of the Resolution to Abolish the Corporal Punishment of Girls . . .* (1866), p. 6.

For similar views, see: William B. Carpenter, *Principles of Human Physiology; With Their Chief Applications to Pathology, Hygiene, and Forensic Medicine* (1850), p. 727; Edward Warren, review of *Etherization in Childbirth,* p. 301; Trotter, *A View of the Nervous Temperament,* p. 46; Wertz and Wertz, *Lying-In,* pp. 109–15; Virginia Drachman, "Women Doctors and the Women's Medical Movement: Feminism and Medicine 1850–1895," unpublished Ph. D. dissertation, State University of New York at Buffalo, 1976, p. 47, quoting Silas Weir Mitchell, *Doctor and Patient* (1888), p. 83.

8. Dubos and Dubos, *The White Plague,* pp. 3–10, 44–66 contains an interesting discussion of the larger topic; see also Welter, "Cult of True Womanhood." For similar views, see Ralph Waldo Emerson, "Woman," *The Complete Writings of Ralph Waldo Emerson* (1929), pp. 1178, 1180; William G. McLoughlin, "Introduction," *American Evangelicals,* p. 18, for the views of Henry Ward Beecher; for the Reverend Mr. John Todd of Pittsfield, Mass., see Barker-Benfield, *Horrors of the Half-Known Life,* p. 200.

Feminine hypersensitivity must not be confused with lack of endurance, however; see below.

9. Trotter, *A View of the Nervous Temperament,* p. 22; Porter, "Medical and Surgical Notes," *AJMS* (1852), 24:29. For similar reports, see Rush, "An Account of the Influence of the Military and Political Events of the American Revolution on the Human Body (1788)," in *Selected Writings,* edited by Runes, p. 327; Adams, *Doctors in Blue,* p. 107; see also ch. 8 note 63 below.

For Plato's attempt to separate manly indifference to pain from true virtue, see Daniel T. Devereux, "Courage and Wisdom in Plato's *Laches,*" *Journal of the History of Philosophy* (April 1977), 15:129–41.

10. Mann, *Lectures on Education,* pp. 313–14.

11. Magendie, *Elementary Compendium of Physiology,* pp. 99, 115; Dickson, "Pain and Death," p. 37; Fülöp-Miller, *Triumph Over Pain,* p. 397. For other references to nineteenth-century medical works on aging, see David Hackett Fischer, *Growing Old in America: The Bland-Lee Lectures Delivered at Clark University* (1977), pp. 188–89, and notes 52–54, and the forthcoming work of Carole Haber.

12. *AJMS* (1852), 24:576.

13. Bigelow in *Trans AMA* (1848), 1:211. For similar views, see Rush, *Selected Writings,* edited by Runes, p. 153. For Bentham's reply that both children and the lower ani-

mals should be protected from pain, see *Animals and Man in Historical Perspective,* edited by Joseph and Barrie Klaits (1974), p. 151: "The question is not, Can they *reason?* nor, Can they *talk?* but, Can they *Suffer?"* emphasis in original.

14. Trotter, *A View of the Nervous Temperament,* p. 126. For convergence of female and child roles, see Kuhn, *Mother's Role in Childhood Education.* See also Sheila M. Rothman, *Woman's Proper Place: A History of Changing Ideals and Practices, 1870 to the Present* (1978); and Buchan's *Domestic Medicine* (1790) as quoted in *OED,* 9:461.

15. Tocqueville, *Democracy in America,* 2:137. For a similar critique of democracy as causing extreme sensitivity to pain, see Trotter, *A View of the Nervous Temperament,* pp. xiii–xiv. Though not discussing pain sensitivity per se, a number of historians have documented the nineteenth-century medical concern that democracy caused a wide range of neurological disorders. See Rothman, *Discovery of the Asylum,* pp. 117–18; Sicherman, "The Paradox of Prudence"; George Rosen, "Social Stress and Mental Disease in the Eighteenth to Twentieth Centuries," *Milbank Memorial Fund Quarterly* (January 1959), 37:5–32. For the contrast with the pro–democratic views of Benjamin Rush, see Manfred J. Wasserman, "Benjamin Rush on Government and the Harmony and Derangement of the Mind," *Journal of the History of Ideas* (October–December 1972), 33:639–42.

Middle-class Victorian reformers assumed that the lower classes were insensitive *both* to their own pains and to those of others; see Turner, *Reckoning with the Beast,* eg., p. 27. "Mean" originally meant "common" (and hence "lower class"); but in mid-nineteenth-century America "mean" first took on the added connotations of "vicious," "brutal," or "cruel"; *OED.*

16. De Forest quoted in Fredrickson, *Inner Civil War,* p. 87. See also Trotter, *A View of the Nervous Temperament,* p. 45. The basic idea is quite old; see, for example, Gouge, *God's Arrows* (1631) quoted in *OED,* 5:333.

17. Garrison, *Garrison's History of Neurology,* p. 435, on alcoholic neuritis and hyperaesthesia, discovered as a syndrome in 1822. For similar comments before 1822, see Trotter, *A View of the Nervous Temperament,* pp. 17, 38–40, 70, 136. Arthur MacDonald, *Criminology* (New York, 1893), p. 80, cited in James B. Gilbert, "Anthropometrics in the U.S. Bureau of Education: The Case of Arthur MacDonald's 'Laboratory,' " *History of Education Quarterly* (Summer, 1977), 17:169–95; Nichols, *Forty Years,* 2d ed. (1874), p. 491.

18. The Grimm collection was first published in 1812 and 1815, including the story of "The Princess on the Pea." See note 6 above for the earlier origins of the tale. Although the stories were not available in English in the 1840s, they may well have been known to those Americans conversant with German Romanticism; see Maria Leach, ed., *Dictionary of Folklore, Mythology and Legend* (1949).

19. W. Tyler Smith, *Parturition, and the Principles and Practice of Obstetrics,* 1st American ed. (Philadelphia: Lea & Blanchard, 1849), quoted in *AJMS* (1849), 17:181; Gunning S. Bedford, *Clinical Lectures on the Diseases of Women and Children,* 8th ed. (New York: William Wood & Company, 1867), pp. 4–8, quoted in Martha H. Verbrugge, "Historical Complaints and Political Disorders," *International Journal of Health Services* (1975), 5:323–33; Dewees, "Examination of Dr. Osburn's Opinion of the Physical Necessity of Pain," p. 280. In what is certainly a typographical error, this paragraph goes on to claim that the poor and hardworking suffer more than the dissipated rich. For a 1622 opinion that nursing was more painful for the rich than for the poor woman, see James Axtell, *The School upon a Hill: Education and Society in Colonial New England* (1976, 1974), p. 80. See also the valuable but oversimplified examination of class and sex in Barbara Ehrenreich and Deirdre English, *Complaints and Disorders: The Sexual Politics of Sickness* (1973). For other examples, see Trotter, *A View of the Nervous Temperament,* p. 300; Wertz and Wertz, *Lying-In,* p. 70; William Sweetser, *Mental Hygiene* (1850), p. 323.

20. Ecclesiastes 1:18; Genesis 2:17, 3:16. Perhaps significantly, Eve, Pandora, and Athena, each of whom introduced a new and painful kind of knowledge, were all women: femininity, sensitivity, and culture have long been correlated concepts. The idea that knowledge causes pain is of course the converse of the idea that learning must be painful, see ch. 3, note 112 above.

21. Horace Mann, *Twelfth Annual Report*, in *The Republic and The School*, pp. 81–84; Mann, *Lectures on Education*, pp. 313–14; John Duffy, "Mental Strain and 'Overpressure' in the Schools: A Nineteenth-Century Viewpoint," *Journal of the History of Medicine and Allied Sciences* (January 1968), 23:63–79; Rothman, *Discovery of the Asylum*, pp. 115–21; Grob, *Mental Institutions in America*, pp. 157–58. For other examples, see Amariah Brigham, *Remarks on the Influence of Mental Cultivation and Mental Excitement Upon Health* (1973 reprint of 1833); June A. Kennard, "Review Essay: The History of [Women's] Physical Education," *Signs* (Summer, 1977), 2:835–42; John R. Betts, "American Medical Thought on Exercise, 1820–60," *Bulletin of the History of Medicine* (March–April 1971), 45:138–52; Betts, "Mind and Body in Early American Thought," *Journal of American History* (March 1968), 54:787–805; Trotter, *A View of the Nervous Temperament*, pp. 36, 91.

22. Smith-Rosenberg and Rosenberg, "The Female Animal," p. 336; Vern Bullough and Martha Voight, "Women, Menstruation, and Nineteenth Century Medicine," *Bulletin of the History of Medicine* (January–February 1973), 47:66–82; for related background, see Joan N. Burstyn, "Catharine Beecher and the Education of American Women," *New England Quarterly* (September 1974), 47:386–403; Burstyn "Education and Sex: The Medical Case Against Higher Education for Women in England, 1870–1900," *Proceedings of the American Philosophical Society* (1973), 117(2):79–84; Jill Ker Conway, "Perspectives on the History of Women's Education in the United States," *History of Education Quarterly* (Spring, 1974), 14:1–12; Kennard, "History of Physical Education."

23. Trotter, *A View of the Nervous Temperament*, pp. 247–48 discusses both possibilities; Dewees, "Examination of Dr. Osburn's Opinion, of the Physical Necessity of Pain."

24. Trotter, *A View of the Nervous Temperament*, pp. 21, 22, 38, 151, 155.

25. Griscom, *Uses and Abuses of Air*, pp. 70, 145, also pp. 53, 64, 155; Trotter, *A View of the Nervous Temperament*, pp. 21, 239.

26. The words are those of Hugh Hodge summarizing Dewees' essays, in Williams, *American Medical Biography*, p. 137; Dewees, "Examination of Dr. Osburn's Opinion, of the Physical Necessity of Pain"; Dewees, *Lessening Pain and Facilitating Parturition*, p. 41; Lyman, *Artificial Anaesthesia*, p. 68; Elizabeth Cady Stanton to Lucretia Mott, October 22, 1852, in *Oven Birds*, p. 260; Trotter, *A View of the Nervous Temperament*, p. 32. The view has survived until the present. For the early twentieth century, see Miller, "Pain, Parturition, and the Profession," p. 22. A 1961 text declared birth pain "part of the price of 'civilization' . . . ," see Woolmer, *Conquest of Pain*, p. 85.

Conversely, the opinion that modern civilized women could not stand the pain of birth played a major role in forwarding the fledgling birth control movement of the nineteenth century. See Smith-Rosenberg and Rosenberg, "Female Animal," pp. 345–46.

27. Simpson quoted in Louise Schneider, "Anaesthesia in Natural Labor," unpublished M.D. thesis, Women's Medical College of Pennsylvania, 1879, pp. 34–35; Stanton to Mott, October 22, 1852, in *Oven Birds*, p. 260. For more of Simpson's view, see Simpson, *Anaesthesia*, pp. 234, 235, 246; for more of Stanton's view, see Wertz and Wertz, *Lying-In*, p. 115. See also John S. Haller, Jr. and Robin M. Haller, *The Physician and Sexuality in Victorian America* (1974), p. 10.

28. See, for example, J. T. Clegg, "Some of the Ailments of Woman Due to Her Higher Development in the Scale of Evolution," *Texas Health Journal* (1890–1891), 3:57–59. I am indebted to Gina Morantz for this reference. See also Flavia Alaya, "Victorian Science

and the 'Genius' of Woman,'' *Journal of the History of Ideas* (April–June 1977), 38:263–64; Hayman, "Economy of Pain," p. 24.

29. J. S. Jewell, "Influence of Our Present Civilization in the Production of Nervous and Mental Disease," *Journal of Nervous & Mental Disease* (1881), 8:4, quoted in Rosenberg, "Science and American Social Thought," p. 143; S. Weir Mitchell, "Civilization and Pain," *Journal of the American Medical Association* (1892), 18:108, quoted in de Moulin, "Bodily Pain in Western Man," p. 541, emphasis added.

30. James Fenimore Cooper, *The Pathfinder, Or, The Inland Sea* (1840, reprinted n.d.), p. 33; Rush, "Medicine Among the Indians of North America: A Discussion," (1774), in *Selected Writings*, p. 259; see also Nathan G. Goodman, *Benjamin Rush, Physician and Citizen* (1934), pp. 288–89. Note that Cooper's explanation depends on "natur' " and Rush's on nurture, a point to be developed below. See also Robert F. Berkhofer, Jr., *The White Man's Indian* (1978), pp. 42, 95, but also p. 11.

31. Samuel Stanhope Smith, *An Essay on the Causes of the Variety of Complexion and Figure in the Human Species*, edited by Winthrop D. Jordan, (1965 reprint of 1810 ed., 1st ed. 1787), p. 72; Wertz and Wertz, *Lying-In*, p. 115; Simpson, *Anaesthesia*, p. 246.

32. Thomas F. Gossett, *Race: The History of an Idea in America* (1963), pp. 47–49; Haller, "The Negro and the Southern Physician," p. 246, quoting *Professional Planter: Practical Rules for the Management and Medical Treatment of Negro Slaves in the Sugar Colonies* (London, 1811), pp. 200–1.

33. Cartwright, "Report on the Diseases and Physical Peculiarities of the Negro Race," *New-Orleans Medical and Surgical Journal* 7 (1851), quoted in James O. Breeden, "States-Rights Medicine in the Old South," *Bulletin of the New York Academy of Medicine* (March–April 1976), 52:358. Note that the word "dysaesthesia" derives from the same root as "anaesthesia." See also Haller, "The Negro and the Southern Physician," pp. 244, 249; Cartwright, "Natural History of the Prognathous Species of Mankind," New York *Day-Book*, November 10, 1857, reprinted in *Slavery Defended: The Views of the Old South*, edited by Eric L. McKitrick (1963), p. 142, discussing general differences in neuroanatomy.

34. Merrill, "Distinctive Peculiarities of the Negro," pp. 16–17, 67.

35. George Frederick Holmes, "Uncle Tom's Cabin," *Southern Literary Messenger* (December 1852), 18:721–31, reprinted in *Slavery Defended*, p. 107. See also Fredrickson, *Black Image*, pp. 57, 76; Rosenberg, "Science and American Social Thought," p. 142; *The Pro-Slavery Argument; as Maintained by . . . Chancellor Harper, Governor Hammond, Dr. Simms, and Professor Dew* (1853), pp. 128–29, also pp. 34, 51, 59.

36. Seale Harris, *Woman's Surgeon: The Life Story of J. Marion Sims* (1950), p. 109; Walter F. Jones, "On the Utility of Applications of Hot Water to the Spine in the Treatment of Typhoid Pneumonia," *Virginia Medical and Surgical Journal* (1854), 3:108–10, quoted in Savitt, *Medicine and Slavery*, p. 299; P. M. Kollock, "An Account of Cholera, as It Prevailed in the City of Savannah . . . ," *Southern Medical Journal* (1836), 1:329–30, quoted in Rosenberg, *Cholera Years*, p. 60. Abolitionist Theodore Dwight Weld charged that " 'public opinion' would tolerate surgical experiments, operations, processes, performed upon [slaves], which it would execrate if performed upon their masters or other whites," quoted in Todd L. Savitt, "The Use of Blacks for Medical Experimentation and Demonstration in the Old South," *Journal of Southern History* (August 1982), 48:341.

These patients all had fevers, which supposedly further stupified the Negro sensibility, and which, according to heroic doctrine, required painful counterirritants.

37. For Rush, see Winthrop Jordan, *White Over Black, American Attitudes Toward the Negro, 1550–1812* (1969, 1968), p. 518; for Lincoln, see Wilson, *Patriotic Gore*, p. 109; for Child, see Walters, *Antislavery Appeal*, p. 64; Tocqueville, *Democracy in America*, 1:345; for Watson and Loguen, see John W. Blassingame, *The Slave Community: Plantation Life in*

the Antebellum South (1972), pp. 196–97. See also Smith, *Variety of Complexion in the Human Species*, p. 169.

Others who cited God's beneficence in proportioning sensitivity to circumstances included Rev. Thomas Morong, *The Beneficence of Pain* (1858), p. 7; *Transactions of the New Hampshire Medical Society* (1865), p. 25.

38. Conversely, Henry J. Bigelow concluded that "an intelligent dog" would equal or surpass "a Bushman or a Digger Indian" in suffering during surgery, *Surgical Anaesthesia*, p. 374.

For Olmstead, see Kenneth M. Stampp, *The Peculiar Institution: Slavery in the Ante-Bellum South* (1956), p. 316; for the London journal, see Flexner, *Doctors on Horseback*, p. 143. See also Smith, *Variety of Complexion in the Human Species*, p. 172. Spanish and other dark-skinned women were also supposedly less sensitive than fair-complexioned females; see, for example, Cora in Cooper's *Last of the Mohicans*.

39. For Nott, see Breedon, "States-Rights Medicine," p. 352, quoting "The Mulatto a Hybrid," *AJMS* (1843), 6:252–56; for sentimental novels, see Fredrickson, *Black Image*, p. 118; Merrill, "Distinctive Peculiarities of the Negro," pp. 69–71; Melville, *White-Jacket*, pp. 274–76; see also Carolyn L. Karcher, "Melville's 'The 'Gees': A Forgotten Satire on Scientific Racism," *American Quarterly* (October 1975), 27:421–42.

40. This identification of particular groups as more or less sensitive remained remarkably unaffected by the vast scientific changes in late nineteenth-century medicine. Two new trends did, however, influence such research: specialization and quantification. Anthropologists like Arthur MacDonald, psychologists Joseph Jastrow and James McKeen Cattell, and the founders of criminology, Cesare Lombroso and Salvatore Ottolenghi, now joined with the medical profession to devise instruments to measure precisely the many alleged group differences in pain perception. For typical reports, see: *Proceedings of the National Conference of Charities and Correction* (1895), 22:474–77; Edgar James Swift, "Sensibility to Pain," *American Journal of Psychology* (1899–1900), 11:312–17; Richard J. Behan, M.D. *Pain: Its Origin, Conduction, Perception and Diagnostic Significance* (1915), pp. 111–15, 123; Seeman, *Man Against Pain*, p. 10; Fülöp-Miller, *Triumph Over Pain*, p. 397; *Mind* (1890), 15:373–80; and notes 17, 28, and 29 above. I am grateful to Judith Walzer Leavitt for the first reference and to Michael Sokal for the last.

On every substantive point but one, these late-nineteenth-century studies confirmed the earlier observations outlined in this chapter. However, some of the Italian criminologists believed women were *less* sensitive than men were; Mary Gibson, "On the Insensitivity of Women: Criminological Experiments in Pre-World War I Italy," unpublished paper, Fifth Berkshire Conference on the History of Women, Vassar College, June 18, 1981. Lombroso himself believed only *criminal* women lacked sensitivity to pain; see *The Female Offender* (1915), p. 138. But his daughter Gina and his follower Ottolenghi later reported *all* women to be less sensitive, a radical break from the accepted wisdom; see Gina Lombroso-Ferrero, *Criminal Man* (1911), p. 292; Behan, *Pain*, p. 113.

Behan also cited a *British Medical Journal* report of 1906, which alleged that the "Hebrew" was the "race" most sensitive to pain, but he dismissed this particular claim as propaganda, p. 112.

Sinclair Lewis in 1947 blasted all such research as racist:

. . . Negroes are not human beings . . . . [E]xperiments at the University of Louisiana have conclusively shown, cocoanuts, sledgehammers and very large rocks may be dropped upon their heads without their noticing anything except that they have been kissed by butterflies. This is called Science.

(But what it really all comes down to is, would you want your daughter to marry a nigger?)

Lewis, *Kingsblood Royal* (New York: Random House, 1947), pp. 66–67, quoted in Judith R. Berzon, *Neither White Nor Black: The Mulatto Character in American Fiction* (1978), p. 30.

41. The question of whether these differences were normal or abnormal is related to but *not* the same as whether they were environmental or hereditary. Most nineteenth-century Americans accepted that environmentally acquired characteristics could become hereditary; thus heredity was not necessarily "normal" or permanent. For a good discussion of these issues, see Rosenberg, "The Bitter Fruit."

42. Cooper, *Pathfinder*, p. 33. Fredrickson, *Black Image*, pp. 81–82. Cartwright, interestingly, was an exception. Though he thought blacks were *permanently* insensible and thus fitted for the status quo, he did not see their condition as *normal* but as the result of hereditary *disease*. Cartwright was exceptional in this position, because he was among the few who held that heredity could not be altered by the environment, at least not for victims of "dysaesthesia."

43. For the distinction between those who sought to make slavery more "humane" and those who sought to abolish it, see, for example, Eugene D. Genovese, *In Red and Black: Marxian Explorations of Southern and Afro-American History* (1971), pp. 49–66.

44. Mann, *Lectures on Education*, pp. 313–14; Wyman, *Progress in School Discipline;* Shattuck, *Report*, p. 267; note 37 above.

45. Henry Watson, quoted in Blassingame, *Slave Community*, pp. 196–97. Such testimony may, of course, have been an attempt to live up to stereotypes held by white benefactors, or it may have been a rationalization of shameful behavior aimed at preserving self-respect. Many blacks had other explanations of their seeming insensitivity; see below.

46. Olga Lengyel, *Five Chimnies: The Story of Auschwitz*, p. 20, as quoted by Stanley M. Elkins, *Slavery: A Problem in American Institutional and Intellectual Life*, 2d ed. (1968), p. 109. I cite this example simply to show that repeated abuse can produce a reaction that the victim experiences as numbness. This parallel does not imply that the plantation was a concentration camp nor that such numbness to physical abuse reflected other aspects of slave personality. I do not intend to claim that Southern slavery was unique in this regard; notes 31–32 above contain similar examples from the West Indies, Europe, and colonial Africa too.

Black physician James McCune Smith believed the psychological mechanism we would call "repression" was at work here, rather than the physiological mechanism of "numbness"; see Blassingame, *Slave Community*, p. 132.

47. Trotter, *A View of the Nervous Temperament*, pp. 27, 145; Dewees, "Examination of Dr. Osburn's Opinion, of the Physical Necessity of Pain," pp. 272, 278. See also Smith, *Variety of Complexion in the Human Species*, p. 172.

48. Rush, "Medicine Among the Indians," in *Selected Writings*, p. 259.

49. Historians have recently become aware of the work of anthropologists in reconstructing the enormous toll of white man's diseases on the Indian during the initial phase of exploration of the New World. This literature is ably summarized by Alfred W. Crosby, "Virgin Soil Epidemics as a Factor in the Aboriginal Depopulation in America," *William and Mary Quarterly*, (April 1976), 3d ser., 33:289–99. Less well quantified is the role of missions, schools, reservations, and other "civilizers" in causing further mortality *after* the initial decimations. Virginia Allen, "The White Man's Road: Physical and Psychological Impact of Relocation on the Southern Plains Indians," *Journal of the History of Medicine and Allied Sciences* (April 1975), 30:148–63.

50. Merrill, "Distinctive Peculiarities of the Negro," pp. 66–67, 4. Recent work by Richard N. Ellis, William B. Skelton, and Thomas C. Leonard has traced some of the ambiguities in the military view of Indian nature. See especially Leonard, "Red, White and Army Blue: Empathy and Anger in the American West," *American Quarterly* (May 1974), 26:176–90.

51. For an interesting example of nonmedical views on the subject, from a profession that at least theoretically was most optimistic about the efficacy of environmental change, see "Natural *Versus* Acquired Habits," *Massachusetts Teacher* (1849), 2:303. In general, see Rosenberg, "Bitter Fruit."

52. For Rush, see Jordan, *White Over Black,* p. 518. See also Winthrop Jordan's introduction to Smith, *Variety of Complexion in the Human Species,* p. lii; John D. Davies, *Phrenology: Fad and Science, A Nineteenth Century Crusade* (1955), p. 145; Trotter, *A View of the Nervous Temperament,* ch. 7.

Both too much and too little sensitivity to pain are still recognized as legitimate medical diseases. The problem is that "too much" and "too little" are relative terms; nineteenth-century theorists were unclear about how much difference was "normal" for different types of people.

53. For example, see *Preamble and Resolution of the Philadelphia County Medical Society,* in *The Female Experience: An American Documentary,* p. 409; Drachman, "Women Doctors," p. 47.

54. Jacobi quoted in Drachman, "Women Doctors," p. 79. For a closely related argument, see Carroll Smith-Rosenberg, "The Hysterical Woman: Sex Roles and Role Conflict in 19th-Century America," *Social Research* (1972), 39:652–78.

55. See ch. 3, note 74 above, and in general, ch. 5, note 99 above. For Dix, in a particularly unflattering light, see Fredrickson, *Inner Civil War,* pp. 109–11.

56. Stanton to Mott, October 22, 1852, in *Oven Birds,* p. 260. The question of whether female sensitivity was an innate virtue or an environmental handicap seriously divided both the feminist medical self-help movement and the ranks of women physicians.

57. Dewees, "Examination of Dr. Osburn's Opinion, of the Physical Necessity of Pain," pp. 272, 280; Dewees, *Lessening Pain and Facilitating Parturition,* pp. 7, 38, 43; Augustus K. Gardner "Physical Decline of American Women," *Knickerbocker* (January 1860), 55:41; see also Drachman, "Women Doctors," p. 82. For Hodge, Meigs, and Ramsbotham, see ch. 3 above. For the curability of birth pain as it directly related to anesthetic use, see ch. 8 below.

58. A good study is Harold D. Langley, *Social Reform in the United States Navy, 1798–1862* (1967); see also Glenn, *Campaigns against Corporal Punishment.* On Melville and Dana, see two insightful articles by Robert F. Lucid, "The Influence of *Two Years Before the Mast* on Herman Melville," *American Literature* (November 1959), 31:243–56; and *"Two Years Before the Mast* as Propaganda," *American Quarterly* (Fall, 1960), 12:392–403. See also Alcott, *Hospital Sketches;* Whitman, "The Wound-Dresser," in *Leaves of Grass,* pp. 252–54; Fredrickson, *Inner Civil War.*

59. For attack on Meigs, see Friend, "Anaesthesia in Labour," p. 6; for Mann, see *Lectures on Education,* pp. 313–14; Dunglison, *Human Physiology* (1850), 2:657. John Stuart Mill's classic essay on *The Subjection of Women* held that women were more sensitive than men, but he too refused to decide between nature and nurture as the cause, 2nd ed. (1911), pp. 131–39, 143.

60. For a good historical overview, see Edel, "Happiness and Pleasure." For a critique of modern approaches, especially Ryles and Wittgenstein, see J. L. Cowan, *Pleasure and Pain: A Study in Philosophical Psychology* (1968). Cowan is hardly definitive but has a good grasp of the medical aspects of the philosophical issues. The slave example is Wittgenstein's. For a version of the argument that the only important aspect of pain is the person's behavior, see B. F. Skinner, *Science and Human Behavior* (1953).

Several quantitative modern studies define sensitivity as the point at which the experimental subject calls his feelings "pain" and endurance as the point at which pain can no longer be tolerated. Supposedly, these studies have found that sensitivity thresholds are relatively constant for different people, while endurance levels are very variable. Yet such studies have major philosophical and methodological problems. For example, what does it mean to say that a subject is in pain if he is evidencing no avoidance behavior? For an introduction to such studies, see W. K. Livingston, "What is Pain?" *Scientific American,* March 1953, reprint no. 407.

Most current studies report that pain endurance varies with sex, occupation, ethnicity, age, race, and religion; Harold Mersky, "The Perception and Measurement of Pain," *Journal of Psychosomatic Research* (1973), 17:253; Richard A. Sternbach and Bernard Tursky, "Ethnic Differences Among Housewives in Psychophysical and Skin Potential Responses to Electric Shock," *Psychophysiology* (January 1965), 1:241–46; *Lancet,* June 19, 1971, p. 1284. As in the nineteenth century, such findings are being used to treat pain differently in different groups of patients; Helen Neal, *The Politics of Pain* (1978), pp. 101, 112.

However, such research has been rightly criticized for glossing over the essential privacy of the pain experience and for showing the clear influence of researcher bias on the results; Wallace E. Lambert, Eva Libman, and Ernest G. Poser, "The Effect of Increased Salience of a Membership Group on Pain Tolerance," *Journal of Personality* (1960), 28:350–57; Gilbert Lewis, "The Place of Pain in Human Experience," *Journal of Medical Ethics* (1976), 4:123. For debate over the validity of pain threshold measurements in general, see Henry K. Beecher, *Measurement of Subjective Responses* (1959); B. Berthold Wolff, "Factor Analysis of Human Pain Responses: Pain Endurance as a Specific Pain Factor," *Journal of Abnormal Psychology* (1971), 78:292; and Mersky, "Perception and Measurement," pp. 251–55.

Recent suggestions that different groups of people may differ in their levels of bodily produced painkillers (endorphins) are exciting but even if conclusively demonstrated would not tell us whether such differences were hereditary or acquired, nor whether they really produce differences in subjective feelings.

For a classic study of ethnic differences in *reactions* to pain that does not attempt to judge whether such reactions reflect differences in *feelings,* see Mark Zborowski, *People in Pain* (1969).

61. *"There can be no question"* that civilized people have more sensitive nerves than do savages, according to one neurologist; Rosenberg, "Science and American Social Thought," p. 143, emphasis added.

62. Cartwright, in Breeden, "States-Rights Medicine," p. 358; *Professional Planter,* in Haller, "The Negro and the Southern Physician," p. 246, emphasis added. Dr. John Harrison wrote that "it is absolutely impossible to form a notion concerning the sensations of others"; yet, in the same journal he declared just as emphatically, "All know that some persons suffer exquisitely, from causes which produce no inconvenience to others." He went on to cite differences in pain sensitivity by sex, age, emotion, and health; "Sensation," *New-Orleans Medical and Surgical Journal* (1849–50), 6:708, 439. John Marshall, *Outlines of Physiology* (1868), p. 336, did maintain sensation was private.

63. Romanticism, with its emphasis on the direct interpersonal awareness of feelings through "sympathy," undoubtedly encouraged nineteenth-century observers to *believe* that they could tell the difference between insensibility and endurance, but that does not tell us much about *how* they actually went about making such determinations.

64. Devereux, "Courage and Wisdom in Plato's *Laches,*" has a few related points of interest; see also *OED.* Conversely, "sensibility" could be a virtue while lack of "endurance" was certainly a defect. However, "sensibility" was ambiguous; especially for men too much of it was also undesirable. See, for example, Rush, *Enquiry into the Effects of Public Punishments,* in *A Plan for the Punishment of Crime,* p. 6.

65. Trotter, *A View of the Nervous Temperament,* pp. 202–3, 250; Duns, *Simpson,* p. 265. For identical sentiments by midcentury Americans, see Dickson, "Pain and Death," p.

59; Sweetser, *Mental Hygiene*, pp. 323–24; *Transactions of the New Hampshire Medical Society* (1865), pp. 22–25.

66. Langston Hughes, "Minstrel Man," *The Dream Keeper* (New York: Alfred A. Knopf, 1932), p. 38, used with permission.

67. Quoted in Blassingame, *Slave Community*, pp. 211–12, from Elizabeth Keckley, *Behind the Scenes* (New York, 1868), p. 34. Such forms of resistance make most sense when no others are available. Compare with the reaction of a modern black writer, Wertz and Wertz, *Lying-In*, p. 169.

68. Fredrickson, *Black Image*, pp. 102–17; Walters, *Antislavery Appeal*, pp. 58–59.

69. For an interesting analysis of Higginson's expectations and discoveries, see Eugene D. Genovese, *Roll, Jordan, Roll: The World the Slaves Made* (1974), p. 640.

70. Linda K. Kerber, "The Abolitionist Perception of the Indian," *Journal of American History* (September 1975), 62:271–95.

71. Smith, *Variety of Complexion in the Human Species*, pp. 128–29, emphasis added; Jefferson, *Notes on Virginia*, in *The Life and Selected Writings of Thomas Jefferson*, edited by Adrienne Koch and William Peden (1944), pp. 210–11, emphasis added. See also: Gossett, *Race*, p. 238; Wilson, *Patriotic Gore*, pp. 282–83.

72. Linda K. Kerber, *Federalists in Dissent: Imagery and Ideology in Jeffersonian America* (1970), p. 71.

73. Whitman spoke with admiration of the heroic endurance of wounded westerners and referred to "the unmistakable western physiognomy." See Whitman, *Specimen Days—The Armies Returning*, in *The Portable Walt Whitman*, p. 575; Lowenfels, *Walt Whitman's Civil War*, p. 113. For AMA statement on the biological differences of Americans and Europeans, see *Trans AMA* (1848), 1:287. In general, see ch. 5, notes 60–63 above, for additional such references.

74. Meigs, *Females and Their Diseases;* compare, for example, p. 50, on women's delicacy and sensitivity, with p. 49, "Men cannot suffer the same pains as women." See also John William Draper, *Human Physiology* (1856), p. 546; Mill, *Subjection of Women*, pp. 131–39.

75. "Woman," *Godey's Lady's Book* (August 1831), 2:110, quoted in Welter, "Cult of True Womanhood."

76. Bowditch, *History of Massachusetts General Hospital* (1851), 387. See also, Welter, "The Feminization of Religion."

77. Gardner, *Our Children*, pp. 250–51, quoted in Barker-Benfield, *Horrors of the Half-Known Life*, p. 283. See also: Samuel Warren, *Passages from the Diary of a Late Physician* (n.d. [1832?]), 1:41–50. I am indebted to Carol Pollard for this citation. For women's greater endurance, see also George H. Napheys, *The Physical Life of Woman: Advice to the Maiden, Wife, and Mother* (1869), pp. 11–12.

78. For Gardner, see *AJMS* (1852), 24:130. For more such examples, see ch. 8, note 16 below. For Gardner's priority, see Kelly and Burrage, *American Medical Biographies*.

79. Most Americans still considered that the defects of the Irish were more a matter of environment than heredity, though they warned such defects would rapidly become hereditary if not corrected soon. A few, like pioneer Massachusetts public health statistician Dr. Edward Jarvis, implied it was already too late. For majority opinion, see Gossett, *Race*, p. 97; for Jarvis, see Katz, *Irony of Early School Reform*, p. 182.

80. Duffy, *A History of Public Health in New York City, 1625–1866*, pp. 582, 588, offers some data; Oscar Handlin, *Boston's Immigrants: A Study in Acculturation* (1971), p. 254, offers another glimpse.

81. See, for example, Erichsen, *Science and Art of Surgery* (1854 ed.), pp. 75, 79. For full discussion, see ch. 8 below.

82. Jordan, *White Over Black,* pp. 293, 283.

83. *Measure for Measure,* Act III, Scene 1, line 76. Dentist J. H. M'Quillen wrote, "There is more of poetic imagination . . . than truthfulness in the assertion," *Dental Cosmos* (1866), 7:633. For similar remarks, see A. B. Crosby, "The Significance of Pain," *Transactions of the New Hampshire Medical Society* (1865), pp. 22, 25, 27.

84. Thomas, "On the Propriety of Anaesthetic Agents," p. 1, emphasis in original; Mott, "Remarks on the Importance of Anaesthesia," p. 86; see also Kidd, *Manual of Anaesthetics,* p. 15. For shared, but unequal, sensitivity, see Ralph Colp Jr., " 'I was born a naturalist': Charles Darwin's 1838 Notes about Himself," *Journal of the History of Medicine and Allied Sciences* (January 1980), 35:11–12. Darwin used the universality of sensation as an argument for common origins of man and beast. See also Paul F. Eve in *Southern Medical and Surgical Journal* (1849), 5:718; Staum, *Cabanis,* p. 223.

85. Wills, *Inventing America,* explains that Jefferson, following the Scottish Common Sense Realists, did believe that all men were created literally equal in their possession of an innate moral sense. For an excellent but brief exposition of the connection between this innate moral sense and pain, see McLoughlin, "Introduction," *American Evangelicals,* pp. 2–4.

86. For Bentham, see ch. 6, note 49 above. For Mann, see *Twelfth Annual Report* in *The Republic and the School.* The electorate, of course, excluded many of those who had differing levels of sensitivity to pain: women, almost all blacks, Indians, aliens, and children.

87. *New York Tribune,* October 7, 1862, quoted in Durden, "Ambiguities in the Antislavery Crusade of the Republican Party," in *The Antislavery Vanguard,* p. 390, emphasis in original. See also James M. McPherson, *The Struggle for Equality: Abolitionists and the Negro in the Civil War and Reconstruction* (1964), ch. 6.

8. INDICATIONS AND CONTRAINDICATIONS

1. William Lawrence to John Collins Warren, February 24, 1848, John C. Warren Papers, vol. 23, item 51.

2. *AJMS* (1851), 22:497–98n.

3. *AJMS* (1851), 22:426; Bryant, *Practice of Surgery,* pp. 488, 928; *Bulletin of the New York Academy of Medicine* (1864), 2:334.

4. Thomas, "On the Propriety of Anaesthetic Agents," p. 7; Sykes, *Essays,* 1:158.

5. *Trans AMA* (1848), 1:211; Warren, *Etherization,* p. 31. For the opposite view, see Hamilton, *Military Surgery,* p. 623.

6. Lyman, *Artificial Anaesthesia,* pp. 73–74; *AJMS* (1851), 22:426. Lyman did caution, "Even with children there should be a certain amount of explanation and persuasion, . . ." before resorting to "abrupt and seemingly violent measures. These little patients, fortunately, are so tolerant of anaesthesia that their fears and their struggles are less dangerous" than would be the case in forcibly anesthetizing an adult, though. Lyman, *Artificial Anaesthesia,* p. 50; this ambiguous (at best) call for restraint was virtually the only caveat against unlimited disciplinary anesthetization of children.

7. *AJMS* (1849), 18:96; Thomas, "On the Propriety of Anaesthetic Agents," p. 7. See also the printed case histories in *AJMS* (1849), 18:401; (1853), 25:224; *Trans AMA* (1848), 1:224—"one of the most obstinate, self-willed patients of his age [twelve] I have met with"; *Ohio Medical and Surgical Journal* (July 1857), 9:530.

8. *Trans AMA* (1848), 1:211.

9. Voorhies, "Chloroformum," p. 18.

10. Lyman, *Artificial Anaesthesia,* p. 48. Lyman apparently believed that the desirable effects of anesthesia varied according to the type of patient, while the *side* effects varied proportionally to the dose—an odd theory but understandable given the newness of nineteenth-

century medical attention to measuring side effects. For a similar example, see "Report of the Medical Society of Virginia," pp. 183, 186. See also: Druitt, *Principles and Practice of Modern Surgery*, p. 592; Philip S. Wales, *Mechanical Therapeutics: A Practical Treatise on Surgical Apparatus, Appliances, and Elementary Operations* (1867), p. 671.

11. Gross, *A System of Surgery*, p. 538; *AJMS* (1851), 21:435; William Thomas Green Morton, "Comparative Value of Sulphuric Ether and Chloroform," *B Med Surg J* (1850), 43:119. See also *Trans AMA* (1848), 1:188; Thomas E. Keys, "John Snow, MD: Anesthetist," *Journal of the History of Medicine and Allied Sciences* (Fall, 1946), 1: 560; Turnbull, *Artificial Anaesthesia*, pp. 108–109; George Hayward, *Surgical Reports and Miscellaneous Papers* (1855), p. 228; *Nashville Journal of Medicine and Surgery* (1879), n.s. 24:7.

12. A handful of physicians did deny that age should influence the use of anesthetics at all; see Smith, "Anaesthetics," p. 29; *AJMS* (1851), 22:329; *AJMS* (1852), 23:193. The latter article cited this view only to refute it.

13. "Report of the Boston Society for Medical Improvement, on the Inhalation of Sulphuric Ether," p. 233; Voorhies, "Chloroformum," p. 19; Erichsen, *Science and Art of Surgery* (1854 ed.), pp. 78, 79; Druitt, *Principles and Practice of Modern Surgery*, p. 592.

14. "Report of the Medical Society of Virginia," p. 183; *Ohio Medical and Surgical Journal* (July 1857), 9:530; Sykes, *Essays*, 1:158; Turnbull, *Artificial Anaesthesia*, p. 302.

15. Lyman, *Artificial Anaesthesia*, p. 48; Warren, *Etherization*, pp. 81–82; *Nashville Journal of Medicine and Surgery* (1879), n.s. 24:7; Kidd, *Manual*, p. 109; Bruno Jaehrig, "Anaesthetics," unpublished M.D. thesis, 1865, University of Michigan, Michigan Historical Collections, Bentley Library, Ann Arbor, p. 9; Frank E. Fletcher, "Chloroform," unpublished M.D. thesis, 1865, University of Michigan, p. 16; William Henry George, "Anaesthetics," unpublished M.D. thesis, 1869, University of Michigan, p. 31.

16. Wyman, *Progress in School Discipline*, p. 6; Todd quoted in Barker-Benfield, *Horrors of the Half-Known Life*, p. 200; Warren, review of *Etherization in Childbirth*, p. 301. See also Warren, *Etherization*, p. 38. Jackson, *Manual*, p. 97, endorses anesthesia for women and children, based in part on their high sensitivity, despite his claim that women are capable of *enduring* surgery better than men are, p. 66.

The question of the painfulness of medical therapy for women is one of the more controversial issues in recent women's historiography. It was raised by Ann Douglas Wood, " 'The Fashionable Diseases': Women's Complaints and Their Treatment in Nineteenth-Century America," *Journal of Interdisciplinary History* (Summer, 1973), 4:25–52. Wood catalogued excruciatingly heroic therapies performed by male doctors on women's sex organs. The claim that physicians were brutal in their treatment of women patients also formed a central thesis of Ehrenreich and English, *Complaints and Disorders*, and Barker-Benfield, *Horrors of the Half-Known Life*. Smith-Rosenberg, "The Hysterical Woman," contained a less extreme version of this thesis. However, these authors made no attempt to compare the painfulness of treatment for women with the painfulness of nineteenth-century treatment of men, a criticism raised by Regina Morantz, "The Lady and Her Physician," in *Clio's Consciousness Raised*, pp. 38–53. One attempt to make such comparison found no difference in the painfulness of therapy for men and women, Gail Pat Parsons, "Equal Treatment for All: American Medical Remedies for Male Sexual Problems, 1850–1900," *Journal of the History of Medicine and Allied Sciences* (January 1977), 32:55–71. While Parsons demonstrated that painful operations similar to those described by Wood and Barker-Benfield were also done on men, she fell short of demonstrating "equal" treatment, in that she made no attempt to estimate the frequency of such treatments, nor did she provide any definition of what "equality" of painfulness might mean.

In this book and in an earlier paper, I have tried to show that, compared to men, women were given generally *less* painful treatment by nineteenth-century male doctors but that this less painful treatment had both medically and politically disadvantageous aspects. Pernick, "Women and the Infliction of Pain in the Practice of 19th Century Professions: The Case of Surgical Anesthesia," unpublished paper given at the Berkshire Conference on the History of Women, June 1976.

17. For women's attraction to homeopathy, see ch. 5, note 84 above.

18. Druitt, *Principles and Practice of Modern Surgery*, p. 592.

19. Horner, "Anaesthetics," p. 30.

20. *AJMS* (1851), 22:498.

21. Gross, *A System of Surgery*, p. 538. See also Wales, *Mechanical Therapeutics*, p. 671.

22. Lyman, *Artificial Anaesthesia*, pp. 48–49.

23. Smith, *The Principles and Practice of Surgery*, 1:171; Smith, *A System of Operative Surgery* (1855), 1:185. Edward R. Squibb suggested two ounces for a strong man, one ounce for a woman or a sensitive man, *New York Medical Journal* (April 1871), 13:403. Such numerical dosage indications were still very rare. Most nineteenth-century anesthetists agreed with John Collins Warren's instructions, "The proper measure of quantity is its influence on the patient, and this influence must be obtained, whether it require drachms or ounces," *Etherization*, p. 77; Jackson, *Manual*, p. 87.

24. Dunglison, *Human Physiology* (1850), 2:659.

25. Lyman, *Artificial Anaesthesia*, p. 49.

26. *AJMS* (1851), 21:435; see also *AJMS* (1852), 22:495; *New-Orleans Medical and Surgical Journal* (1851–52), 8:424–25. The slightly altered source of the quote is Thomas Nunneley, *On Anaesthesia and Anaesthetic Substances Generally* (1849), p. 374.

27. Voorhies, "Chloroformum," p. 20. In fact, the "Report of the Medical Society of Virginia," p. 192, thought that anesthetics might be useful therapeutically to treat hysterical fits.

28. "Report of the Boston Society for Medical Improvement on the Inhalation of Sulphuric Ether," p. 231. See also Voorhies, "Chloroformum," p. 20; *AJMS* (1867), 53:165–66. For soldiers, see notes 63–75, this chapter. One author claimed that sex was unimportant in anesthetization, though the reviewer for the *AJMS* dissented (1852), 23:193.

29. *AJMS* (1851), 22:488.

30. Simpson, *Anaesthesia*, p. 246, emphasis added; see also p. 234. Lyman, *Artificial Anaesthesia*, p. 68.

31. Gregory, *Man-Midwifery*, p. 43.

32. Lyman, *Artificial Anaesthesia*, p. 68. Charles T. Jackson reported using anesthesia on "an American Indian," though it would seem he considered the case quite unusual and noteworthy. See Jackson, *Southern Medical and Surgical Journal* (January 1853), 9:5–20, reprinted in *Milestones in Anesthesia*, p. 123.

33. Miller, "Pain, Parturition, and the Profession," p. 28. Toni Morrison, *The Bluest Eye* (New York: Holt, Rinehart and Winston, Inc., 1970), p. 97; Wertz and Wertz, *Lying-In*, p. 169. Lombroso reported that prostitutes often did not require anesthesia, even for leg amputations, *The Female Offender*, p. 139. However, Kidd attributed medical unwillingness to anesthetize poor women to physicians' reluctance to spend time with nonremunerative cases, *Manual*, p. 100.

34. See, for example, the case of Dennis P., MGH Records, vol. 31, admitted April 6, 1847, discussed in ch. 11 below. Also, see *AJMS* (1851), 22:489–90, for a similar case in Ireland.

35. Vogel, "Patrons, Practitioners, and Patients."

36. Voorhies, 'Chloroformum," pp. 7–8; *New York Medical Journal* (1872), 16:154.

37. "Report of the Standing Committee for 1847," *Transactions of the Medical Society of New Jersey* (1766–1858), 1:412.

38. Voorhies, "Chloroformum," p. 7. Only one commentator cited expense as a consideration; see John P. Reynolds in *Semi-Centennial of Anaesthesia*, p. 55; see also note 33 above.

39. "Report of the Medical Society of Virginia," p. 186; Turnbull, *Artificial Anaesthesia*, p. 109; *Western Lancet* (1853), 14:658; *New-Orleans Medical and Surgical Journal* (1851–52), 8:279. For the general influence of nationality, see also Jackson, *Manual*, p. 97; and Kidd, *Manual*, p. 23.

40. J. F. Smithcors, "History of Veterinary Anesthesia," *Textbook of Veterinary Anesthesia*, edited by Lawrence R. Soma (1971), pp. 1–23, esp. 8, 12, 19–20; for exceptions, see pp. 16–17.

41. *AJMS* (1851), 22:496; L[ouis] Lewin, *The Untoward Effects of Drugs. A Pharmacological and Clinical Manual* (1883), p. 174; Kidd, *Manual*, p. 84.

42. Lyman, *Artificial Anaesthesia*, p. 49; Turnbull, *Artificial Anaesthesia*, pp. 208–209. However, the Medical Society of Virginia thought ether might also be useful in *treating* delirium tremens, "Report," p. 192; see also L. P. Yandell, "On the Progress of Etherization," *Western Journal of Medicine and Surgery* (1849), 3:1–36; and ch. 4, note 31 above.

43. Clarke, "Anaesthesia in Surgery," pp. 12–13; Jackson, *Manual*, p. 96; *Nashville Journal of Medicine and Surgery* (1879), n.s. 24:7; *Dental Cosmos* (1869), 11:49; *AJMS* (1867), 53:169, attributed the discovery of this danger to Nelaton.

44. Smith, *A System of Operative Surgery*, 1:185. For similar comments and observations, see "Report of the Medical Society of Virginia," p. 183; W. T. G. Morton, *Remarks on the Proper Mode of Administering Sulphuric Ether by Inhalation* (1847), reprinted in *Milestones in Anesthesia*, p. 59; C. T. Jackson, "On Anesthetic Agents," in *Milestones in Anesthesia*, p. 123.

Modern researchers agree that habitual alcoholics are much harder to anesthetize; see Mostert, "States of Awareness During General Anesthesia," pp. 71–72.

45. Voorhies, "Chloroformum," p. 24.

46. "Report of the Boston Society for Medical Improvement on the Inhalation of Sulphuric Ether," p. 232. For the only exception, see John Snow, "A Lecture on the Inhalation of Vapour of Ether in Surgical Operations," *Lancet* (May 29, 1847), 1:551–54, in *Milestones in Anesthesia*, p. 82.

47. See ch. 3, note 55 above.

48. *AJMS* (1851), 22:271, 272, emphasis in original.

49. *AJMS* (1851), 22:493. The first was cautiously negative; the second, cautiously positive.

50. *B Med Surg J* (1847), 35:520.

51. Elizabeth D., admitted April 27, 1847, MGH Records, vol. 31.

52. Dupierris, "Reduction of Femoral Dislocation," p. 291.

53. "Report of the Boston Society for Medical Improvement on the Inhalation of Sulphuric Ether," p. 232. For the University of Michigan, see these unpublished M.D. theses: Samuel Perky, "Chloroform," (1862), p. 28; Walker, "Anaesthesia and Anaesthetics," (1862), p. 26; Jaehrig, "Anaesthetics," (1865), pp. 19–20; George, "Anaesthetics," (1869), p. 15. See also Voorhies, "Chloroformum," pp. 19–20; and *AJMS* (1851), 21:239.

54. Druitt, *The Principles and Practice of Modern Surgery*, p. 592; Warren, *Etherization*, pp. 14–17; Sykes, *Essays*, 1:158. On a related point, J. F. B. Flagg thought the use of ether should be proportional to "the amount of *dread*" felt by the patient, *Ether and Chloroform*, p. 166; for fear as a *contra*indication, see Lyman, *Artificial Anaesthesia*, p. 50; Chapin, "Chloroform," pp. 13–15; Kidd, *Manual*, p. 84 (chloroform).

55. See, for examples: *AJMS* (1851), 21:238–39; Lyman, *Artificial Anaesthesia,* p. 49; "Report of the Medical Society of Virginia," p. 196; *New York Medical Gazette* (May 1, 1851), 2:104, clipping in Hamilton Case Book, 3:214 (chloroform only); Warren, *Etherization,* pp. 81–82; *New-Orleans Medical and Surgical Journal* (1851–52), 8:424 (primarily chloroform); *Nashville Journal of Medicine and Surgery* (1879), n.s. 24:6–7 (chloroform only). University of Michigan students throughout the mid-nineteenth century were taught not to use ether or chloroform in brain, heart, or lung diseases: Perky, "Chloroform," (1862), p. 28; Walker, "Anaesthesia and Anaesthetics," (1862), p. 26; Alexander Gunn, "Chloroform," (1864), pp. 13–14; Jaehrig, "Anaesthetics," (1865), p. 9; Muir, "Anaesthesia," (1871), pp. 15–16. For the related debate over whether anesthesia caused or cured insanity, see ch. 4, note 32 above.

For a survey of modern theory, see Daniel E. N. Evans, "Anaesthesia and the Epileptic Patient: A Review," *Anaesthesia* (1975), 30:34–45, in which dangers are pointed out and ether is concluded to be the safest agent when anesthetization of the epileptic must be done.

56. In addition to virtually all the sources in note 55 above, see also: Jackson, *Manual,* p. 97; Clarke, *Manual,* p. 272 (chloroform only); Sackrider, "Ether and Chloroform," p. 28; "Report of the Standing Committee for 1847," *Transactions of the Medical Society of New Jersey* (1766–1858), 1:412; "Report of the Boston Society for Medical Improvement on the Inhalation of Sulphuric Ether," pp. 232–33; *AJMS* (1852), 23:193; Flagg, *Ether and Chloroform,* p. 47; Horner, "Anaesthetics," pp. 21, 27; Thomas, "On the Propriety of Anaesthetic Agents," p. 6; Chapin, "Chloroform," p. 27.

There were a few dissenters who held anesthesia safe for heart disease: *AJMS* (1867), 53:169 (chloroform); Barker, "Anaesthetics in Midwifery" (1862), p. 299 (ether more acceptable than chloroform).

57. Lyman, *Artificial Anaesthesia,* p. 50; "Report of the Boston Society for Medical Improvement on the Inhalation of Sulphuric Ether," p. 233.

58. Chloroform only: *Nashville Journal of Medicine and Surgery* (1879), n.s. 24:6; Muir, "Anaesthesia," p. 26.

59. Horner, "Anaesthetics," pp. 21, 27; *AJMS* (1851), 21:239; (1852), 23:193; Kidd, *Manual,* p. 84; Samuel K. Crawford, "Chloroform, in Relation to Medical Jurisprudence," unpublished M.D. thesis, University of Michigan, 1861, p. 22.

60. See ch. 3, note 55 above.

61. For prohibition: Lyman, *Artificial Anaesthesia,* p. 49; Porter, "Medical and Surgical Notes," *AJMS* (1852), 24:29; *New York Medical Gazette* (May 1, 1851), 2:104, in Hamilton Case Book, 3:214 (chloroform only); Hamilton, *Military Surgery,* pp. 613–14, 622; Samuel D. Gross, *A Manual of Military Surgery,* (1862), p. 81; *Dental Cosmos* (1869), 11:49.

Against prohibition: "Report of the Boston Society for Medical Improvement on the Inhalation of Sulphuric Ether," p. 232; Erichsen, *Science and Art of Surgery* (1860 ed.), p. 32; Bryant, *Practical Surgery,* pp. 925, 927, 933 (chloroform only).

62. Hemorrhage contraindication: *AJMS* (1851), 21:498; Barker, "Anaesthetics in Midwifery," (1862), p. 300; George, "Anaesthetics," p. 15; Muir, "Anaesthesia," pp. 15–16. The idea dates back to Humphry Davy's first 1800 suggestion that laughing gas might be used as an anesthetic "during surgical operations in which no great effusion of blood takes place," Fülöp-Miller, *Triumph Over Pain,* p. 65.

Plethora contraindication: *AJMS* (1852), 23:193; *Dental Cosmos* (1869), 11:48; Smith, "Anaesthetics," p. 32; and ch. 5, note 11 above.

63. Porter, "Medical and Surgical Notes," *AJMS* (1852), 24:29; and (1852), 23:33. Almost a century later, Harvard's distinguished anesthesiologist Henry K. Beecher discovered a similar insensibility to pain and indifference to anesthesia among troops seriously wounded in the Second World War. Beecher's widely discussed report became an important element in the development of several major new theories of pain perception. Henry K. Beecher, "Pain in

Men Wounded in Battle,'' *Bulletin of the United States Army Medical Department* (1946), 5:445–54.

64. Porter, ''Medical and Surgical Notes,'' *AJMS* (1852), 23:33; Jaehrig, ''Anaesthetics,'' p. 16; Langley, *Social Reform in the Navy*.

65. *Western Lancet* (1848), 7:128; *B Med Surg J* (July 1847), 36:466–67; *New York Herald*, July 9, 1847, p. 1; George Winston Smith and Charles Judan, eds., *Chronicles of the Gringos: The U.S. Army in the Mexican War, 1846–1848* (1968), pp. 347–50.

66. Porter, ''Medical and Surgical Notes,'' *AJMS* (1852), 23:33; (1852), 24:29–30.

67. Smith and Judan, *Chronicles of the Gringos*, pp. 349–50.

68. Anesthetists like John Snow were particularly insistent in trying to distinguish courage under fire from courage under the knife; they declared that even the bravest soldier would rather face the sword than the surgeon and pointed out that bravery took place in the heat of battle while surgery took place in the depression afterward. See, for example, Snow, ''Lecture on Ether,'' in *Milestones in Anesthesia*, p. 88.

69. Mott, *Pain and Anaesthetics;* Chisholm, *Manual*, p. 433; George H. B. Macleod, *Notes on the Surgery of the War in the Crimea* (1862), pp. 123–26. Of course, part of the change was probably due to a change in the public perception of the social class origins of soldiers and sailors, with a perceived rise in middle-class enlistments in the early days of the Civil War.

70. Alcott, *Hospital Sketches*, pp. 37–38: ''ether was not thought necessary that day, so the poor souls had to bear their pains as best they might.'' See also Oliver Wendell Holmes, *Touched With Fire: Civil War Letters and Diary of Oliver Wendell Holmes* (1946), pp. 23–33, quoted in Howe, *Holmes: The Shaping Years*, I, 104: ''near the entrance a surgeon calmly grasping a man's finger and cutting it off—both standing—while the victim contemplated the operation with a very grievous mug''; Wiley, *Johnny Reb*, pp. 265–66, 269.

71. Fülöp-Miller, *Triumph Over Pain*, pp. 307–9.

72. *Sanitary Commission Document No. 57*, p. 8.

73. William Thomas Green Morton, ''The First Use of Ether as an Anesthetic at the Battle of the Wilderness in the Civil War,'' *Journal of the American Medical Association* (April 23, 1904), 42:1068–73.

74. *Sanitary Commission Document No. 57*, pp. 9, 12.

75. For standardization, see Fredrickson, *Inner Civil War*, ch. 7; for Hammond's intentions in general, see Brieger, ''Therapeutic Conflicts.''

76. Snow, ''Inhalation of Ether,'' in *Milestones in Anesthesia*, p. 89; Lyman, *Artificial Anaesthesia*, pp. 93–98; Warren, *Etherization*, p. 54; Jackson, *Manual*, p. 93. However, for an attack on these uses as unethical, see *AJMS* (1850), 19:260.

77. For a random example, see Henry H. Smith, *Minor Surgery; or, Hints on the Every-Day Duties of the Surgeon* (1859), p. 315. See also *AJMS* (1850), 19:100; *Trans AMA* (1848), 1:222.

78. For some typical examples, see: *AJMS* (1851), 22:497–98; (1850), 19:258; *Western Lancet* (1847), 6:182; (1848), 7:362; Sargent, *On Bandaging and Minor Surgery* (1856), pp. 261–62; Druitt, *Principles and Practice of Modern Surgery*, p. 594; Lyman, *Artificial Anaesthesia*, p. 48. For a recent historian who reads similar sources as implying that ''almost all'' patients were being anesthetized by the 1850s, see Youngson, *Scientific Revolution*, p. 121.

79. Pp. 315–26.

80. Thompson, ''Anaesthesia,'' p. 7. See also: *AJMS* (1851), 21:498; Turnbull, *Artificial Anaesthesia*, p. 98; Warren, *Etherization*, p. 33; *AJMS* (1850), 19:258–59; Warren, review of *Etherization in Childbirth*, p. 314; *Western Lancet* (1847), 6:182; J. R. Maltby, ''Francis Sibson, 1814–1876,'' *Anaesthesia* (1977), 32:59.

81. Lyman, *Artificial Anaesthesia*, pp. 48, 73–74, emphasis added. The spokes-

men for "professional" dentistry generally agreed with such assessments, at least until the reintroduction of nitrous oxide in the 1880s. For an exception, a *professional* dentist who denied that oral surgery was too minor for anesthesia, see Flagg, *Ether and Chloroform*, p. 166.

The use of general anesthesia in dentistry is still an issue of extreme volatility. For a stinging denunciation of the public for demanding such anesthesia, see Gabor Czoniczer, "The Role of the Patient in Modern Medicine," *Man and Medicine* (1978), 3(1):19. Czoniczer, an M.D., phrases his attack little differently from John Wesley Thompson's nineteenth-century arguments. For a (somewhat) calmer appraisal of the issue, see "General Anesthesia by Dentists Unacceptable," *Anesthesiology* (1978), 48:384–85. While Czoniczer echoes the nineteenth-century view that dental pain is too minor to justify anesthesia, *Anesthesiology* argues that modern local anesthetics can relieve dental pain adequately and that dentists are unskilled in the use of general anesthetics.

The *St. Louis Medical and Surgical Journal* criticized the French for using anesthesia in opening abscesses (1850), 7:151. For a modern claim that evulsion of the toenail is "one of the most painful operations in surgery," see *Journal of the American Podiatry Association* (July 1979), 69:415.

82. *AJMS* (1851), 22:426; see also notes 1–2 above, this chapter.

83. Gross, *A System of Surgery*, p. 536; Smith, *Minor Surgery*, p. 315; Clarke, *Manual*, p. 272; Sykes, *Essays*, 1:114; Jaehrig, "Anaesthetics," p. 19; George, "Anaesthetics," p. 30. John Collins Warren disapproved of anesthetics in minor head and neck surgery but did not prohibit them in mouth and throat operations, *Etherization*, pp. 73, 84. For a full debate see *AJMS* (1851), 21:491–98.

84. R. G. Gordon Jones, "A Short History of Anaesthesia for Hare-Lip and Cleft Palate Repair," *British Journal of Anaesthesia* (1971), 43:796–802, esp. 797; *AJMS* (1863), 46:305–313; Bryant did, however, allow chloroform, for younger cleft patients and for older harelip repairs, *Practice of Surgery*, pp. 234, 249.

85. *AJMS* (1851), 22:490; Turnbull, *Artificial Anaesthesia*, p. 113; Clarke, *Manual*, p. 272.

86. See ch. 3, notes 114–16 above. For eyes: D. Hayes Agnew, quoted by William Campbell Posey and Samuel Horton Brown, *The Wills Hospital of Philadelphia* (1931), p. 208, also p. 99; Turnbull, *Artificial Anaesthesia*, p. 113; Kidd, *Manual*, p. 202; Jaehrig, "Anaesthetics," p. 19. For the view that anesthesia was not contraindicated in eye operations, see "Report of the Medical Society of Virginia," p. 191.

For hernia contraindication: Warren, *Etherization*, p. 28; Kidd, *Manual*, p. 82; Samuel Fenwick, "Statistical Inquiry into the Effects of Chloroform," *American Medical Gazette and Journal of Health* (October 1857), 8:594. I am grateful to James Cassedy for tracking down this last citation for me. Bryant, *Practice of Surgery*, p. 925, did allow anesthesia in such operations.

For a view that anesthetics should not be contraindicated in bladder stones, see J. Mason Warren, "Lithotomy and Lithotrity, With the Use of Ether in those Operations," *AJMS* (1849), 18:47–59.

87. Turnbull, *Artificial Anaesthesia*, pp. 113–14;

88. This section is limited to the indications and contraindications presented by authorities who accepted the use of obstetric anesthesia in at least some circumstances. For a full discussion of the pros and cons of obstetric anesthesia, see chs. 3 and 4 above.

89. Morton, *Remarks on Administering Ether*, in *Milestones in Anesthesia*, p. 56.

90. Horner, "Anaesthetics," p. 30, for a man's view of control; Rebecca L. Fussell, "Anaesthetics," unpublished M.D. thesis, Female Medical College of Pennsylvania, February 1858, p. 15, for a woman's view. See also: Barker, "Anaesthetics in Midwifery" (1857), p. 263; Perky, "Chloroform," p. 34.

91. Wertz and Wertz, *Lying-In*, pp. 117–18.

92. *Trans AMA* (1848), 1:230, emphasis in original.

93. Wertz and Wertz, *Lying-In*, ch. 3.

94. Napheys, *Physical Life of Woman*, pp. 199–200; Friend, "Anaesthesia in Labour," pp. 6, 14–16; Mordecai, "Effects of Chloroform," p. 19; Warren, *Etherization*, p. 68; Barker, "Anaesthesia in Midwifery," (1862), pp. 288–89, 293; Bedford, *Principles and Practice*, p. 734; Jaehrig, "Anaesthetics," p. 21.

95. J. V. C. Smith, editor of the *B Med Surg J*, quoted by Gregory, *Man-Midwifery*, p. 43. John P. Reynolds, in 1897, ruled that "Ether, when properly given in normal obstetrics, never contents the patient. She incessantly cries for more," *Semi-Centennial of Anaesthesia*, p. 53. In the most extreme version of this viewpoint, one British surgeon held, "It was wrong to give it to women who would not die without it," *AJMS* (1849), 18:277.

96. Lyman, *Artificial Anaesthesia*, pp. 68–69.

97. See ch. 3, notes 64–80, 84–103; ch. 4, notes 12, 13, 22; and ch. 5, notes 9–13 above.

98. "Report on Obstetrics and Diseases of Women," *Illinois State Medical Society*, p. 96; Barker, "Anaesthetics in Midwifery," (1862), p. 268; Storer, "Absolute Safety," and *B Med Surg J* (1863), 69:249–58; *The Stethoscope* (1855), 5:422–35. For attacks on the distinction between "pathological" and "physiological" labor pains, see: *Westminster Review* (1859), 71:69; *New-Orleans Medical and Surgical Journal* (1851–52), 8:281; *AJMS* (1849), 18:181.

99. "Report of the Standing Committee for the Year 1849," *Transactions of the Medical Society of New Jersey* (1766–1858), 1:455.

100. Barker, "Anaesthetics in Midwifery," (1862), p. 287; *Transactions of the New Hampshire Medical Society* (1862), p. 32.

101. Lyman, *Artificial Anaesthesia*, p. 69; *AJMS* (1851), 21:249; Wertz and Wertz, *Lying-In*, pp. 117–18.

102. For use of anesthesia on the "phlegmatic," see Hamilton, *Military Surgery*, p. 623; for "lymphatic" males, see Jaehrig, "Anaesthetics," p. 9.

103. Dickson, "Pain and Death," p. 59; *New York Medical Journal* (April 1871), 13:403.

104. See ch. 4, notes 35–37 above.

105. Erichsen, *Science and Art of Surgery* (1854 ed.), p. 79; Thompson, "Anaesthesia," p. 10. See also Henry, "Etherization, as a Surgical Remedy," p. 10; *AJMS* (1853), 25:519; Posey and Brown, *Wills Hospital*, p. 208; Bryant, *Practical Surgery*, p. 185; see also note 54 above.

106. *New-Orleans Medical and Surgical Journal* (1851–52), 8:428, quoting the British anesthetist John Snow, emphasis in original.

107. See ch. 6, notes 29–32 above.

108. In addition to note 106 above, see Barker, "Anaesthesia in Midwifery," (1862), p. 298; Metcalfe, "Chloroform," p. 149.

9. IDEOLOGY AND ACTION

1. Kelly and Burrage, *American Medical Biographies*.

2. *Timespan:*

MGH—November 7, 1846, to October 16, 1847. In a study currently underway, I intend to compare these early records with cases from 1854–55 and 1859–60 and with similar data from the New York Hospital. However, a large proportion of these records omitted data on anesthetic usage; for a discussion of this problem see ch. 1, notes 7 and 8 above.

Pa. H.—October 16, 1853, to October 15, 1862, with an apparent gap in the records for 1860–61. Anesthetic use at the Pa. H. began in July 1853; these dates were selected to avoid any seasonal variations in comparision with MGH data. See also ch. 1, note 6 above.

Hamilton—July 1849 to February 1877.

    Completeness:

MGH—One hundred and thirty cases; includes all operations, major and minor, performed in the timespan covered, with the exception of seven cases for which the records conflict concerning anesthesia. See ch. 1, note 7 above.

Pa. H.—Sixty-nine cases; includes only major limb amputations for fractures. Includes all cases for which anesthetic data were recorded. See ch. 1, note 6 above.

Hamilton—One hundred thirty-seven cases, major and minor procedures. Unlike the hospital records, however, Hamilton states explicitly that he did not keep records of all operations; in many types of operations he seems to have favored "unusual" cases in his recording while in other places he states explicitly that the examples listed are representative or typical. Only in the case of amputations and other bone surgery does he appear to have been attempting comprehensiveness. I did not tabulate cases for which no social data were provided nor cases of cataract removal, for which Hamilton never used anesthetics. Military surgery cases were also excluded for reasons discussed in ch. 1, note 10 above.

    3. 43/130 or 33.1 percent. Of course, most of the anesthesia literature appeared after these early Massachusetts General patients were treated. Thus, these particular cases were not "following" the textbooks; rather, these cases reflect and are products of the same professional attitudes and ideas that helped shape the textbooks.

    4. One likely exception is Theophilus P., admitted November 16, and subjected to a leg amputation the same day. P. was an immigrant, run over by a railroad train while drunk. The actual case records make no mention of anesthesia and imply very strongly that none was given; "During operation patient made no complaint." Nor was P. listed in the tabulation of anesthetized cases in *Trans AMA* (1848), 1:215. But in the tabulation presented in *AJMS* (1851), 21:180, he was listed as having received ether. Thus, in accordance with my procedure of eliminating cases where the records conflict, he was dropped from the tabulation used in this study. Note that, according to the professional literature, an adult male immigrant drunk was the least likely candidate for anesthetization.

    5. 28/130 or 21.5 percent. For calling breast removals "amputations," see Erichsen, *Science and Art of Surgery* (1854 ed.), p. 82.

    6. Removal of jaw bone sections accounted for 5 of the 130 operations! Perhaps this is a reflection of poor dental hygiene; perhaps it was a side effect of calomel poisoning, and/or a result of syphilis.

    7. 43/102 or 42.2 percent. The difference between amputations and minor surgery is significant at better than .01 level.

    8. A twelve-year-old girl, admitted June 6, 1855, operated on by J. Mason Warren, for repair of a cleft soft palate, MGH Records vol. 64 West, p. 198. However, one of the seven 1846–47 cases is tabulated as having received ether for repair of a double harelip, although the actual case record mentions nothing about anesthesia. The patient, Henrietta B, age five months, was admitted October 9, 1847, MGH Records vol. 32 East.

    9. See ch. 8, note 13 above.

    10. For "a certain class of navigators, and labourers," as forming a separate category regarding anesthesia, see ch. 8, note 36 above.

    11. In cataract operations, however, Hamilton consistently withheld anesthesia, see note 2 above. "Major limbs" are arms, legs, hands, and feet.

    12. Samuel X. Radbill, "Hospitals and Pediatrics, 1776–1976," *Bulletin of the History of Medicine* (Summer 1979), 53:288–89, notes that the Pennsylvania Hospital was unique

among American general hospitals, in that it "abhorred children." Children's Hospital of Pennsylvania, founded in 1855, thus received almost all the young patients requiring hospitalization in mid-nineteenth-century Philadelphia.

13. Unfortunately, the ethnicity of these patients was not indicated in the available records.

14. Regina Markell Morantz and Sue Zschoche, "Professionalism, Feminism, and Gender Roles: A Comparative Study of Nineteenth-Century Medical Therapeutics," *Journal of American History* (December 1980), 67:587. Table 15 was calculated by me, on the basis of data provided to me by Dr. Morantz. I am deeply indebted to her for sharing these data; however I assume full responsibility for the calculations and conclusions.

The data were drawn from the records of the Boston Lying-In Hospital from 1887–1899, and the New England Hospital for Women, 1873–1899. Unlike the other data discussed in this chapter, these statistics are based on a sample, rather than on complete tabulations. The sample was taken by counting every fifth case, using the records of every other year. All records located at Countway Library of Medicine, Boston.

15. Unfortunately, the records contain only three cases identified as "color^d"; though several additional cases almost undoubtedly were black people, the identifications could not be made positively.

Another recent study contains data that indicate Dr. Stephen W. Williams used chloroform more often on women than on men, though these are therapeutic, not surgical cases. Laurie MacLeod, "The Dyspepsia Generation: An Investigation into the Causes and Cures of Sickness in the Early Nineteenth Century; . . . ." unpublished senior thesis, Hampshire College, Amherst, Massachusetts, 1977, pp. 81–84, 99. From these data, I have calculated that 78 percent of Williams' chloroform prescriptions, in cases where the sex of the patient was recorded, were for women, but women comprised only 59.2 percent of the total number of patients for whom he prescribed. Put another way, 6.2 percent of the prescriptions for women, and only 2.5 percent of the prescriptions for men, were for chloroform. These data would seem to support my findings; however more information is needed on exactly how Williams was using the drug. I am indebted to Robert Gross of Amherst College for showing me this paper and to Laurie MacLeod for permission to cite it.

16. Thus, for example, in table 10 A, knowing that a given amputee was a woman, child, or old person enables us to predict with certainty that they received anesthesia. In technical terms, if table 10 A were broken down into 2x2 contingency tables, a unidirectional measure of strength of association, such as Goodman and Kruskal's Tau (T_b) would be 1.00, for the proportional reduction of error.

17. By using a much larger group of patient records, I hope to be able to detect the influence of much finer grained distinctions among patients. See note 2 above. A modern study has discovered exactly such a pattern in present-day medical treatment of pain in men and women patients; see K. J. Armitage, L. J. Schneiderman, and R. A. Bass, "Response of Physicians to Medical Complaint in Men and Women," *Journal of the American Medical Association* (May 18, 1979), 241:2186–87. But for an opposing view, see L. M. Verbrugge and R. P. Steiner, "Physician Treatment of Men and Women Patients: Sex Bias or Appropriate Care?" *Medical Care* (1981), 19:609–32.

18. Again, using the data in table 10 A to construct 2 x 2 tables, a *two-way* test of strength of association, such as $\emptyset^2$, would be very low (as would T_a). Knowing age, sex, and whether the patient received an amputation, does not greatly improve our ability to predict anesthetic use for most patients, only for the exceptional ones. Despite the disappearance of one cell in each of the tables, the overall unexplained variation remains high. For a brief general discussion of such situations, see Hubert M. Blalock, Jr., *Social Statistics* (1960), pp. 231–33.

10. WHY DOCTORS STILL DIFFERED

1. Ch. 1, notes 6–8 above.
2. Ch. 7, note 38 above.
3. Bigelow, "Inaugural Lecture," p. 226.
4. Chisholm, *Manual of Military Surgery*, p. 432.
5. Bragg, "Anaesthetics," p. 4; Kidd, *Manual*, p. 202.
6. Dunglison to John Collins Warren, January 29, 1848, John C. Warren Papers, vol. 23, item 40.
7. Kelly and Burrage, *American Medical Biographies*. Youngson, *Scientific Revolution*, p. 227, notes correctly that there were young and old on each side.
8. Warren, the oldest, used anesthetics in more than 90 percent of his operations after November 1846; Bigelow, the youngest, used anesthetics in less than 60 percent between 1846 and 1847. The other surgeons were in between.
9. It is not always possible to tell from the records which were the most complex operations; however, two classes of operations that were generally long and tedious and required great dexterity were the removal of tumors (excepting lip and skin tumors) and the ligature of major arterial aneurisms. For the three older surgeons (John C. Warren, George Hayward, and Solomon Townsend), such operations comprised 23.8, 18.8, and 19.2 percent of their case load respectively. Of the three new appointees, only J. Mason Warren did any such operations; they comprised only 13.3 percent of his case load.

Pooling the results, 6.25 percent of the case load for the three youngest surgeons consisted of tumors and arterial ligatures; for the three oldest the figure was 20.64 percent; the difference is significant at .01. (Excluding three operations in which the surgeon was not recorded, total N was 127.)

10. Friend, "Anaesthesia in Labour"; Voorhies, "Chloroformum"; Bragg, "Anaesthetics"; Mordecai, "Effects of Chloroform"; Thompson, "Anaesthesia"; Clarke, "Anaesthesia in Surgery"; Harvey, "Ether, in Surgical Operations"; Henry, "Etherization, as a Surgical Remedy"; the exception was Horner, "Anaesthetics."

11. Pa. H. Fracture Books. From October 16 to October 15. The exceptions were 1853–1854 and 1860–1861.

1852–61	37/60	62 percent
1861–63	34/37	92 percent

J. Forsythe Meigs, *A History of the First Quarter of the Second Century of the Pennsylvania Hospital . . .* (1877), p. 95. Both Norris and Peace did perform anesthetic surgery. They seem to have used the new painkillers less often than younger surgeons did, though the surgeon's name was not recorded frequently enough to be sure.

12. Hamilton Case Books. From July to June (based on the anniversary of his first use of chloroform).

1850–54	22/39	56.4 percent
1854–58	21/41	51.2 percent
1858–62	12/13	92.3 percent
1862–66	16/16	100.0 percent
1866–70	16/20	80.0 percent
1870–74	5/6	83.3 percent

The 1867–74 period did not differ from the 1850–58 period, nor from the cumulated career data presented with regard to the relation of age, sex, and type of operation to anesthetization. When Hamilton returned to partial use of anesthesia, he returned to the same patterns of selective use.

13. See, for example, Simpson to Ramsbotham, July 23, 1848; January 14, 1851; April 21, 1852, in Ramsbotham Papers. For more on the Edinburgh-London rivalry, see Youngson, *Scientific Revolution*, pp. 85, 220. Flagg, *Ether and Chloroform*, p. 32; Morton, *Letheon Circular*, p. 67; Oliver Wendell Holmes, *An Introductory Lecture delivered at the Massachusetts Medical College, November 3, 1847* (1847), pp. 20–23; Hodges, *Introduction of Ether*, p. 61; see also Bigelow in *B Med Surg J* (April 1848), 38:233–56.

14. Most previous histories of anesthetic adoption have ignored the crucial difference between these two variables, assuming that once a surgeon tried ether for the first time, he would immediately begin using it in all operations.

15. Ch. 1, notes 2, 4 above.

16. *Trans AMA* (1848), 1:215–19.

17. Ch. 1, note 8 above, for citation and a caveat.

18. See table 6.

19. Ch. 1, notes 6–8, and text accompanying note 1, this chapter.

20. Bond, in *B Med Surg J* (December 1846), 35:446. Even generally pro-anesthetic comments regarded the innovation as a "Yankee dodge"; see Liston in "Notes on the Discovery of Surgical Anesthesia," John C. Warren Papers, vol. 23, item 1.

21. Flagg, *Ether and Chloroform*, p. 21.

22. *Annalist* (January 1847), 1:189. See also Morton, *Letheon Circular*, p. 87, for a reply to the "Yankee" slur; *Phil Med Ex*, (May 1847), n.s. 3:318.

23. Holmes, *Introductory Lecture*, p. 23, also pp. 20, 22.

24. Holmes, *Introductory Lecture*, p. 21.

25. *Summary of the Transactions of the College of Physicians of Philadelphia* (1846–1849), 2:155.

26. Leonard K. Eaton, "Medicine in Philadelphia and Boston, 1805–1830," *Pennsylvania Magazine of History and Biography* (January 1951), 75:66–75.

27. Bowditch, *History of Massachusetts General Hospital* (1851); Eaton, "Medicine in Philadelphia and Boston"; *Trans AMA* (1848), 1:18, 250–53; F. P. Henry, *Standard History of the Medical Profession of Philadelphia* (1897); Thomas G. Morton and Frank Woodbury, *A History of the Pennsylvania Hospital, 1751–1895* (1897); George W. Norris, *The Early History of Medicine in Philadelphia* (1886); Williams, *America's First Hospital;* George W. Corner, *Two Centuries of Medicine: A History of the School of Medicine of the University of Pennsylvania* (1965); Joseph Carson, *A History of the Medical Department of the University of Pennsylvania, from its Foundation in 1765* (1869); James Fyfe Gayley, *A History of the Jefferson Medical College of Philadelphia* (1858); R. W. Downie, "Pennsylvania Hospital Admissions, 1751–1850," *Transactions and Studies of the College of Physicians of Philadelphia* (1964), 32:20–35.

28. Eaton, "Medicine in Philadelphia and Boston," pp. 70, 72.

29. Harrington, *Harvard Medical School;* Bowditch, *History of Massachusetts General Hospital* (1851); Hodges, *Introduction of Ether;* Samuel A. Green, *The History of Medicine in Massachusetts: A Centennial Address Before the Massachusetts Medical Society at Cambridge, June 7, 1881* (1881); Henry R. Viets, *A Brief History of Medicine in Massachusetts* (1930); Dirk J. Struik, *Yankee Science in the Making* (1962), pp. 281–84.

Simpson claimed that opposition to anesthesia was linked to opposition to contagionism in puerperal fever; see Simpson to Ramsbotham, July 23, 1848, in Ramsbotham Papers. There likely is validity in such charges, though there were anticontagionists like Channing who strongly favored anesthesia; see Tilton, *Amiable Autocrat*, p. 174.

30. Holmes, *Introductory Lecture*, pp. 8–9, emphasis in original.

31. *Trans AMA* (1848), 1:283–88, a report by Holmes et al. on medical journals of the various regions.

32. Richard H. Shryock, "Medical Practice in the Old South," in *Medicine in America: Historical Essays,* pp. 49–70; Martha Carolyn Mitchell, "Health and the Medical Profession in the Lower South, 1845–1860," *Journal of Southern History* (November 1944), 10:424–46; John Duffy, "Medical Practice in the Ante Bellum South," *Journal of Southern History* (February 1959), 25:53–72; Duffy, "Sectional Conflict and Medical Education in Louisiana," *Journal of Southern History* (August 1957), 23:289–306; Duffy, "A Note on Ante Bellum Southern Nationalism and Medical Practice," *Journal of Southern History* (May 1968), 34:266–76; Numbers and Warner, "Maturation of Medical Science."

33. For historical studies, see: Allan Pred, "Large City Interdependence and the Preelectronic Diffusion of Innovation in the United States," *Geographical Analysis* (April 1971), 3:165–81; and Rondo Cameron, "The Diffusion of Technology as a Problem in Economic History," *Economic Geography* (July 1975), 51:217–30.

For contemporary studies that helped me clarify concepts and approach, see: James S. Coleman, Elihu Katz, and Herbert Menzel, *Medical Innovation: A Diffusion Study* (1966); Everett M. Rogers and George M. Beal, "The Importance of Personal Influence in the Adoption of Technological Change," *Social Forces* (May 1958), 36:329–35; Elihu Katz, Martin L. Levin, and Herbert Hamilton, "Traditions of Research on the Diffusion of Innovation," *American Sociological Review* (April 1963), 28:237–52; Elihu Katz and Paul Lazarsfeld, *Personal Influence: The Part Played by People in the Flow of Mass Communication* (1955); Diana Crane, *Invisible Colleges: Diffusion of Knowledge in Scientific Communities* (1972); Elina Hemminki, "Review of the Literature on the Factors Affecting Drug Prescribing," *Social Science and Medicine* (1975), 9:111–15.

34. Bigelow, for example, spoke of "the wide-spread influence" that the Pennsylvania Hospital "exerts upon their own section of the country, and upon the large community of which they are the scientific centre," *B Med Surg J* (April 1848), 38:237. For the role of Europe, see ch. 3, note 32 above; Warren, *Etherization,* p. iii.

35. For Horner, see Eckenhoff, *Anesthesia from Colonial Times,* p. 26; see Dunglison to John Collins Warren, January 29, 1848; and Horner to John Collins Warrren, January 18, 1848; John C. Warren Papers, vol. 23, items 40, 33. For confirmation of my impressions concerning Warren's Philadelphia correspondence, see Eaton, "Medicine in Philadelphia and Boston," p. 74.

36. Flagg, *Ether and Chloroform,* pp. 30–31; for family connections, see *DAB.*

37. Fülöp-Miller, *Triumph Over Pain,* ch. 12, "Ships for Europe," conveys very well the immense importance of this European communication. See also the comments of Metcalfe, "Purity and Use of Chloroform," pp. 140–41; and Edward Everett to Henry Holland, November 14, 1846, December 31, 1846, February 1, 1847, Everett Papers, vol. 80, reel 27, items 56–57, 159–60, 199.

In his autobiography, Warren claimed he immediately wrote "letters to the South" (meaning Philadelphia?), as well as articles to London and Paris. However, Warren's personal influence "to the South" appears to have been confined to a small circle of friends, Warren, *Life of John Collins Warren,* 1:385.

38. Flexner, *Doctors on Horseback,* pp. 281–82; Metcalfe, "Purity and Use of Chloroform," pp. 140–41n; Howard Dittrick, "The Introduction of Anesthesia into Ohio," *Ohio Archaeological and Historical Quarterly* (1941), 50:345.

39. Ch. 3, note 32 above. *B Med Surg J* (1847), 36:109. "Instructer" *sic.*

40. *Trans AMA* (1848), 1:220–21; Kelly and Burrage, *American Medical Biographies.* See also Horner to John Collins Warren, January 18, 1848, John C. Warren Papers, vol. 23, item 33.

41. *Trans AMA* (1848), 1:220–21.

42. To make such estimates would require information on the surgical patient pop-

ulation, *before* and after anesthesia; I have not been able to locate such records for the Philadelphia clinics. They do exist for the MGH and Pa. H.; see ch. 11 below for analysis.

43. Sanford V. Larkey and Janet B. Koudelka, "Medical Societies and Civil War Politics," *Bulletin of the History of Medicine* (January–February 1962), 36:1–12; the uniqueness of AMA unity was first noted by Carl Russell Fish, as quoted by Clement Eaton, *A History of the Southern Confederacy* (1954), p. 23.

44. Horner, "Anaesthetics." Eaton does, however, claim that Confederate surgeons were prejudiced against ether and preferred chloroform, though he does not give a reason or a citation; Eaton, *Southern Confederacy*, p. 102. One surviving thesis by an English student was not counted.

45. Boland, *The First Anesthetic*.

46. Ahlstrom, *Religious History of the American People*, chs. 15, 16, and pp. 466–68; Bozeman, "Antebellum Presbyterian Thought."

47. Flagg, *Ether and Chloroform*, pp. 145, 147; Parrish to J. Mason Warren, February 29, 1848, John C. Warren Papers, vol. 26; Kelly and Burrage, *American Medical Biographies*. Summary of the Transactions of the College of Physicians of Philadelphia (1846–1849), 2:156.

48. For trenchant comments, see Flagg, *Ether and Chloroform*, pp. 34–35; for an example of what Flagg was talking about, see the reaction of Thomas E. Bond, in J. A. Taylor, *History of Dentistry* (1922), p. 85.

49. *Medical Gazette*, August 20, 1870, clipping in Hamilton Case Book, 8:44; the reference is undoubtedly to the *B Med Surg J*. Thus, the great paradox of American medical nationalism: America was highly dependent on European approval, yet also intensely nationalistic. See Eckman, "Anglo-American Hostility"; also Thomas N. Bonner, "The Social and Political Attitudes of Midwestern Physicians 1840–1940: Chicago as a Case History," *Journal of the History of Medicine and Allied Sciences* (April 1953), 8:140. For similar comments by Dr. Lyman B. How, see *Transactions of the New Hampshire Medical Society* (1869), pp. 40–41.

50. *AJMS* (1867), 53:184; *Buffalo Medical and Surgical Journal* (April 1862), 17:276–78.

51. *New York Medical Journal* (April 1871), 13:389, 409.

52. *AJMS* (1861), 41:357–71 (F. D. Lente); *Medical and Surgical Reporter* (1866), 14:395–96 (Erastus Wilson); (1866), 14:5–6 (J. M. Carnochan); (1872), 27:436–38 (J. S. Wight).

53. Not surprisingly, the change coincided precisely with the 1867 resignation of Dr. Moses Gunn, the University's first professor of surgery. Gunn used chloroform, at least through 1862 (Perky, "Chloroform," p. 43) but had begun using the "A.C.E." mixture by 1867 (Smith, "Anaesthetics," p. 43). However, at least one of Gunn's successors in the 1868–1872 period, Alpheus Benning Crosby, was a prominent advocate of chloroform (Kelly and Burrage, *American Medical Biographies*).

54. William James Herdman, "Record of Surgical Clinics from January 1st to March 21, 1875," unpublished M.D. thesis, University of Michigan, 1875.

55. Turner, "Anaesthetics," p. 20. Dr. Crosby resigned from the Michigan faculty in 1871, to replace his father as professor at Dartmouth; Shaw, *Encyclopedic History*, vol. 2, part 5, p. 939.

11. A CRITICAL EVALUATION

1. Rothstein, *American Physicians*, p. 252.

2. Bowditch, *History of Massachusetts General Hospital* (1851), p. 215.

3. Warren, *Etherization*, p. 4; J. Collins Warren, *Influence of Anaesthesia*, pp. 24–29.

4. Bigelow, *Inaugural Address*, p. 240; ch. 3, notes 117–25 above; Youngson, *Scientific Revolution*, p. 97; Sykes, *Essays*, 1:150.

5. Rothstein, *American Physicians*, p. 252; Samuel D. Harvey, "Effect of the Introduction of Anesthesia Upon Surgery," *Journal of the American Dental Association* (November 1945), 32:1354. Guy's Hospital in London performed 101 operations over 12 months in 1846–47; during only a 6 month period of 1853 they performed 135 procedures; Greene, "Development of Surgery," p. 8.

One recent study does reject the notion that anesthesia led to a rush of surgery, at least for the Glasgow Royal Infirmary in Scotland; Hamilton, "Nineteenth-Century Surgical Revolution," p. 32. However, Hamilton's data show a 25 percent rise in surgery following anesthesia, from 151 to 188 operations a year, over the period 1842–50. While this increase is less than the 51 percent boom in a comparable period following antisepsis, it was hardly inconsiderable by 1840s standards. Furthermore, interpretation of these figures is limited by the failure to control for changes in the numbers of patients admitted.

6. The increases in Boston's immigrant and pauper populations both outstripped the increase in amputations over these years; Handlin, *Boston's Immigrants*, pp. 256, 242. For a detailed assessment of the role of industrialization, see the next section of this chapter below. On the expansion of the Massachusetts General Hospital, see Bowditch, *History of Massachusetts General Hospital*, 2nd ed., with a Continuation to 1872 (1872), pp. 197–201, 202, 203.

7. The major difficulty was the lack of widespread understanding of the use of statistical controls; the concept that in order to understand the effects of a drug, it was necessary to keep records on those cases for which the drug was *not* administered. This and other errors, and the ideological basis for them, were discussed in chs. 5 and 6 above, especially ch. 5, note 32.

8. One variable these figures still do not control for is the possibility that, with a new wing to fill, the patients admitted after 1847 were on average "less sick" than those admitted before. If so, that would make the actual rise in operations per admission even more dramatic than these figures indicate. See Bowditch, *History of Massachusetts General Hospital* (2nd ed.), p. 209, for an indication that this probably was the case.

9. From October 16, 1852, to October 15, 1853, 22 of 245 fracture cases admitted received amputations (9 percent); the figure remained almost constant over the next decade, dropping slightly to 26 of 371 cases (7 percent) by the corresponding period 1862–63. Pa. H. Fracture Books.

10. In 1859, the rate was still just over 23 percent (243/1353; 319/1463; 386/1660), NYH Records. These NYH data are preliminary results of a large multivariate analysis currently in progress; see ch. 1, note 8. If a slightly different indicator, the total number of operations per patient admitted, is used, the increase becomes more apparent; from 22 percent in 1845–46, to 29 percent in 1847–48, and 33 percent in 1859–60 (297/1353; 429/1463; 549/1660).

Charles Rosenberg reports a much lower operation per admission rate, 7.4 percent, for the single month of October 1858, "And Heal the Sick," p. 444. Perhaps that month was atypical; more likely his figure excludes many "minor" procedures often not reported as operations in the published hospital tabulations, see ch. 8 above.

11. While the average absolute number of amputations per year for the entire period 1821–1846 was 5.0, for the period 1840–46, it was only 3.5, despite the fact that the patient population had increased. Calculated from data in *AJMS* (1851), 21:178–83; and Rothstein, *American Physicians*, p. 252.

12. And also his inexplicable inclusion of 1846–1850 in the pre-anesthetic period. Controlling for admissions, the pre-anesthetic proportion was 1.4/15.9 or 0.088. After anes-

thesia, the proportion was 6.8/39.6 or 0.172. Virtually identical results are obtained even without controlling for admissions.

13. For the lack of change in composition of the patient population, see note 51 below.

14. The quote is from *AJMS* (1852), 23:455. For charges of opponents, see ch. 3, notes 117–25; for sexual aspects, see also ch. 8, note 16 above.

15. The latter type were sometimes called "normal ovariotomies"; the operations were also called oöphorectomies.

16. For Atlee, see *AJMS* (1849), 18:346; *Ohio Medical and Surgical Journal* (1849), 2:38–39. For Gardner, see *AJMS* (1852), 24:130. For both, see Kelly and Burrage, *American Medical Biographies*.

There were a few pioneer ovariotomists, such as Charles Wallace Clay of England, who preferred to operate without anesthesia, as late as 1863; *B Med Surg J* (1863), 69:176; Hamilton, *Military Surgery*, p. 617.

17. Kidd, *Manual*, p. 96; also Bryant, *Practice of Surgery*, p. 928.

18. For a sample of opposition, see *AJMS* (1851), 22:140; *Transactions of the New Hampshire Medical Society* (1866), pp. 18–19; Lawrence D. Longo, "The Rise and Fall of Battey's Operation: A Fashion in Surgery," *Bulletin of the History of Medicine* (Summer, 1979), 53:244–67.

19. The first was Elizabeth S. G., admitted August 30, 1847, MGH Records, vol. 31. The second was Mary A. B., admitted September 3, 1847, MGH Records, vol. 33 W.

20. Hayward, *Surgical Reports*, p. 236; also Bryant, *Practice of Surgery*, p. 928.

21. Such does not appear to have been the case with animals. Anesthesia seemingly fostered a large increase in experimental animal surgery, at least according to the anecdotal accounts of both supporters and opponents. See: William H. Welch, "The Influence of Anaesthesia Upon Medical Science," in *The Semi-Centennial of Anaesthesia*, pp. 57–68; French, *Antivivisection*, pp. 32–33, 40, 68; Fülöp-Miller, *Triumph Over Pain*, p. 407; Whipple, *Evolution of Surgery*, p. 38; and the comments of *Punch* quoted by Weller, "*Punch*, on Anaesthesia," p. 1270.

It is likely that anesthesia led to a somewhat greater increase in experimentation after a few years than it did in the initial year of its use, though such a delayed reaction is hard to demonstrate statistically. My concern here, however, has been to judge the extent to which the immediate postanesthetic boom was experimental.

22. Rothstein, *American Physicians*, p. 252. The charges were especially frequent during the Civil War. For examples of claims that Civil War surgeons overoperated, in part owing to the conquest of pain, and for judicious assessment of such criticism, see: Adams, *Doctors in Blue*, pp. 108, 116–18; H. H. Cunningham, *Doctors in Gray: The Confederate Medical Service* (1960), pp. 225–30; and Stewart Brooks, *Civil War Medicine* (1966), pp. 97–98. These authors generally agree that Civil War surgery was more "conservative" than nineteenth-century critics charged. For more dramatic accounts, see Gordon W. Jones, "Wartime Surgery," *Civil War Times Illustrated* (1963), 2(2):7–8, 28–30, especially 28; "University of Pennsylvania Alumni in the Civil War," *Medical Affairs* (Spring, 1961), 2:10.

The issue was especially controversial in obstetrics. For a debate over whether anesthetics led to greater surgical interference in childbirth, see the running dispute conducted by Charles C. Hildreth and Thad A. Reamy of Ohio: *AJMS* (1866), 51:361–64; *Philadelphia Medical and Surgical Reporter* (1867), 16:21–26, 110–112, 277–84.

23. Mark V. Pauly, "What is Unnecessary Surgery?" *Milbank Memorial Fund Quarterly* (Winter, 1979), 57:95–117; see ch. 5 above.

Many other conflicts of medical doctrine contributed to the lack of consensus on the necessity and legitimacy of surgery. For example, "solidists" generally favored more frequent operations than did "humoralists."

24. For a more detailed explanation, see the following section on industrial accidents. In addition, accident victims were, on the whole, poorer than other patients at most nineteenth-century hospitals, since, in emergencies only, hospital managers waived the requirement that patients be certified as "deserving" before admission as charity cases. For Boston, see Vogel, *Invention of the Hospital;* for Philadelphia, see the Admissions and Discharge Records, Pennsylvania Hospital Historical Library, Philadelphia, in which patients were recorded in one of three categories: Paying, Free, or "Received-Accident."

25. Between October 16, 1845, and October 15, 1846, cases admitted within a week of their initial symptoms accounted for 7 of the 11 deaths of surgical patients, though they comprised only 66 of the 221 surgical admissions. The difference of proportions is significant at the .05 level. MGH Records, vols. 29–30.

26. In theory this restraint was due to the belief that such patients were too weakened by their injuries to stand the operation; see ch. 3, note 55 above. However other reasons may have included a system of triage in which doctors decided that such cases were "hopeless" and a waste of time or the possibility that surgeons avoided such cases in order not to depress their "batting average" or recovery rate. I have seen no evidence either for or against these latter two speculations.

27. Controlling for admissions, emergencies constituted 6.1/26.1 or 23.4 percent of pre–anesthetic surgery, and 23.6/70.6 or 33.4 percent of postanesthetic surgery. (Without controlling for admissions, the corresponding proportions are 4/31 or 12.9 percent and 21/95 or 22.1 percent.)

Of course, the increase in surgery following the discovery of anesthesia almost certainly included an increase in the absolute *number* of "unnecessary" operations. But, more importantly, these figures indicate that anesthesia probably decreased the *proportion* of operations that were "unnecessary."

28. Turnbull, *Artificial Anaesthesia,* p. 15, believed surgeons everywhere followed this pattern.

29. Bryant, *Practice of Surgery,* p. 928, for excisions; Warren, *Etherization,* p. 60, for lithotrity; Barker, "Anaesthetics in Midwifery," (1862), p. 264, for Caesarian section; *Westminster Review* (1859), 71:81.

At MGH, excisions, resections, and bone pinning increased immediately following 1846, but amputations increased even more. And the number of reconstructive bone operations remained a tiny fraction (4/293) of surgery that year.

A recent study claims to detect no major changes in the kinds of operations done, before and after anesthesia, at the leading American and British hospitals, Greene, "Development of Surgery." His data, based on an 1870 tabulation rather than on the original patient records, list no reconstructive bone surgery at all at the MGH from 1821–1870, although the patient records clearly indicate otherwise. Furthermore, at Guy's Hospital in London, bone excisions jumped from 2 percent of all surgery in 1845, to 13 percent in 1853, and remained at 15 percent through 1861–68; in the same period amputations fell from 25 percent to 18.5 and 18 percent. Also at Guy's, ovariotomies jumped following anesthesia, from 0.5 percent of all operations in 1843–44, to nearly 3 percent in 1861–68, Greene, "Development of Surgery," pp. 8–9.

30. For ether: Eliza Cope Harrison, ed., *Philadelphia Merchant: The Diary of Thomas P. Cope, 1800–1851* (1978), p. 533 (May 1, 1848, 1:10,000); *Westminster Review* (1859), 71:77 (1:16,216); Turnbull, *Artificial Anaesthesia,* p. 32 (1885, 1:23,000); Lewin, *Untoward Effects of Drugs,* p. 184 (1883, 1:30,000).

For chloroform: Turnbull, *Artificial Anaesthesia,* p. 93 (1885, 1:2,500); *Chicago Medical Examiner* (1868), 9:657 (Edward Andrews, 1:3,600); *New York Medical Journal* (1871), 13:389, 409 (Edward R. Squibb, 1:5,800); Walker "Anaesthesia and Anaesthetics," p. 37 (1862, 1:10,000). Note the growing confidence in ether, and fear of chloroform, over time.

For early attempts to assess the long-term effects, see: *AJMS* (1848), 16:33–43; (1851), 21:178–83; (1852), 23:450–55; *Medical Communications of the Massachusetts Medical Society* (1864), 10:229. The statistics are my conversion to percentages of the data in *AJMS* (1852), 23:453.

Simpson presented data to show that anesthesia lowered the death rate from amputation in several European hospitals. His figures were occasionally cited in the American literature but never duplicated in an American hospital. For citations, see "Report of Medical Society of Virginia," p. 191; Henry, "Etherization, as a Surgical Remedy," p. 9. On Simpson's data, see Youngson, *Scientific Revolution*, pp. 89, 115.

31. Rothstein, *American Physicians*, pp. 251–52; converted to percentages and deaths per hundred by me.

32. Duffy, "Science and Medicine," p. 123.

33. For the former explanation, see Porter, "Medical and Surgical Notes," *AJMS* (1852), 24:30; also *AJMS* (1852), 23:452, 455; and ch. 3, notes 45–55, 63 above.

For the latter explanation, see *Western Lancet* (1848), 7:365; and ch. 3, notes 117–25 above.

For Erichsen's view, that anesthesia led to more surgery, hence more crowded wards; crowding considered as a direct cause of infection, see Erichsen, *Science and Art of Surgery* (1860), p. 30; Harvey, "Effect of Anesthesia," p. 1354. For especially full discussion of these issues, see: *Bulletin of the New York Academy of Medicine* (1864), 2:327–45.

34. J. Collins Warren, *Influence of Anaesthesia*, pp. 24–29. See Rothstein, *American Physicians*, p. 252, for modern endorsement of similar views.

35. *AJMS* (1851), 21:182.

36. Norris, "Statistical Account of the Cases of Amputation," *Pennsylvania Hospital Reports* (1868), 1:149.

37. *Trans AMA* (1848), 1:215–17.

38. Gross, *System of Surgery*, 1:535. For a homeopathic endorsement, see Gilchrist, *Syllabus*, p. 21.

39. FitzWilliam Sargent, the only nineteenth-century American to test the relative roles of accidents and anesthesia statistically, reached a different conclusion from mine, *AJMS* (1852), 23:450–55. For the MGH data, he did all the right calculations yet simply and baldly misread the results. In general, Sargent's statistical logic and technique were far in advance of his contemporaries, especially in his use of a statistical control for an intervening variable and in his scrupulous care in recounting the actual data himself. Yet his cumbersome use of fractions rather than percentages and his lack of a method of testing statistical significance seemingly led him astray in his interpretation of the MGH data.

Likewise, Sargent's analysis of the New York Hospital data on this question does not show what he claims to show. He claims that anesthesia caused a rise in the death rate because, even with accidents controlled for, the surgical death rate rose after 1848. However, he does not distinguish those who received anesthetics from those who did not after 1848. While the available data are not good enough to say for sure who did not get anesthetics, comparing those who are definitely recorded as having received anesthetics with those for whom no anesthetic administration was recorded indicates that the death rate was lower for the anesthetized.

Sargent's inclusion of the Pennsylvania Hospital in his data is misleading, since anesthetics had not yet been introduced there; there is no reason to believe that practice at the three hospitals was similar enough to use the Pennsylvania data as a control on the New York and Boston data the way Sargent has done. My study of the fracture cases at the Pa. H. does reveal a higher death rate among those given anesthesia, even when accidents are taken into account. (In fact, almost all these cases were due to accidents.) But the difference is not statistically significant.

Sargent's study was replicated in England by Dr. James Arnott, *AJMS* (1867), 53:164; see Youngson, *Scientific Revolution,* p. 115, for a seemingly garbled version, with no citation. See also Hamilton, *Military Surgery,* p. 621; Jaehrig, "Anaesthetics," p. 17.

40. MGH accident admissions fell off sharply in the mid-1860s because of the opening of Boston City Hospital.

The immediate postanesthesia years were also the peak accident years in New York and Philadelphia. The Philadelphia casualty rate jumped more sharply between 1846 and 1859 than in any other comparable period from 1839 to 1901; Roger Lane, *Violent Death in the City: Suicide, Accident, and Murder in Nineteenth-Century Philadelphia* (1979), p. 36. New York Hospital noted that the number of emergency accident victims admitted in 1849 was double that of any previous year, *State of the New York Hospital and Bloomingdale Asylum, for the Year 1849* (1849).

One recent study of surgery in nineteenth-century Glasgow, Scotland, suggests that the unprecedented peak in amputation deaths between 1849 and the 1860s was due to the worsening nutritional status of the patients. However, the data presented also show that 1846–1855 witnessed the sharpest increase in compound fractures of any period from 1842–1899; Hamilton, "Nineteenth Century Surgical Revolution," pp. 33, 36.

41. *Westminster Review* (1859), 71:80. So far as I can tell, Fenwick's study was never fully published in this country. What is clearly only the second half was reprinted in the relatively obscure *American Medical Gazette* (October 1857), 8:592–600; I am extremely grateful to Jim Cassedy for finding this for me. In addition to distinguishing trauma and disease statistics for five separate kinds of amputations, Fenwick also presented data on eight other specific kinds of surgery. He concluded that only in hernia did the postanesthetic death rate compare unfavorably with earlier years.

For the beginning of modern anesthesia case records in 1894, see Henry K. Beecher, "The First Anesthesia Records (Codman, Cushing)," *Surgery, Gynecology and Obstetrics* (1940), 71:689–93. I am grateful to Susan Reverby for this citation.

Punch, January 30, 1847, quoted by Weller, "*Punch,* on Anaesthesia," p. 1270.

42. For nineteenth-century opinion that this was the case, see Gross, *System of Surgery,* 1:535; Hurd, "Anaesthetics," p. 31; Turner, "Anaesthetics," pp. 8–9.

43. From 2 of 5 cases to 5 of 16 cases. F. F. Cartwright claims similar results at King's College Hospital in England, though his data are confusing and incompletely documented, "Antiseptic Surgery," in *Medicine and Science in the 1860s,* edited by F. N. L. Poynter (1968), p. 82.

44. The greatest rise in unnecessary interventions may have been in obstetrics; however, I have not been able to locate any data on the pre-1846 use of obstetrical instruments to serve as a statistical control.

45. For Sargent's acceptance of this calculus, see *AJMS* (1852), 23:450–51. For dissenters, see ch. 5, notes 133–34 above.

46. Bowditch, *History of Massachusetts General* (1st ed.), p. 215.

47. Lester Noble, "When Ether Was A New Miracle," edited by Robert S. Gillcash, *Journal of the Maine Medical Association* (May 1963), 54:102.

48. MGH Records, vols. 29–33.

49. Bowditch, *History of Massachusetts General* (2nd ed.), p. 209. In 1847, there were 212 surgical outpatients, *Annual Report of the Trustees of Massachusetts General Hospital and McLean Asylum* (1859), p. 7.

50. Mott, "Remarks on the Importance of Anaesthesia," p. 86; Warren, *Etherization;* see also Francis R. Packard, *The Pennsylvania Hospital of Philadelphia* (1938), p. 56.

51. There was a rise in the proportion of children admitted, but the numbers were not large enough to affect the overall age distribution of the patient population.

52. K. G. Huston, *Resuscitation—An Historical Perspective* (1976); *Stethoscope and Virginia Medical Gazette* (1852), 2:681–84; Lewin, *Untoward Effects of Drugs*, pp. 178–79. For Morton's Bromfield House operations see Bigelow, *Surgical Anaesthesia*, p. 163.

53. Berlant, *Profession and Monopoly*, p. 86.

54. Ch. 5, note 52 above.

55. Reynell Coates, *Introductory Lecture to the Class of the Female Medical College of Pennsylvania, 1860* (1861). I am indebted to Gina Morantz for this document and for those cited in notes 60–62 and 70–71 below. Coates was paraphrasing an argument with which he disagreed.

56. Edmund Andrews, "The Surgeon," *Chicago Medical Examiner* (1861), 2:587–90; reprinted in *Medical America*, ed. by Brieger, p. 178, emphasis in original.

57. Scholten, "Importance of the Obstetrick Art," p. 441, quoting Walter Channing, *Remarks on the Employment of Females as Practitioners in Midwifery* (Boston, 1820), pp. 4–7, emphasis in original. This booklet may actually have been the work of John Ware.

58. Trotter, *A View of the Nervous Temperament*, p. 164.

59. Nichols, "Woman the Physician," p. 3; Gregory, *Man-Midwifery*, p. 43; Stanton to Mott, October 22, 1852, in *Oven Birds*, p. 260.

60. Quoted by R. T. Trall, "Allopathy *Adversus* Woman," *The Water-Cure Journal* (1852), 13:87. Gardner was speaking of the defects of women obstetricians.

61. (October 1850), 2:77. For other examples, see Morantz, "The 'Connecting Link.' "

62. Samuel Gregory, "Female Physicians," *The Living Age* (April–June 1862), 73:243, 244.

63. *Announcement of the Female Medical College of Pennsylvania, 1851*, 2nd announcement (1851), p. 9. I am indebted to Gina Morantz for this citation. Blackwell, *Pioneer Work*, p. 199. Emily did not become a full-time surgeon, though she in turn served as preceptor for the first woman who did, Mary Thompson. See Kelly and Burrage, *American Medical Biographies*.

64. In addition to the small sample size, another methodological problem in interpreting this evidence is the "ecological fallacy" involved in comparing cases at two different hospitals. Though Professor Morantz attempted to control for relevant intervening variables in the patient populations at the two hospitals, it is possible that in some unrecorded or unmeasurable way, women doctors attracted a disproportionate share of those types of patients who would have received anesthesia from physicians of either sex. Further, the dates of the two samples are not identical.

65. See note 59 above.

66. Lasch, "Woman Reformer's Rebuke."

67. " 'Twas But A Babe," reprinted in *Oven Birds*, p. 59. For the general romantic hostility to utilitarianism, see Miller, "The Romantic Dilemma in American Nationalism and the Concept of Nature," in *Nature's Nation*, pp. 199–201.

68. Blackwell, *Pioneer Work*, p. 56.

69. Blackwell, *Pioneer Work*, p. 102.

70. S. R. Adamson [Sarah Adamson Dolley] to Elijah F. Pennypacker, February 3, 1850, Archives of the Medical College of Pennsylvania, Philadelphia.

71. Marie E. Zakrzewska, *Introductory Lecture . . . Before the New England Female Medical College at the Opening of the Term 1859–60* (1859), pp. 5–6. Emphasis in original. For a fascinating modern study of this issue, see Lynn R. Davidson, "Sex Roles, Affect, and the Woman Physician: A Comparative Study of the Impact of Latent Social Identity Upon the Role of Women and Men Professionals," unpublished Ph.D. dissertation, New York University, 1975.

72. Alcott, *Hospital Sketches*, pp. 37–38, 87–88. For a good exposition of Catharine Beecher's attempt to reconcile belief in professional training for women with belief in woman's innate feminine talents for healing and other professional duties, see Parker, "Introduction," *Oven Birds*, pp. 31–32.

73. Alcott, *Hospital Sketches*, p. 86.

74. For an interesting example, compare the role of woman as terrified observer in Thomas Eakins' "The Gross Clinic" (1875) with the calm, starched, detached nurse in Eakins' post-Listerian "The Agnew Clinic" (1898). *The Art of Philadelphia Medicine* (1965), pp. 64–70. Philip A. Kalisch and Beatrice J. Kalisch, *The Advance of American Nursing* (1978), pp. 181–83.

75. Greene, *Anesthesiology and the University*, p. 15.

76. See ch. 3, notes 113–145; ch. 4, notes 33–45 above. Portions of this section appeared in Pernick, "Patient's Role," pp. 21–28.

77. *AJMS* (1849), 18:401; 96; see also *AJMS* (1853), 25:556, and ch. 8, note 7 above.

78. Simpson, *Account of a New Anaesthetic Agent*, in *Milestones in Anesthesia*, pp. 99–100.

79. Ether was not used, because the operation was for harelip. Patient admitted June 19, 1854, MGH Records, vol. 64 W. For other examples of children anesthetized for control, see MGH Records, vol. 88 W, admitted October, 1859, p. 37; NYH Case Books, vol. 18, 1 S.D., discharged July, 1854, patient number 659.

80. Jackson, *Manual*, pp. 104–7. Ironically, Jackson himself ended his days a patient at McLean. Individual case records are confidential, so history will never know whether Jackson ever received anesthetic tranquilization. The term "tranquilization" was Superintendent Dr. John E. Tyler's, quoted by Jackson, p. 107.

81. For an overview, see *American Journal of Insanity* (1865), 22:58–61, 76–81; Henry K. Beecher, "Anesthesia's Second Power: Probing the Mind," *Science* (1947), 105:164–66. For similar use in a general hospital, see NYH Case Books, 1859 1 S.D., discharged June 24, 1859, patient number 1003, entry of April 29, 1859. On origins of modern tranquilizers, see Anne E. Caldwell, "The History of Psychopharmacology; Its Relation to Anesthesiology," *Diseases of the Nervous System* (December 1967), 28:816–20. See also ch. 4, note 32 above.

82. See ch. 8, notes 17–20 above, and Pernick, "Patient's Role," p. 23, n. 69, and passim.

83. MGH Records, vol. 31 admitted April 7, 1847; Warren, *Etherization*, p. 37. MGH Records, vol. 65 E, p. 18, admitted February 24, 1855; both her legs were amputated against her will; she died March 7. For another similar case, see MGH Records, vol. 63 E, p. 236, admitted January 24, 1855.

Physicians generally argue that pain and disease themselves deprive us of rational autonomy whether or not a physician is present. In other words, a person sick or in pain is "not himself." The physician thus does not usurp the patient's autonomy but rather carries out the decision the patient would have made, if the patient had been free of the duress and pain of illness. See Samuel W. Bloom, *The Doctor and His Patient: A Sociological Interpretation* (1965, 1963). Since Bloom's analysis, any number of criticisms have been voiced, especially in the works of Eliot Freidson, Elliot A. Krause, and Eric J. Cassell. It is my belief that pain and illness do deprive us of much of our rational decisionmaking capability but that *medical* criteria are not the only appropriate values to consider in assessing who is "competent" to make decisions; Pernick, "Patient's Role."

84. For example, "Death Produced by the Fear of Dying," *Journal of Health* (Philadelphia) (1831–32), 3:39.

85. *Transactions of the New Hampshire Medical Society* (1864), pp. 38–39. The

AJMS warned that a doctor who told a patient about the risks of chloroform would likely cause the patient to die of fear (1867), 53:175.

86. *AJMS* (1851), 22:498; Horner, "Anaesthetics," p. 30. The quote is from Dr. George T. Elliot, in Barker, "Anaesthetics in Midwifery," (1862), pp. 295, 304.

87. Jonathan Dawson, "The 'Gross Outrage,' " *Ohio Medical and Surgical Journal* (1857), 9:333–34.

88. Campbell, "Anaesthesia," p. 11; Turnbull, *Artificial Anaesthesia*, p. 158.

89. This patient was also undergoing alcohol withdrawal, MGH Records, vol. 65 E, p. 20, admitted February 24, 1855. The second case was also delirious from a fracture, MGH Records, vol. 88 W, admitted July 13, 1860.

Conversely, there were cases in which patients who requested anesthesia were denied it, Wiley, *Johnny Reb*, p. 266.

90. *Carpenter v. Blake*, 60 Barb. 488 (N.Y. Sup. Ct., 1871); 75 N.Y. 12 (1878). For extensive discussion, see Pernick, "Patient's Role," pp. 10–28.

91. Transcript published in *Lancet* (1866), part 2, pp. 561–64.

92. Turner, "Anaesthetics," p. 33.

93. See, for example: James D. admitted March 12, 1847, MGH Records, vol. 31; "Mr. P." Hamilton Case Book, 8:147; Thomas W., Hamilton Case Book, vol. 6, February 1857; Mrs. R., Hamilton Case Book, 12:38; Thomas K., admitted September 5, 1853, Pa. H. Fracture Books. The first two men were stated to be immigrants; the other two men had Irish last names. See also ch. 3, note 22 above for additional cases in which the patient's reasons were recorded.

94. MacQuitty, *Battle for Oblivion*, p. 94.

95. "The Patient's Consent to an Operation and the Surgeon's Discretion," *The Medical Record* (New York) (December 1880), 18:715, reports a case that still upheld the view of the patient as *non compos mentis*. In *Mohr v. Williams*, 95 Minn. 261, 104 N.W. 12 (1905), the court seemed to hold that patients should be consulted about midoperative decisions. However, in *Bennan v. Parsonnet*, 83 N.J.L. 20, 83 Atl. 948 (1912) and *McGuire v. Rix*, 118 Neb. 434, 225 N.W. 120 (1929), this obligation was removed in recognition of anesthetization.

96. "It Knew no Medicine—," *Poems*, edited by Johnson, 2:426. Johnson dates the manuscript c. 1862.

97. Illich, *Medical Nemesis*, presents the basic argument. I agree with his observations on this point, but his belief that the problem originated in a professional conspiracy is historically unfounded. For Bishop Lawrence, see *Outlook* (1904), 76:873, quoted in Turner, *Reckoning With the Beast*, p. 82. For similar statements, see Hayman, "Economy of Pain," pp. 18–19; *Lancet* (1886), part 1, p. 845; the concept that pain relievers lower endurance is much older than anesthesia; see the Spanish mystic Saint Teresa of Avila, quoted in Steven F. Brena, *Pain and Religion* (1972), p. 31.

98. Thompson, "Anaesthesia"; *Western Lancet* (1848), 7:364; *Semi-Centennial of Anaesthesia*, p. 53. For such exceptions as Elizabeth Cady Stanton, see ch. 3 above.

99. Van Buren, "Anaesthesia," p. 50. For an example of the use of discretionary anesthetization to reward a cooperative patient, see *AJMS* (1851), 22:271.

100. For two very different views, see Ben-David, "Scientific Productivity"; Bernhard J. Stern, *Society and Medical Progress* (1941). Other important historical treatments include Daniel H. Calhoun, *The Intelligence of a People* (1973); Shryock, *American Medical Research;* Youngson, *Scientific Revolution;* and Brooke Hindle, *Emulation and Invention* (1981). See also Dennis J. Palumbo and Richard A. Styskal, "Professionalism and Receptivity to Change," *American Journal of Political Science* (May 1974), 18:385–94.

For nineteenth-century opinion, see Hodges, *Narrative*, p. 126, and ch. 3, note 40 above.

101. Olmsted, *Magendie*, pp. 244–47.

102. See also Turner, *Reckoning with the Beast*, p. 82.

103. During the Revolution, Benjamin Rush had observed how the bureaucratic structure of the British hospital system "mechanically forced happiness and satisfaction upon our countrymen perhaps without a single wish in the officers of the hospital to make their situation comfortable"; letter to John Adams quoted in Eric T. Carlson, "Benjamin Rush on Revolutionary War Hygiene," *Bulletin of the New York Academy of Medicine* (July–August 1979), 55:622. For America's war hospitals, see Fredrickson, *Inner Civil War*.

104. "Report of Boston Society for Medical Improvement on the Inhalation of Sulphuric Ether," p. 230; Lawrence G. Blochman, *Doctor Squibb: The Life and Times of A Rugged Idealist* (1958).

105. *The Complete Poems of Emily Dickinson*, edited by Thomas H. Johnson (1960), p. 123, no. 269.

106. Binney regarded anesthesia "as one of the great metaphysical discoveries of the age"; Binney to John Collins Warren, January 18, 1848, and also April 28, 1849, John C. Warren Papers, vol. 23, items 32, 75. Edward Everett to John Collins Warren, January 28, 1848, and Isaac P. Davis to John Collins Warren, January 23, 1848, both John C. Warren Papers, item 36. Warren evidently sent Binney's letter to Everett and Davis for comment; Everett agreed mildly with Binney; Davis was more noncommittal. Others who wrote on the mind-body implications include Kidd, *Manual*, pp. 24, 27; Jackson, *Manual*, p. 77; Flagg, *Ether and Chloroform*, p. 52. For other accounts, see Mostert, "States of Awareness During General Anestheisa," p. 75; Shedlin and Wallechinsky, *Laughing Gas*, pp. 77–81; see also the speculation by Kern, *Anatomy and Destiny*, p. 78.

Others tried to comprehend the larger materialist-antimaterialist implications; Warren, *Etherization*, pp. 12–13; *AJMS* (1867), 53:164. The discovery of a regular progression of stages of anesthesia also helped prepare the foundation for Henry Head's later theories about the evolutionary hierarchy of the nervous system. See for example *Westminster Review* (1859), 71:72; Hurd, "Anaesthetics," p. 9.

107. Everett to Warren January 28, 1848; Binney to Warren January 18, 1848; Samuel Parkman to John Collins Warren, January 7, 1848, John C. Warren Papers, vol. 23, items 32, 36, and 25 respectively. *AJMS* (1851), 21:254–55. "Letheon" was named for Lethe, the "waters of forgetfulness" at the entrance to Hades. See also Warren, *Etherization*, pp. 93–94.

108. Shryock, *Medicine and Society in America*, pp. 49–51.

109. *AJMS* (1852), 23:358. See also *AJMS* (1851), 22:123. For a good discussion of related concepts, see Rosenberg, "Therapeutic Revolution."

110. Robinson, *Victory Over Pain*, p. 245.

111. Turnbull, *Artificial Anaesthesia*, p. 16.

112. Dickson, "Pain and Death," p. 61.

113. On heroic surgery see English, *Crile*, pp. 20–46. Edmund D. Pellegrino, "The Sociocultural Impact of Twentieth-Century Therapeutics," in *The Therapeutic Revolution*, edited by Morris J. Vogel and Charles E. Rosenberg (1979), pp. 245–66.

114. Throughout this book I have attempted to point up current parallels and divergences in the footnotes. For the revival of interest in "individualized" pain therapy, see Helen Neal, *The Politics of Pain* (1978), especially pp. 101–112; and ch. 7, note 60 above.

115. "A Woman Waits for Me," in *Leaves of Grass*, p. 106. "Love is never more truly exercised than in inflicting necessary pain," Orcutt, *Discipline of the School*, p. 7.

116. Letter 34, January 1843, *Letters From New York*, in *Oven Birds*, p. 92. Emphasis in original.

For an important current debate on this issue, see Samuel Gorovitz and Alasdair

MacIntyre, "Toward a Theory of Medical Fallibility," *Journal of Medicine and Philosophy* (March 1976), 1:51–71; Michael D. Bayles and Arthur Caplan, "Medical Fallibility and Malpractice," *Journal of Medicine and Philosophy* (September 1978), 3:169–86.

AFTERWORD

1. Of course, not all professions involved the infliction of pain, nor do all occupations that inflict pain rely on an ideology of professionalism to regulate their behavior.

"Affective neutrality," which includes the ability to witness and inflict suffering without becoming emotionally involved, formed a central tenet of Talcott Parsons' classic functionalist definition of professionalism, see "The Professions and Social Structure," in *Essays in Sociological Theory* (1954), pp. 34–49; and "Social Structure and Dynamic Process: The Case of Modern Medical Practice," in *The Social System* (1951), pp. 428–79. Robert Merton first revised this definition to take into account the need to balance affective neutrality with positive compassion. See Robert King Merton, "Some Preliminaries to a Sociology of Medical Education," in *The Student-Physician: Introductory Studies in the Sociology of Medical Education,* edited by Merton, George C. Reader, and Patricia L. Kendall (1957), pp. 71–79.

2. Noel Parry and José Parry, *The Rise of the Medical Profession: A Study of Collective Social Mobility* (1976). This ahistorical focus is found in even the most historically sophisticated sociological studies, such as Berlant, *Profession and Monopoly;* Margali Sarfatti Larson, *The Rise of Professionalism: A Sociological Analysis* (1977).

Among the few sociological attempts to discuss changes over time in professionalism are: A. M. Carr-Saunders and P. A. Wilson, *The Professions* (1933); Philip Elliott, *The Sociology of the Professions* (1972); and Reader, *Professional Men.*

3. For a view of professional attributes, including systematic knowledge and a service ideal, see William J. Goode, "The Theoretical Limits of Professionalization," in *The Semi-Professions and their Organization,* edited by Amitai Etzioni (1969), pp. 277–78.

On monopoly and bureaucracy, see Berlant, *Profession and Monopoly;* Larson, *Rise of Professionalism;* Eliot Freidson, *Profession of Medicine: A Study of the Sociology of Applied Knowledge* (1970); and Freidson, *Professional Dominance: The Social Structure of Medical Care* (1970); also Max Weber, *From Max Weber: Essays in Sociology,* translated by H. H. Gerth and C. Wright Mills (1946).

4. Ernest Greenwood, "Attributes of a Profession," *Social Work* (July 1957), 2:45–55; Wilbert E. Moore, *The Professions: Roles and Rules* (1970); Bernard Barber, "Some Problems in the Sociology of the Professions," in *The Professions in America,* edited by Kenneth S. Lynn and the editors of *Daedalus* (1965), pp. 15–34.

5. Goode, "Limits of Professionalization," p. 292.

6. Walter Metzger, "What is a Profession?" Columbia University Program of General and Continuing Education in the Humanities, *Seminar Reports* (1975), 3(1).

7. G. Harries-Jenkins, "Professionals in Organizations," in *Professions and Professionalization,* edited by J. A. Jackson (1970), p. 58.

8. Rosen, *Specialization of Medicine;* Stevens, *American Medicine,* pp. 3–4, 45–54.

9. *AJMS* (1852), 24:20; *B Med Surg J* (1847), 37:33. Medical schools had additional reasons to oppose medical societies, see ch. 2 above.

10. Berlant, *Profession and Monopoly,* shows that most historical versions of professionalism have included monopoly as an important feature; however he also provides examples of some that did not. He uses this finding to claim that monopoly represents a more adequate model of professionalism than functionalism does. I use his finding to emphasize that

neither the Parsonian nor the Weberian model account for all the variations in the content of past professional values.

For a sophisticated and sensitive account of the various nineteenth-century professional positions on monopoly in medicine, see Ramsey, "Politics of Professional Monopoly."

11. See Parsons, "Professions and Social Structure," and *The Social System*, pp. 428–79.

12. Merton, Reader, and Kendall, eds., *The Student-Physician*, pp. 71–79; Berlant, *Profession and Monopoly;* Everett C. Hughes, "Professions," in *The Professions in America*, edited by Lynn, pp. 6–7.

13. Everett C. Hughes, "Professions," pp. 6–7; J. A. Jackson, ed., *Professions and Professionalization* (1970), p. 6. See also Louis Lasagna, "The Conflict of Interest Between Physician as Therapist and As Experimenter" (1975), 26 pp.

14. Elliott, *Sociology of Professions*, pp. 91, 142–44.

15. M. Jeanne Peterson, *The Medical Profession in Mid-Victorian London* (1978), p. 37. Peterson's work is less presentist than many others. For example, she footnotes Sheldon Rothblatt's caution that the term "profession" has changed in meaning over time.

16. Carlo M. Cipolla, "The Professions: The Long View," *Journal of European Economic History* (1973), 2:37–52; Carr-Saunders and Wilson, *The Professions; OED*.

17. Burton Bledstein, *The Culture of Professionalism: The Middle Class and the Development of Higher Education in America* (1976), pp. 87–88; Haskell, *Emergence of Professional Social Science*, pp. 18, 27–28.

18. Thomas Bender, "The Cultures of Intellectual Life: The City and the Professions," in *New Directions in American Intellectual History*, edited by John Higham and Paul K. Conkin (1979), p. 183; Borrowman, *Liberal and Technical;* Calvert, *Mechanical Engineer*. See also William R. Johnson, *Schooled Lawyers: A Study in the Clash of Professional Cultures* (1978); Metzger, "What is a Profession?"; Gelfand, *Professionalizing Modern Medicine;* and Nathan Reingold, "Definitions and Speculations: The Professionalization of Science in America in the Nineteenth Century," in *The Pursuit of Knowledge in the Early American Republic*, edited by Alexandra Oleson and Sanborn C. Brown (1976), pp. 33–69.

19. The standard collection on the process of professionalization is Howard M. Vollmer and Donald Mills, eds., *Professionalization* (1966). Very few of the selections avoid the problem of judging past practitioners' behavior as if they had been trying to conform to today's ideals.

20. See note 18 above; also Thomas Kuhn, title essay in *The Essential Tension: Selected Studies in Scientific Tradition and Change* (1977).

21. In separate and independent studies published in the late 1970s, both philosopher Stephen Toulmin and I suggested different versions of the above hypothesis. Toulmin, "The Meaning of Professionalism: Doctors' Ethics and Biomedical Science," in *Knowledge, Value and Belief*, edited by H. Tristram Engelhardt, Jr. and Daniel Callahan (1977), pp. 254–78; and Pernick, "Medical Professionalism" (1978). Of course, this hypothesis can be proven only by empirical historical research, as Toulmin carefully acknowledges.

BIBLIOGRAPHY

Primary Source Materials

MANUSCRIPT PATIENT RECORDS

Countway Library of Medicine, The Harvard Medical School, Boston, Massachusetts. Rare Books Room. Massachusetts General Hospital, Surgical Records, Vols. 29–33 (1845–47); Vols. 62–67 (1854–55); Vols. 84–89, 91 (1859–60).

National Library of Medicine, History of Medicine Division. Bethesda, Maryland. Frank H. Hamilton Case Books.

New York Hospital, Medical Archives, New York. New York Hospital Surgical Case Books, First and Second Surgical Divisons, 1845–46; 1847–48; 1859–60; First Surgical Division, 1854–55.

Pennsylvania Hospital Historical Library, Philadelphia, Pennsylvania. Admissions and Discharge Records, 1840–51.

—— Fracture Books, 1852–69.

MANUSCRIPT M.D. THESES

Locations are abbreviated as follows:

FMCPA   Female Medical College of Pennsylvania Archives, Archives and Special Collections on Women in Medicine, Florence A. Moore Library, Medical College of Pennsylvania, Philadelphia.

HMC Hahnemann University Archives and History of Medicine Collection, Philadelphia.
UM University of Michigan Medical Theses, Bentley Library, Michigan Historical Collections, Ann Arbor.
UPA University of Pennsylvania Library, Philadelphia.

Bragg, Jonathan C. "Anaesthetics." January 1857. UPA.
Campbell, Clarence T. "A Thesis on Anaesthesia." February 1866. HMC.
Chapin, E. Jennie. "Chloroform." 1866. FMCPA.
Clarke, Edward. "Anaesthesia in Surgery." January 1860. UPA.
Crawford, Samuel K. "Chloroform, in Relation to Medical Jurisprudence." 1861. UM.
Criley, John M. "Anaesthesia in Labor." 1869. HMC.
Fletcher, Frank E. "Chloroform." 1865. UM.
Friend, Nathaniel. "Anaesthesia in Labour." January 1857. UPA.
Fussell, Rebecca L. "Anesthetics." February 1858. FMCPA.
George, William Henry. "Anaesthetics." 1869. UM.
Giles, Charles Henry. "The Origin Nature and Use of Pain." 1883. HMC.
Gunn, Alexander. "Chloroform." 1864. UM.
Harvey, John, Jr. "Ether, in Surgical Operations." 1851. UPA.
Henry, Charles F. "Etherization, As a Surgical Remedy." February 1853. UPA.
Herdman, William James. "Record of Surgical Clinics from January 1st to March 21, 1875." 1875. UM.
Horner, Edward H. "Anaesthetics." February 1855. UPA.
Hurd, Edward Homer. "Anaesthetics." 1867. UM.
Jaehrig, Bruno. "Anaesthetics." 1865. UM.
James, Bushrod W. "An Essay on the Progress of Surgery." February 1857. HMC.
McClelland, James H. "An Inaugural Dissertation on Anaesthesia in Labor." February 1867. HMC.
Mordecai, Edward R. "The Effects of Chloroform on the System and Its Therapeutical Applications." February 1849. UPA.
Muir, Daniel Henry. "Anaesthesia." 1871. UM.
Mulheron, John Jolliffe. "Pain." 1869. UM.
Perky, Samuel. "Chloroform." 1862. UM.
Ridings, James H. "An Essay on Anaesthetics." January 1868. HMC.
Riggs, John Upton. "Anaesthetics." 1868. UM.
Sackrider, Charles H. "Ether and Chloroform." 1856. UM.
Schneider, Louise. "Anaesthesia in Natural Labor." 1879. FMCPA.
Seelye, Mary T. "Relief of Pain as a Therapeutical Agent." 1870. FMCPA.
Smith, Stillman Hiram. "Anaesthetics." 1868. UM.
Thomas, Eliza L. S. "On the Propriety of Anaesthetic Agents in Surgical Operations." February 1855. FMCPA.
Thompson, John Wesley. "Anaesthesia." January 1860. UPA.
Turner, James. "Anaesthetics in Surgery and Parturition." 1871. UM.
Voorhies, Alfred Hunter. "Chloroformum." February 1860. UPA.

Wade, John K. "Anaesthetics in Labor." 1882. HMC.
Walker, I. R. "Anaesthesia and Anaesthetics." 1862. UM.

OTHER MANUSCRIPT COLLECTIONS

Boston Public Library. Boston School Committee Papers, 1845–1867.
Countway Library of Medicine, The Harvard Medical School, Boston, Massachusetts. Rare Books Room. Albert Blodgett Papers.
—— "Ether Material," donated by William Sturgis Bigelow to the Treadwell Library and from there donated to the Massachusetts General Hospital.
—— Edward Jarvis Papers.
—— Abel Peirson Papers.
—— John Ware Papers.
Harvard School of Business, Boston, Massachusetts. Business Archives. Folders, "Drug, Misc., Printed."
Illinois State Historical Library, Springfield, Illinois. Samuel Willard Papers.
Massachusetts Historical Society, Boston. Jacob Bigelow Papers.
—— George B. Emerson Papers.
—— Edward Everett Papers.
—— William B. Fowle Papers.
—— Samuel G. Howe Papers.
—— Charles T. Jackson Papers.
—— Horace Mann Papers.
—— John D. Philbrick Papers.
—— George C. Shattuck Papers.
—— Warren Family Papers.
Medical College of Pennsylvania, Philadelphia. Archives.
National Library of Medicine, History of Medicine Division. Bethesda, MD. Francis Henry Ramsbotham Papers.
Pennsylvania State University College of Medicine, Hershey, Pennsylvania. Special Collections, George Harrell Library. Manuscript Notes of Lecture by Henry H. Smith, taken by John Hainson Rodgers, n.d., in the margin of Smith, *Syllabus of the Lectures on the Principles and Practice of Surgery, Delivered in the University of Pennsylvania.*

PERIODICALS AND JOURNALS

American Institute of Homeopathy. *Proceedings.* 1847.
American Journal of Insanity. Vol. 22 (1865).
American Journal of the Medical Sciences. N.S., Vols. 11 (1846)–53 (1867).
American Medical Association. *Transactions.* Vols. 1 (1848)–12 (1859).
The Annalist; A Record of Practical Medicine (New York). Vols. 1 (1846)–2 (1848).
Boston Medical and Surgical Journal. Vols. 35 (1846)–65 (1861).
Brooklyn Daily Eagle. October 1846–October 1848.
Buffalo Medical Journal. Vol. 3 (1847–48).
College of Physicians of Philadelphia. *Summary of the Transactions.* Vol. 2 (1846–49).

——— *Transactions.* Vols. 7 (1846–49)–2 Ser., 1 (1850–53).
Common School Journal (Massachusetts). Vol. 3 (1841).
Dental Cosmos. Vols. 6 (1866)–11 (1869).
Eclectic Medical Journal. N.S. Vols. 1 (1849)–2 (1850).
Hahnemannian Monthly. Vol. 4 (1869).
Homoeopathic Medical Society of New York. *Transactions.* 1864–67.
Massachusetts Eclectic Medical Society. *Publications.* 1860–72.
Massachusetts Medical Society. *Medical Communications.* Vols. 7 (1842)–10 (1864).
Massachusetts Teacher. Vols. 1 (1848)–5 (1852).
Medical Examiner (Philadelphia). Vols. 2 (1846)–5 (1849).
Medical Society of New Jersey. *Transactions.* Vol. 1 (1766–1858).
Medical Society of the State of New York. *Transactions.* Vol. 1 (1847–49).
New-Orleans Medical and Surgical Journal. Vol. 8 (1851–52).
New York Academy of Medicine. *Bulletin.* Vol. 2 (1864).
——— *Transactions.* Vol. 1 (1847–57).
New York Herald. July 9, 1847.
New York Journal of Medicine and the Collateral Sciences. Vols. 3 (1847)–3d Ser.,
    8 (1960).
New York Post. March 8, 1844.
New York Teacher. Vols. 1 (1852–53)–6 (1856–57).
New York Teachers' Advocate. Vols. 1 (1845)–3 (1848).
North American Journal of Homeopathy. Vol. 1 (1851).
Ohio Medical and Surgical Journal. Vol. 2 (1849).
Pennsylvania State Medical Association. *Proceedings.* Vol. 1 (1848).
The Practical Educator and Journal of Health (various titles). Vols. 1 (1846)–3 (1848).
The Presbyterian (Philadelphia). Vols. 17 (1847)–18 (1848).
St. Louis Medical and Surgical Journal. Vol. 7 (1850).
Southern Medical and Surgical Journal. N.S. Vol. 5 (1849).
Western Journal of Medicine and Surgery. Vol. 3 (1849).
Western Lancet and Hospital Reporter. Vols. 6 (1847)–9 (1849).
Westminster Review. Vols. 71 (1859), 96 (1871).

ARTICLES AND BOOKS

Many of the periodicals listed above contained scores of articles used in this study. Only those articles cited by author in the text are itemized separately below. Materials that are readily available in scholarly reprint editions are so cited.

Alcott, Louisa May. *Hospital Sketches.* Edited by Bessie Z. Jones. John Harvard
    Library. Cambridge: Belknap Press of Harvard University Press, 1960, 1863.
Alcott, William A. "Healing Wounds." *The Teacher of Health and the Laws of the
    Human Constitution* (1843), 1:180–84.
Allen, P. W. "On the Advantages of Anaesthesia and the Relative Value of Its Dif-
    ferent Agents." *Eclectic Medical Journal* (October 1850), 2:433–38.
Andrews, Edmund. "The Surgeon." *Chicago Medical Examiner* (1861), 2:587–90.
    Reprinted in *Medical America in the Nineteenth Century: Readings from the Lit-

erature, pp. 176–81. Edited by Gert H. Brieger. Baltimore and London: Johns Hopkins Press, 1972.

Announcement of the Female Medical College of Pennsylvania, 1851. Philadelphia: Clarkson & Scattergood, 1851.

Annual Report of the Trustees of Massachusetts General Hospital and McLean Asylum. Boston: 1846–1880.

Atlee, Washington Lemuel. *The Surgical Treatment of Certain Fibrous Tumours of the Uterus, Heretofore Considered beyond the Resources of Art.* Philadelphia: T. K. and P. G. Collins, 1853.

Bacon, Francis. *Essays,* No. 30. Edited by Henry Morley. New York: A. L. Burt, n.d.

Barker, B. Fordyce. "On the Use of Anaesthetics in Midwifery." *Transactions of the New York Academy of Medicine* (1857), 2:251–68.

—— "On the Use of Anaesthetics in Midwifery" [different article from the above], *Bulletin of the New York Academy of Medicine* (1862), 1:287–313, 345–55.

Barker, S. W. "Anesthesia." *Harper's* (1865), 31:453–58.

Bartlett, Elisha. *An Inquiry into the Degree of Certainty in Medicine.* Philadelphia: Lea and Blanchard, 1848.

Barry, William. "The Ethics of Pain." *The Living Age* (1898), 219:861–64.

Beach, W[ooster]. *The American Practice Condensed.* New York: James M'Alister, 1847.

Bedford, Gunning S. *The Principles and Practice of Obstetrics.* 3d ed., revised and enlarged. New York: William Wood, 1863.

Beecher, Catharine. *Letters to the People on Sickness and Happiness.* New York: Harper, 1855.

Beecher, Henry Ward. *The Sermons of Henry Ward Beecher in Plymouth Church, Brooklyn, "Plymouth Pulpit." First Series.* New York: J. B. Ford, 1870. *Fifth Series.* New York: J. B. Ford, 1872.

Behan, Richard J. *Pain: Its Origin, Conduction, Perception and Diagnostic Significance.* New York: D. Appleton, 1915.

Bell, Benjamin. *A System of Surgery.* 2d ed. Philadelphia: Budd & Bartram, 1802.

Bell, John. *A Treatise on Baths.* 2d ed. Philadelphia: Lindsay & Blakiston, 1859.

Bennan v. Parsonnet, 83 N.J.L. 20, 83 Atl. 948 (1912).

Bigelow, Henry Jacob. "A History of the Discovery of Modern Anaesthesia." *A Century of American Medicine, 1776–1876,* pp. 75–112. Philadelphia: Henry C. Lea, 1876.

—— "Inaugural Lecture, Introductory to the Course on Surgery, Delivered Before the Medical School of Harvard University, Boston, 1849." *Surgical Anaesthesia: Addresses and Other Papers,* pp. 222–58. Boston: Little, Brown, 1900.

—— "Insensibility During Surgical Operations Produced by Inhalation." *Boston Medical and Surgical Journal* (1846), 35:309–17.

Bigelow, Jacob. *Brief Expositions of Rational Medicine.* Boston: Phillips, Sampson, 1858.

—— *Nature in Disease, and Other Writings.* Boston: Ticknor and Fields, 1854.

Billings, John Shaw. "Progress of Medicine in the Nineteenth Century." *Annual Re-*

port of the Board of Regents of the Smithsonian Institution for the Year Ending June 30, 1900, pp. 637–44. Washington, D.C.: GPO, 1901.

Blackwell, Elizabeth. *Pioneer Work in Opening the Medical Profession to Women.* London & New York: Longmans, Green, 1895. Reprinted with a new introduction. New York: Schocken Books, 1977.

Blau, Joseph L., ed. *Social Theories of Jacksonian Democracy: Representative Writings of the Period 1825–1850.* The American Heritage Series. Indianapolis: Bobbs-Merrill, 1954.

Boling, William M. "Remarks on the Use of Anaesthetic Agents, More Especially in Parturition." *New-Orleans Medical and Surgical Journal* (1851–52), 8:275–307, 411–45.

Bowditch, Nathaniel Ingersoll. *History of Massachusetts General Hospital.* Boston: John Wilson and Son, 1851.

—— *History of Massachusetts General Hospital.* 2d ed., with a Continuation to 1872. Boston: Printed by the Trustees, 1872.

Bowditch, Vincent Y. *Life and Correspondence of Henry Ingersoll Bowditch.* 2 Vols. Cambridge: Harvard Univeristy Press, 1902.

Brieger, Gert H., ed. *Medical America in the Nineteenth Century: Readings from the Literature.* Baltimore and London: Johns Hopkins Press, 1972.

Brigham, Amariah. *Observations on the Influence of Religion Upon the Health and Physical Welfare of Mankind.* Boston: Marsh, Capen & Lyon, 1835.

—— *Remarks on the Influence of Mental Cultivation and Mental Excitement Upon Health.* 2d ed. Boston: Marsh, Capen & Lyon, 1833. Delmar, N.Y.: Scholar's Facsimilies and Reprints, 1973.

Brock, Arthur John, M.D. "Introduction." *Galen On the Natural Faculties.* Cambridge: Harvard University Press, 1963, 1916.

Browning, Elizabeth Barrett. *The Complete Works.* Edited by Charlotte Porter and Helen A. Clarke. New York: Thomas Y. Crowell, 1900.

Bryant, Thomas. *The Practice of Surgery.* Philadelphia: Henry C. Lea, 1873.

Bullard, J. Arthur. "Some Thoughts About Doctors and Homeopathic Doctors and Homeopathy." *The Medical Counselor* (November 1903), 22:353–55.

[Burnham, Walter]. "Chloroform: Its Advantages Over Ether As An Anaesthetic Agent." *Publications of the Massachusetts Eclectic Medical Society,* 1860–1872, pp. 35–45.

Caldwell, Charles. *Autobiography.* Edited by Harriot W. Warner. New York: Da Capo Press, 1968. Reprint of 1855 edition.

Carpenter v. Blake, 60 Barb. 488 (N.Y. Sup. Ct., 1871); 75 N.Y. 12 (1878).

Carpenter, William B. *Principles of Human Physiology; With Their Chief Applications to Pathology, Hygiene, and Forensic Medicine.* 4th American ed. Philadelphia: Lea and Blanchard, 1850.

Cartwright, Samuel A. "Diseases and Peculiarities of the Negro Race." *De Bow's Review* (1851), 2:64–69, 209–13, 331–36, 504–08.

—— "Natural History of the Prognathous Species of Mankind." *Day-Book* (New York), November 10, 1857. Reprinted in *Slavery Defended: The Views of the Old South,* pp. 139–47. Edited by Eric L. McKitrick. Englewood Cliffs, N.J.: Prentice-Hall, 1963.

—— "Report on the Diseases and Physical Peculiarities of the Negro Race." *New-Orleans Medical and Surgical Journal* (1851), 7:691–715.

Channing, Walter. *Anaesthetics in Obstetrics*. Boston: Ticknor and Co., 1848.

Chipley, W. S. "Memoranda on Anesthetics." *American Journal of Insanity* (1865), 22:76–81.

Chisholm, J. Julian. *A Manual of Military Surgery for the Use of Surgeons in the Confederate States Army*. Richmond: West & Johnson, 1862.

Clark, J. H. "On the Constitutional Effects of Anaesthetic Agents." *New York Journal of Medicine* (1856), 3d Ser., 1:181–89.

Clarke, W. Fairlie. *A Manual of the Practice of Surgery*. New York: William Wood, 1879.

Clegg, J. T. "Some of the Ailments of Woman Due to Her Higher Development in the Scale of Evolution." *Texas Health Journal* (1890–1891), 3:57–59.

Coates, Reynell. *Introductory Lecture to the Class of the Female Medical College of Pennsylvania, 1860*. Philadelphia: Merrihen & Thompson, 1861.

Cole, Frank, [ed.] *Milestones in Anesthesia: Readings in the Development of Surgical Anesthesia, 1665–1940*. Lincoln: University of Nebraska Press, 1965.

Cooper, James Fenimore. *The Pathfinder, Or, The Inland Sea* (1840). Garden City, N.Y.: Dolphin Books, Doubleday, n.d.

—— *The Prairie; A Tale*. Philadelphia: Carey, Lea & Carey, 1827.

Cooper, Samuel. *A Dictionary of Practical Surgery*. From the 4th London ed. New York: Collins and Hannay, 1822. Vol. 2.

Crompton, Dickinson. "Reminiscences of Provincial Surgery." *Guy's Hospital Reports* (1887), 29:144.

Crosby, A. B. "The Significance of Pain." *Transactions of the New Hampshire Medical Society* (1865), pp. 18–37.

Davis, Nathan Smith. *History of the American Medical Association from Its Organization up to January, 1855*. Philadelphia: Lippincott, Grambo, 1855.

—— *History of Medical Education and Institutions in the United States from the First Settlement of the British Colonies to the Year 1850*. Chicago: S. C. Griggs, 1851.

"Deaths From the Administration of Ether." *The Medical Gazette* (New York), August 20, 1870. Clipping in Frank H. Hamilton Case Books, National Library of Medicine, 8:44.

Dewees, William Potts. *An Essay on the Means of Lessening Pain, and Facilitating Certain Cases of Difficult Parturition*. Philadelphia: John H. Oswald, 1806.

—— "An Examination of Dr. Osburn's Opinion, of the Physical Necessity of Pain and Difficulty in Human Parturition," *Philadelphia Medical Museum* (1805), 1:270–84.

Dickinson, Emily. *The Complete Poems*. Edited by Thomas H. Johnson. Boston: Little, Brown, 1960.

—— *The Poems*. Edited by Thomas H. Johnson. 3 vols. Cambridge, Mass.: Harvard University Press, 1963.

Dickson, S. H. "An Introductory Lecture, delivered before the Medical Class of Jefferson College, Philadelphia, on Pain and Death." *Charleston Medical Journal and Review* (1860), 15:33–64.

Dixon, Edward H. *Woman and Her Diseases, from the Cradle to the Grave: Adapted Exclusively to Her Instruction in the Physiology of Her System.* . . . 10th ed. Philadelphia: G. G. Evans, 1859.

Dorsey, John Syng. *Elements of Surgery.* Vol. 2. Philadelphia: Edward Parker, 1813.

Draper, John William. *Human Physiology.* New York: Harper, 1856.

Druitt, Robert. *The Principles and Practice of Modern Surgery.* New and revised American from the 8th enlarged and improved London ed. Philadelphia: Blanchard and Lea, 1860.

Dunglison, Robley. *Human Physiology.* Vol. 2. Philadelphia: Carey & Lea, 1832.

—— *Human Physiology.* Vol. 2. Philadelphia: Lea and Blanchard, 1850.

Dupierris, Martial. "Reduction of a Femoral Dislocation of Six Months' Standing, by Manipulation." *North American Medico-Chirurgical Review* (Philadelphia) (1857), 1:290–94.

Earle, A. Scott, ed. *Surgery in America: From the Colonial Era to the Twentieth Century: Selected Writings.* Philadelphia and London: W. B. Saunders, 1965.

Eliot, T. S. "Four Quartets." *Complete Poems and Plays, 1909–1950.* New York: Harcourt, Brace & World, 1952.

Elwell, John J. *A Medico-Legal Treatise on Malpractice and Medical Evidence.* 3d ed., revised and enlarged. New York: Baker, Voorhis, 1871.

Emerson, Ralph Waldo. *Emerson on Education.* Edited by Howard Mumford Jones. Classics in Education No. 26. New York: Teachers College Press of Columbia University, 1966.

—— *Essays, First Series.* New and revised ed. Boston: Houghton, Mifflin and Company, 1888.

—— "Woman." *The Complete Writings,* pp. 1178–84. New York: Wm. H. Wise, 1929.

Erichsen, John. *The Science and Art of Surgery.* Edited by John H. Brinton. Philadelphia: Blanchard and Lea, 1854.

—— *The Science and Art of Surgery.* Improved American ed., from the 2d Enlarged and Revised London ed. Philadelphia: Blanchard and Lea, 1860.

Eve, Paul F. "Mesmerism." *Southern Medical and Surgical Journal* (1845), N.S. 1:167–92.

—— "Report of Operations performed under Anaesthetic Agents." *Southern Medical and Surgical Journal* (1849), N.S. 5:278–81.

An Extract from the Report of the Directors of Massachusetts State Prison, . . . Reviewing Certain Parts of the Second Annual Report of the Prison Discipline Society, to which is Added, the Report of the Physician of Massachusetts State Prison. Boston: Dutton and Wentworth, 1827.

Ezorsky, Gertrude, ed. *Philosophical Perspectives on Punishment.* Albany: State University of New York Press, 1972.

"Female Physicians." *The Water-Cure Journal* (January 1860), 29:3–4.

Fenwick, Samuel. "Statistical Inquiry into the Effects of Chloroform." *American Medical Gazette and Journal of Health* (October 1857), 8:592–600.

Finney, Charles Grandison. *Lectures on Revivals of Religion.* Edited by William G. McLoughlin. John Harvard Library. Cambridge, Mass.: Belknap Press of Harvard University Press, 1960. Reprint of 1835 edition.

Flagg, J. F. B. *Ether and Chloroform: Their Employment in Surgery, Dentistry, Midwifery, Therapeutics, Etc.* Philadelphia: Lindsay and Blakiston, 1851.

Flint, Austin. "Conservative Medicine." *American Medical Monthly* (1862), 18:1–24. Reprinted in *Medical America in the Nineteenth Century: Readings from the Literature*, pp. 134–42. Edited by Gert H. Brieger. Baltimore and London: Johns Hopkins Press, 1972.

—— "Remarks on the Numerical System of Louis." *New York Journal of Medicine and Surgery* (1841), 4:283–303.

Francis, John Wakefield. *Old New York: or Reminiscences of the Past Sixty Years.* New York: W. J. Widdleton, 1865.

Galen. *On the Natural Faculties.* Translated by Arthur John Brock, M.D. Cambridge: Harvard University Press, 1963, 1916.

Gamble, Samuel D. "On the Influence of Pain in the Production of Death." *Southern Medical and Surgical Journal* (1838), 2:712.

Gardner, Augustus K. "Physical Decline of American Women." *Knickerbocker* (January 1860), 55:37–52.

Gayley, James Fyfe. *A History of the Jefferson Medical College of Philadelphia.* Philadelphia: J. M. Wilson, 1858.

Gibson, William. *The Institutes and Practice of Surgery.* 2d ed. Philadelphia: Carey, Lea & Carey, 1827.

Gilchrist, J. G. *A Syllabus of Lectures on Surgery.* Ann Arbor, Mich.: John Moore, 1877.

Grace, M. B. "Christ and Mothers." *Presbyterian Magazine* (1851), 1:181–83.

Gregory, Samuel. "Female Physicians." *The Living Age* (April–June 1862), 73:243–49.

—— *Man-Midwifery Exposed and Corrected; . . . Together With Remarks on the Use and Abuse of Ether, and Dr. Channing's "Cases of Inhalation of Ether in Labor."* Boston: George Gregory, 1848.

Griscom, John H. *The Uses and Abuses of Air. . . .* New York: J. S. Redfield, Clinton Hall, 1850. New York: Arno & The New York Times, 1970.

Gross, Samuel D. "The Factors of Disease and Death After Injuries, Parturition, and Surgical Operations." *Reports and Papers, American Public Health Association* (1874–1875), 2:400–14. Reprinted in *Medical America in the Nineteenth Century: Readings from the Literature*, pp. 190–97. Edited by Gert H. Brieger. Baltimore and London: Johns Hopkins Press, 1972.

—— *A Manual of Military Surgery.* 2d ed. Philadelphia: J. B. Lippincott, 1862.

—— *A System of Surgery.* 4th ed. Vol. 1. Philadelphia: Henry C. Lea, 1866.

Haller, Albrecht von. "A Dissertation on the Sensible and Irritable Parts of Animals." Translated by Owsei Temkin. *Bulletin of the History of Medicine* (October 1936), 4:651–99.

Hamilton, Frank Hastings. *A Treatise on Military Surgery and Hygiene.* New York: Balliere Brothers, 1865.

Harris, George Washington. *Sut Lovingood's Yarns.* Edited by M. Thomas Inge. New Haven, Conn.: College and University Press, 1966.

Harrison, Eliza Cope, ed. *Philadelphia Merchant: The Diary of Thomas P. Cope, 1800–1851.* South Bend, Ind.: Gateway Editions, 1978.

Harrison, John. "Sensation." *New-Orleans Medical and Surgical Journal* (1850), 6:425–42, 561–82, 697–712.

Harrison, John P. "On the Physiology, Pathology, and Therapeutics of Pain." *Western Lancet* (1849), 9:349–54.

Hartshorne, E. *Remarks on the Case of Dr. B.* Philadelphia: Lindsay and Blakiston, 1854.

Hayman, Rev. Henry. "The Economy of Pain." *Bibliotheca Sacra* (1888), 45:1–31.

Hayward, George. *Surgical Reports and Miscellaneous Papers.* Boston: Phillips, Sampson and Company, 1855.

Hill, Benjamin. *Lectures on the American Eclectic System of Surgery.* Cincinnati: W. Phillips, 1850.

Hilton, John. *On Rest and Pain.* 2d ed. New York: William Wood, 1879.

Hippocrates. Translated by W. H. S. Jones. Vol. 4. London: William Heinemann, 1931.

Hodges, Richard Manning. *A Narrative of Events Connected with the Introduction of Sulphuric Ether into Surgical Use.* Boston: Little, Brown and Company, 1891.

Holland, Josiah Gilbert. *Bitter-Sweet; A Poem.* 15th ed. New York: C. Scribner, 1863.

Holmes, George Frederick. "Uncle Tom's Cabin." *Southern Literary Messenger* (December 1852), 18:721–31. Reprinted in *Slavery Defended: The Views of the Old South,* pp. 99–110. Edited by Eric L. McKitrick. Englewood Cliffs, N.J.: Prentice-Hall, 1963.

Holmes, Oliver Wendell. *Currents and Countercurrents in Medical Science.* Boston: Ticknor and Fields, 1861.

—— *Elsie Venner: A Romance of Destiny.* Boston: Houghton, Mifflin, 1891, 1861.

—— *An Introductory Lecture delivered at the Massachusetts Medical College, November 3, 1847.* Boston: William D. Ticknor, 1847.

—— *Medical Essays, 1842–1882.* Boston: Houghton, Mifflin, 1891.

Holmes, Oliver Wendell, Jr. *Touched With Fire: Civil War Letters and Diary of Oliver Wendell Holmes.* Cambridge: Harvard University Press, 1946.

"Homicides by Chloroform." *Boston Medical and Surgical Journal* (February 17, 1870), N.S. 5:113–14.

Hooker, Worthington. *Physician and Patient; or, a Practical View of the Mutual Duties, Relations and Interests of the Medical Profession and the Community.* New York: Baker and Scribner, 1849. New York: Arno Press & The New York Times, 1972.

[Howe, Samuel Gridley.] *Report of a Minority of the Special Committee of the Boston Prison Discipline Society, Appointed at the Annual Meeting, May 27, 1845.* Boston: William D. Ticknor, 1846.

Hughes, Langston. *The Dream Keeper.* New York: Knopf, 1932.

Huxley, Aldous. *Brave New World.* New York: Bantam Books, 1960, 1932.

J. C. R. "Anaesthesia." *American Journal of the Medical Sciences* (January 1867), 53:157–90.

Jackson, Charles T. *A Manual of Etherization.* Boston: J.B. Mansfield, 1861.

—— "On Anesthetic Agents." *Milestones in Anesthesia: Readings in the Development of Surgical Anesthesia, 1665–1940,* pp. 116–29. Edited by Frank Cole. Lincoln: University of Nebraska Press, 1965.

Jefferson, Thomas. *The Life and Selected Writings.* Edited by Adrienne Koch and William Peden. New York: London House, 1944.
—— *The Portable Thomas Jefferson.* Edited by Merrill D. Peterson. New York: Viking Press, 1975.
Jones, Walter F. "On the Utility of Applications of Hot Water to the Spine in the Treatment of Typhoid Pneumonia." *Virginia Medical and Surgical Journal* (1854), 3:108–10.
Kidd, Charles. *A Manual of Anaesthetics.* New ed. London: Henry Renshaw, 1859.
King, John. *American Eclectic Obstetrics.* Cincinnati: Moore, Wilstach, Keys, 1855.
Lamb, Charles. *The Best Letters.* Edited by Edward Gilpin Johnson. Chicago: A.C. McClurg, 1892.
Lente, Frederick D. "Anesthesia in Surgery. How Its Dangers Are To Be Avoided." *New York Journal of Medicine* (1855), N.S. 15:195–201.
—— "The Remote Effects of Anaesthesia on the System." *New York Journal of Medicine* (1856), 3d Ser., 1:354–57.
Lerner, Gerda, ed. *The Female Experience: An American Documentary.* American Heritage Series. Indianapolis: Bobbs-Merrill, 1977.
Letterman, Jona[than]. "Circular Letter of October 30, 1862." *Reports on the Operations of the Inspectors and Relief Agents of the Sanitary Commission, after the Battle of Fredericksburg . . .* , pp. 6–8. Sanitary Commission Document No. 57. Washington, D.C.: United States Sanitary Commission, 1862.
Lewin, L[ouis]. *The Untoward Effects of Drugs: A Pharmacological and Clinical Manual.* 2d ed., revised and enlarged. Detroit: George S. Davis, 1883.
Liston, Robert. *Practical Surgery.* 2d American from the 3d London ed. Philadelphia: Thomas, Cowperthwait, 1842.
Lombroso, Caesare. *The Female Offender.* New York: D. Appleton, 1915.
Lombroso-Ferrero, Gina. *Criminal Man.* New York: G. P. Putnam, 1911.
Lyman, Henry M. *Artificial Anaesthesia and Anaesthetics.* New York: William Wood, 1881.
Lynck, John. "Alcohol as an Anaesthetic." *Cincinnati Lancet and Observer* (May 1876), 37:409–16.
McGuire v. Rix, 118 Neb. 434, 225 N.W. 120 (1929).
McKitrick, Eric L., ed. *Slavery Defended: The Views of the Old South.* Englewood Cliffs, N.J.: Prentice-Hall, 1963.
Macleod, H. B. *Notes on the Surgery of the War in the Crimea.* Philadelphia: Lippincott, 1862.
McLoughlin, William G., ed. *The American Evangelicals, 1800–1900: An Anthology.* New York: Harper & Row, 1968.
M'Quillen, J. H. "Action of Anaesthetics on the Blood Corpuscles." *Dental Cosmos* (1869), 11:113–19.
—— "Pain—Its Beneficent Uses, and Means of Alleviation." *Dental Cosmos* (1866), 7:631–35.
Magendie, F[rançois]. *An Elementary Compendium of Physiology.* Translated by E. Milligan. Philadelphia: James Webster, 1824.
Mann, Horace. *Horace Mann On the Crisis in Education.* Edited by Louis Filler. Yellow Springs, Ohio: Antioch Press, 1965.
—— *Lectures on Education.* Boston: Ide & Dutton, 1855.

—— *Life and Works.* 4 Vols. Boston: Lee and Shepard, 1891.

—— *The Republic and The School: Horace Mann On the Education of Free Men.* Edited by Lawrence A. Cremin. Classics in Education, No. 1. New York: Teachers College Press, 1957.

—— *The Study of Physiology in the Schools.* New York: J. W. Schermerhorn, 1869.

Marshall, John. *Outlines of Physiology.* Philadelphia: Henry C. Lea, 1868.

Meigs, Charles D. *Females and Their Diseases.* Philadelphia: Lea and Blanchard, 1848.

Meigs, J. Forsythe. *A History of the First Quarter of the Second Century of the Pennsylvania Hospital.* Philadelphia: Collins, 1877.

Melville, Herman. *White-Jacket, or The World in a Man-of-War.* Edited by Hennig Cohen. New York: Holt, Rinehart and Winston, 1967, 1850.

Merrill, A. P. "An Essay on Some of the Distinctive Peculiarities of the Negro Race." *Memphis Medical Recorder* (1855), 4:1–17, 65–77, 130–39, 321–30.

Metcalfe, J. T. "On the Purity and Use of Chloroform." *Transactions of the New York Academy of Medicine* (1847–1857), 1:139–58.

Mill, John Stuart. *The Subjection of Women.* 2d ed. New York: Frederick A. Stokes, 1911.

—— *Utilitarianism.* Edited with Critical Essays, by Samuel Gorovitz. Indianapolis: Bobbs-Merrill, 1971.

Mitchell, Silas Weir. "The Birth and Death of Pain." *The Complete Poems of S. Weir Mitchell,* p. 416. New York: Century, 1914.

—— *Doctor and Patient.* Philadelphia: J. B. Lippincott, 1887.

—— *Injuries of Nerves and Their Consequences.* Philadelphia: J. B. Lippincott, 1872.

Mobley, Wm. Frost. *American Broadsides.* Catalog One. Wilbraham, Mass.: privately printed, 1980.

Mohr v. Williams, 95 Minn. 261, 104 N.W. 12 (1905).

"The Moral Limit in the Use of Anaesthetics." *American Ecclesiastical Review* (1890), 3:198–204.

Morong, Rev. Thomas. *The Beneficence of Pain.* Iowa City: Jerome, Duncan & Crouse, 1858.

Morton, William Thomas Green. "Comparative Value of Sulphuric Ether and Chloroform." *Boston Medical and Surgical Journal* (1850), 43:110–19.

—— "The First Use of Ether as an Anesthetic at the Battle of the Wilderness in the Civil War." *Journal of the American Medical Association* (April 23, 1904), 42:1068–73.

—— *Morton's Letheon Circular.* 5th ed. Boston: [privately printed, 1847].

—— *Remarks on the Proper Mode of Administering Sulphuric Ether by Inhalation.* Boston: Dutton and Wentworth, 1847. Reprinted in part in *Milestones in Anesthesia: Readings in the Development of Surgical Anesthesia, 1665–1940,* pp. 45–60. Edited by Frank Cole. Lincoln: University of Nebraska Press, 1965.

Mott, Valentine. *Pain and Anaesthetics: An Essay Introductory to a Series of Surgical and Medical Monographs.* Prepared by Request of the Sanitary Commission. 2d ed. Washington, D.C.: M'Gill & Witherow, 1863.

—— "Remarks on the Importance of Anaesthesia from Chloroform in Surgical Operations, Illustrated by Two Cases." *Transactions of the New York Academy of Medicine* (1847–1857), 1:85–95.

Napheys, George H. *The Physical Life of Woman: Advice to the Maiden, Wife, and Mother.* Philadelphia: George MacLean, 1869.

"Natural *Versus* Acquired Habits." *Massachusetts Teacher* (1849), 2:303.

Nevius, Laird W. *The Discovery of Modern Anaesthesia: By Whom Was it Made? A Brief Statement of Facts.* New York: Cooper Institute, 1894.

New York State Assembly. *Documents.* 53d sess. (1830) Vol. 3, No. 217; 55th sess. (1832) Vol. 3, Nos. 185, 244, 246, 249, 250, 251, 261, 272; 63d sess. (1840) Vol. 8, No. 346; 67th sess. (1844) Vol. 3, No. 60; 82nd sess. (1859), Vol. 3, No. 157.

—— *Journal.* 55th sess. (1832), 108, 173, 319, 509, 564, 570; 67th sess. (1844), 1042, 1162.

New York State Senate. *Documents.* 67th sess. (1844), Vol. 1, No. 31, Vol. 2, No. 55; 73d sess. (1850), Vol. 3, No. 80.

—— *Journal.* 67th sess. (1844), 219, 634–35.

Nichols, M[ary] Gove. "Woman the Physician." *Water-Cure Journal* (October 1851), 12:3.

Nichols, T. L. *The Curse Removed: A Statement of Facts Respecting the Efficacy of Water Cure in the Treatment of Uterine Diseases, and the Removal of the Pains and Perils of Pregnancy and Childbirth.* New York: Water-Cure Journal, 1850.

—— *Forty Years of American Life.* London: John Maxwell, 1864.

—— *Forty Years of American Life.* 2d ed. London: Longmans, Green, 1874.

[Noble, Lester.] "When Ether Was a New Miracle." [Edited by] Robert S. Gillcash. *Journal of the Maine Medical Association* (May 1963), 56:101–03.

Norris, Frank. *McTeague.* Garden City N.Y.: Doubleday, Page, 1924.

—— *A Man's Woman.* New York: Doubleday & McClure, 1900.

Norris, George W. *The Early History of Medicine in Philadelphia.* Philadelphia: Collins, 1886.

—— "Statistical Account of the Cases of Amputation Performed at the Pennsylvania Hospital From January 1, 1850, to January 1, 1860. . . ." *Pennsylvania Hospital Reports* (1868), 1:149–64.

Novotny, Ann, and Carter Smith, *Images of Healing.* New York: Macmillan, 1980.

Nunneley, Thomas. *On Anaesthesia and Anaesthetic Substances Generally.* London: n.p., 1849.

Orcutt, Hiram. *The Discipline of the School.* Washington, D.C.: GPO, 1881, 1871.

Osler, William. *Aequanimitas; With Other Addresses.* 2d ed. London: H. K. Lewis, 1906.

Otis, George A. and D. L. Huntington, *Medical and Surgical History of the War of the Rebellion.* Part 3 of Vol. 2. Washington, D.C.: GPO, 1883.

[Packard, Frederick Adolphus.] A Citizen of Pennsylvania. *An Inquiry into the Alleged Tendency of the Separation of Convicts, One from the Other, to Produce Disease and Derangement.* Philadelphia: E. C. & J. Biddle, 1849.

Paget, Sir James. "The Discovery of Anesthesia." *Eclectic Magazine* (1880), 94:219–22.

"Painless Operations in Surgery." *Littell's Living Age* (June 1847), 13:481–96.

Parker, Gail Thain, ed. *The Oven Birds: American Women on Womanhood, 1820–1920.* Garden City, N.Y.: Anchor Books, Doubleday, 1972.

Pascalis, Felix. "Remarks on the Theory of Pain." *American Medical and Surgical Journal* (1826), 1:79–89.

"The Patent Ether Vapour Inhaler." *Patent Journal and Investor's Magazine*, January 23, 1847, pp. 578–80. Reprinted in *Milestones in Anesthesia: Readings in the Development of Surgical Anesthesia, 1665–1940*, pp. 42–45. Edited by Frank Cole. Lincoln: University of Nebraska Press, 1965.

"The Patient's Consent to an Operation and the Surgeon's Discretion." *The Medical Record* (New York) (December 1880), 18:715.

Pearson, John. *Principles of Surgery*. Boston: Stimpson & Clapp, 1832.

Peck, G. W. "On the Use of Chloroform in Hanging." *American Whig Review* (September 1848), 8:283–96.

Percival, Thomas. *Percival's Medical Ethics*. Edited by Chauncey D. Leake. Baltimore: Williams & Wilkins, 1927.

Poe, Edgar Allan. *The Complete Works*. Edited by James A. Harrison. Vol. 5. New York: John D. Morris, 1902.

Porter, John B. "Medical and Surgical Notes of Campaigns in the War With Mexico." *American Journal of the Medical Sciences* (1852), 23:13–37; (1852), 24:13–30; (1853), 25:25–42.

Preamble and Resolution of the Philadelphia County Medical Society Upon the Status of Women Physicians, with A Reply by a Woman. Philadelphia: Stuchey, 1867. Reprinted in part in *The Female Experience: An American Documentary*, pp. 408–12. Edited by Gerda Lerner. American Heritage Series. Indianapolis: Bobbs-Merrill, 1977.

Proceedings of the National Conference of Charities and Correction (1895), 22:474–77.

The Pro-Slavery Argument; as Maintained by . . . Chancellor Harper, Governor Hammond, Dr. Sims, and Professor Dew. Philadelphia: Lippincott, Grambo, 1853.

"Report of a Committee of the Boston Society for Medical Improvement, on the Alleged Dangers Which Accompany the Inhalation of the Vapor of Sulphuric Ether." *Boston Medical and Surgical Journal* (October 1861), 65:229–43.

"Report of the Committee of the Medical Society of Virginia, On the Utility and Safety of Anaesthetic Agents." *The Stethoscope and Virginia Medical Gazette* (April 1851), 1:181–98.

"Report on Obstetrics and Diseases of Women," *Ninth Annual Meeting of the Illinois State Medical Society* (1859), pp. 87–101.

Rice, Nathan P. *Trials of a Public Benefactor*. New York: Pudney and Russell, 1859.

Rogers, Stephen. "Can Chloroform be Used to Facilitate Robbery?" *Papers Read Before the Medico-Legal Society of New York*. First series, 3d illustrated ed. New York: Medico-Legal Journal Association, 1889.

Roget, P. M. *Outlines of Physiology*. First American, revised. Philadelphia: Lea and Blanchard, 1839.

"Routine Practice." *Boston Medical and Surgical Journal* (January 11, 1883), 108:42–43.

Rush, Benjamin. "Commonplace Book." *The Autobiography of Benjamin Rush, His "Travels Through Life," together with His* Commonplace Book *for 1789–1813*.

Edited by George W. Corner. Princeton, N.J.: Published for the American Philosophical Society by Princeton University Press, 1948.

—— *An Enquiry into the Effects of Public Punishments Upon Criminals and Upon Society.* Philadelphia: Joseph James, 1787. Reprinted in *A Plan for the Punishment of Crime: Two Essays*, pp. 1–17. Edited by Negley K. Teeters. Philadelphia: The Pennsylvania Prison Society, 1954.

—— *Letters.* Edited by Lyman H. Butterfield. Vol. 2. Princeton, N.J.: Princeton University Press, 1951.

—— *Medical Inquiries and Observations.* 4th ed. Vol. 1. Philadelphia: M. Carey and B. & T. Kite, 1815.

—— *The Selected Writings.* Edited by Dagobert D. Runes. New York: Philosophical Library, 1947.

—— *Sixteen Introductory Lectures to Courses of Lectures Upon the Institutes and Practice of Medicine.* Philadelphia: Bradford and Inskeep, 1811.

Sargent, F[itz]W[illiam]. *On Bandaging and Other Operations of Minor Surgery.* Philadelphia: Lea and Blanchard, 1848.

—— *On Bandaging and Other Operations of Minor Surgery.* Philadelphia: Blanchard and Lea, 1856.

The Semi-Centennial of Anaesthesia. Boston: Massachusetts General Hospital, 1897.

[Shattuck, Lemuel.] *Report of the Sanitary Commission of Massachusetts, 1850.* Boston: Dutton and Wentworth, 1850. Reprinted Cambridge, Mass.: Harvard University Press, 1948.

Simpson, James Y. *Anaesthesia, Or the Employment of Chloroform and Ether in Surgery, Midwifery, Etc.* Philadelphia: Lindsay & Blakiston, 1849.

—— *Anaesthesia in Surgery; Does it Increase or Decrease the Mortality Attendant Upon Surgical Operations?* Edinburgh: Sutherland & Knox, 1848.

—— *Answer to the Religious Objections Advanced Against the Employment of Anaesthetic Agents in Midwifery and Surgery.* Edinburgh: Sutherland & Knox, 1847.

—— *Ovariotomy; Is It or is It Not an Operation Justifiable upon the Common Principles of Surgery? Are or are Not Capital Operations in Surgery Justifiable to the Extent Generally Practiced?* Edinburgh: Sutherland & Knox, 1846.

Sims, J. Marion. *The Story of My Life.* New York: D. Appleton, 1884. New York: Da Capo Press, 1968.

Smith, Henry H. *Minor Surgery; or, Hints on the Every-Day Duties of the Surgeon.* Reprinted from the 3d ed. Philadelphia: Blanchard & Lea, 1859.

—— *The Principles and Practice of Surgery.* Vol. 1. Philadelphia: J. B. Lippincott, 1863.

—— *A System of Operative Surgery.* 2d ed. Vol. 1. Philadelphia: Lippincott, Grambo, 1866.

—— *A Treatise on the Practice of Surgery.* Philadelphia: J. B. Lippincott, 1856.

Smith, Mayo G. *A Treatise on the Inhalation of Ether for the Prevention of Pain.* Boston: J. P. Jewett, 1848.

Smith, Samuel Stanhope. *An Essay on the Causes of the Variety of Complexion and Figure in the Human Species.* Edited by Winthrop D. Jordan. John Harvard Library. Cambridge, Mass.: Belknap Press of Harvard University Press, 1965. Reprint of 1810 ed. 1st ed. 1787.

Smith, Stephen. "The Comparative Results of Operations in Bellevue Hospital." *Medical Record* (1885), 28:427–31. Reprinted in *Medical America in the Nineteenth Century: Readings from the Literature*, pp. 201–09. Edited by Gert H. Brieger. Baltimore and London: Johns Hopkins Press, 1972.

—— *Handbook of Surgical Operations*. New York: Ballière Brothers, 1862.

—— "The Physician as Citizen." *Doctor in Medicine; and Other Papers on Professional Subjects*, pp. 149–53. New York: William Wood, 1872.

—— "Reminiscences of Two Epochs: Anaesthesia and Asepsis." *Bulletin of the Johns Hopkins Hospital* (1919), 30:273–78.

Snow, Ellen M. "Duties of Physicians." *Water-Cure Journal* (1856), 21:56.

Snow, John. "A Lecture on the Inhalation of Vapour of Ether in Surgical Operations." *Lancet* (May 29, 1847), 1:551–54. Reprinted in *Milestones in Anesthesia: Readings in the Development of Surgical Anesthesia, 1665–1940*, pp. 79–81. Edited by Frank Cole. Lincoln: University of Nebraska Press, 1965.

Squibb, Edward R. "Anaesthetics." *New York Medical Journal* (1871), 13:385–412.

[Stanton, Elizabeth Cady.] Letter to Lucretia [Mott]. October 22, 1852. *The Oven Birds: American Women on Womanhood, 1820–1920*, p. 260. Edited by Gail Thain Parker. Garden City, N.Y.: Anchor Books, Doubleday, 1972.

Stillé, Moreton. *The Psychical Effects of Ether Inhalation*. Philadelphia: Lindsay and Blakiston, 1854.

State of the New York Hospital and Bloomingdale Asylum. New York: Mahlon Day, 1840–1842; Egbert, Hovey & King, 1844–1852; Wm. C. Bryant, 1853–1862.

Storer, H. R. "As to the Practically Absolute Safety of Profoundly Induced Anaesthesia in Childbirth, as Compared with its Employment in General Surgery." *Edinburgh Medical Journal* (1877), 22:741–43.

—— *Eutokia: A Word to Physicians and to Women Upon the Employment of Anaesthetics in Childbirth*. Boston: A. Williams, 1863.

Sweetser, William. *Mental Hygiene*. New York: George P. Putnam, 1850.

Swift, Edgar James. "Sensibility to Pain." *American Journal of Psychology* (1899–1900), 11:312–17.

Thatcher, James. *American Medical Biography*. New York: Da Capo Press, 1967. Reprinted from 1828 ed.

Tocqueville, Alexis de. *Democracy in America*. 2 Vols. New York: Vintage Books, Random House, 1945.

Trall, R. T. "Allopathy *Adversus* Woman." *The Water-Cure Journal* (1852), 13:86–87.

—— *The Hydropathic Encyclopedia*. New York: Samuel R. Wells, 1873.

Trotter, Thomas. *A View of the Nervous Temperament; Being a Practical Inquiry Into the Increasing Prevalence, Prevention, and Treatment of Those Diseases Commonly Called Nervous, Bilious, Stomach & Liver Complaints. . . .* Troy, N.Y.: Wright, Goodenow, & Stockwell, 1808.

Turnbull, Laurence. *The Advantages and Accidents of Artificial Anaesthesia: A Manual of Anaesthetic Agents*. 2d ed., revised and enlarged. Philadelphia: P. Blakiston, 1885.

"The Ultimate Effects of Anaesthetics with Special Reference to Major Operations," *Bulletin of the New York Academy of Medicine* (1864), 2:327–45.

Van Buren, Peter. "Anaesthesia." *Transactions of the Medical Society of the State of New York*, 1858, pp. 49–84.
Van Buren, William H. "Amputation at the Hip-Joint." *Transactions of the New York Academy of Medicine* (1847–1857), 1:123–38.
Veysey, Laurence, ed. *The Perfectionists: Radical Social Thought in the North, 1815–1860*. New York: John Wiley, 1973.
Wales, Philip S. *Mechanical Therapeutics: A Practical Treatise on Surgical Apparatus, Appliances, and Elementary Operations*. Philadelphia: Henry C. Lea, 1867.
Walker, J. B. F., "Is It Wicked To Be Sick?" *The Water-Cure Journal* (1861), 31:60–61.
Warren, Edward. Review of *A Treatise on Etherization in Childbirth*, by Walter Channing. *North American Review* (April 1849), 68:300–14.
Warren, J. Collins. *Influence of Anaesthesia on the Surgery of the Nineteenth Century*. Boston: privately printed, 1906.
Warren, J. Mason. "Lithotomy and Lithotrity, With the Use of Ether in those Operations." *American Journal of the Medical Sciences* (1849), 18:47–59.
Warren, John Collins. *Etherization; With Surgical Remarks*. Boston: William D. Ticknor, 1848.
—— "Inhalation of Ethereal Vapor for the Prevention of Pain in Surgical Operations." *Boston Medical and Surgical Journal* (1846), Vol. 35. Reprinted in *Surgery in America: From the Colonial Era to the Twentieth Century: Selected Writings*, pp. 160–66. Edited by A. Scott Earle. Philadelphia and London: W. B. Saunders, 1965.
—— "On the Use of Anaesthetics." *Transactions of the American Medical Association* (1850), 3:385–87.
[Warren, Samuel.] *Passages from the Diary of a Late Physician*. From the 5th London ed. New York: Harper & Bros., [1832?].
Wayland, Francis. *The Elements of Moral Science*. Edited by Joseph Blau. John Harvard Library. Cambridge, Mass.: Belknap Press of Harvard University Press, 1963.
Welch, William H. "The Influence of Anaesthesia Upon Medical Science." *The Semi-Centennial of Anaesthesia*, pp. 57–68. Boston: Massachusetts General Hospital, 1897.
Welter, Rush, ed., *American Writings on Popular Education of the Nineteenth Century*. Indianapolis: Bobbs-Merrill, 1971.
Whitman, Walt. *Leaves of Grass*. New York: New American Library, 1958.
—— *Memoranda During the War*. Bloomington: Indiana University Press, 1962, reprint of 1875 edition.
—— *The Portable Walt Whitman*. Edited by Mark Van Doren. New York: Viking, 1945.
Williams, Stephen W. *American Medical Biography, Or Memoirs of Eminent Physicians. . . .* Greenfield, Mass.: L. Merriam, 1845. New York: Milford House, 1967.
Williams, William Carlos. *The Farmers' Daughters: The Collected Stories*. New York: New Directions, 1961.
Wilson, John Stainbach. "The Negro—His Peculiarities as to Disease." *American Cotton Planter and the Soil of the South* (1859), N.S. 3:229.

Wright, Martha Coffin to Ellen Wright Garrison. October 31, 1869. Reprinted in *The Female Experience: An American Documentary*, p. 80. Edited by Gerda Lerner. American Heritage Series. Indianapolis: Bobbs-Merrill, 1977.

Wyman, Morrill. *Progress in School Discipline: Remarks of Dr. Morrill Wyman, of Cambridge, in Support of the Resolution to Abolish the Corporal Punishment of Girls. . . .* Cambridge, Mass.: James Cox, 1866.

Yandell, L. P. "On the Progress of Etherization." *Western Journal of Medicine and Surgery* (1849), 3:1–36.

Young, Edward J. *Words Commemorative of Henry Bigelow, M.D. . . .* Boston: Nichols and Noyes, 1866.

Zakrzewska, Marie E. *Introductory Lecture . . . Before the New England Female Medical College at the Opening of the Term 1859–60*. Boston: J. M. Hewes, 1859.

Secondary Sources

Aaron, Daniel. *The Unwritten War; American Writers and the Civil War*. London: Oxford University Press, 1975, 1973.

Abel-Smith, Brian. *The Hospitals, 1800–1948: A Study in Social Administration in England and Wales*. Cambridge: Harvard University Press, 1964.

Ackerknecht, Erwin H. "Anticontagionism Between 1821 and 1867." *Bulletin of the History of Medicine* (September–October 1948), 22:562–93.

—— "Aspects of the History of Therapeutics." *Bulletin of the History of Medicine* (September–October 1962), 36:389–419.

—— "Diathesis: The Word and the Concept in Medical History." *Bulletin of the History of Medicine* (Fall, 1982), 56:317–25.

—— "Elisha Bartlett and the Philosophy of the Paris Clinical School." *Bulletin of the History of Medicine* (January–February 1950), 24:43–60.

—— *Medicine at the Paris Hospital, 1794–1848*. Baltimore: Johns Hopkins Press, 1967.

Adams, George Worthington. *Doctors in Blue: The Medical History of the Union Army in the Civil War*. New York: Collier Books, 1961, 1952.

Ahlstrom, Sidney E. *A Religious History of the American People*. New Haven, Conn.: Yale University Press, 1972.

Alaya, Flavia. "Victorian Science and the 'Genius' of Woman." *Journal of the History of Ideas* (April–June 1977), 38:261–80.

Allen, Virginia R. "Health and Medical Care of the Southern Plains Indians, 1868–1892." Ph.D. dissertation, Oklahoma State University, 1973.

Altman, L. K. "Auto-Experimentation: An Unappreciated Tradition in Medical Science." *New England Journal of Medicine* (1972), 286:346–52.

Amundsen, Darrel. "The Physician's Obligation To Prolong Life: A Medical Duty Without Classical Roots." *The Hastings Center Report* (August 1978), 8:23–30.

Archer, W. Harry. "The History of Anesthesia." *The History of the Development of*

Anesthesia, Oral Surgery and Hospital Dental Service in the United States of America, pp. 385–401. By Archer, Milton B. Asbell, and William B. Irby. Pittsburgh: n.p., 1971.
—— "Life and Letters of Horace Wells, Discoverer of Anesthesia." Journal of the American College of Dentistry (1944–1945), 11–12:81–210.
Arieli, Yehoshua, Individualism and Nationalism in American Ideology. Cambridge: Harvard University Press, 1964.
Ariès, Philippe. "Death Inside Out." Hastings Center Studies (May 1974), 2:3–18.
—— "The Reversal of Death: Changes in Attitudes toward Death in Western Societies." American Quarterly (December 1974), 26:536–60.
Aring, Charles D. "Gentility and Professionalism." Journal of the American Medical Association (February 4, 1974), 227:512.
Armitage, K. J., L. J. Schneiderman, and R. A. Bass. "Response of Physicians to Medical Complaint in Men and Women." Journal of the American Medical Association (May 18, 1979), 241:2186–87.
The Art of Philadelphia Medicine. Philadelphia: Philadelphia Museum of Art, 1965.
Aspiz, Harold. Walt Whitman and the Body Beautiful. Urbana: University of Illinois Press, 1980.
Atwater, Edward C. "The Medical Profession in a New Society, Rochester, New York (1811–1860)." Bulletin of the History of Medicine (May–June 1973), 47:221–35.
Austin, Anne L. The Woolsey Sisters of New York: Civil War and a New Profession, 1860–1900. Philadelphia: American Philosophical Society, 1971.
Averill, James H. Wordsworth and the Poetry of Human Suffering. Ithaca, N.Y.: Cornell University Press, 1980.
Axtell, James. The School Upon a Hill: Education and Society in Colonial New England. New York: W. W. Norton, 1976, 1974.
Bakan, David. Disease, Pain, Sacrifice. Chicago: University of Chicago Press, 1968.
Bankoff, George. Conquest of Pain: The Story of Anaesthesia. London: MacDonald, [1946].
Banner, Lois W. "Religious Benevolence as Social Control: Critique of an Interpretation." Journal of American History (June 1973), 60:23–41.
Barber, Bernard. "Compassion in Medicine: Towards New Definitions and New Institutions." New England Journal of Medicine (October 21, 1976), 295:939–43.
—— "Some Problems in the Sociology of the Professions." The Professions in America, pp. 15–34. Edited by Kenneth S. Lynn and the editors of Daedalus. Boston: Houghton Mifflin, 1965.
Barker-Benfield, G[raham] J. The Horrors of the Half-Known Life. New York: Harper & Row, 1976.
Bayles, Michael D. and Arthur Caplan. "Medical Fallibility and Malpractice." Journal of Medicine and Philosophy (September 1978), 3:169–86.
Becker, Howard Saul; B. Geer; Everett C. Hughes; and Anselm Strauss. Boys in White: Student Culture in Medical School. Chicago: University of Chicago Press, 1961.
Beecher, Henry K. "Anesthesia's Second Power: Probing the Mind." Science (1947), 105:164–66.

—— "The First Anesthesia Records (Codman, Cushing)." *Surgery, Gynecology and Obstetrics* (1940), 71:689–93.

—— *Measurement of Subjective Responses.* New York: Oxford University Press, 1959.

—— "Pain in Men Wounded in Battle." *Bulletin of the United States Army Medical Department* (1946), 5:445–54.

—— *Research and the Individual.* Boston: Little, Brown, 1970.

Beecher, Henry K. and Donald P. Todd. *A Study of the Deaths Associated with Anesthesia and Surgery.* Springfield, Ill.: Charles C Thomas, 1954.

Ben-David, Joseph. "Scientific Productivity and Academic Organization in Nineteenth Century Medicine." *American Sociological Review* (December 1960), 25:828–43.

Bender, Thomas. "The Cultures of Intellectual Life: The City and the Professions." *New Directions in American Intellectual History,* pp. 181–95. Edited by John Higham and Paul K. Conkin. Baltimore: Johns Hopkins University Press, 1979.

Bendix, Reinhard. *Work and Authority in Industry.* New York: John Wiley, 1956.

Benedict, Michael Les. "Contagion and the Constitution: Quarantine Agitation from 1859–1866." *Journal of the History of Medicine and Allied Sciences* (April 1970), 25:177–93.

Berger, Peter L. *Pyramids of Sacrifice: Political Ethics and Social Change.* Garden City, N.Y.: Anchor Press, Doubleday, 1976, 1974.

Berkhofer, Robert F., Jr. *The White Man's Indian: Images of the American Indian from Columbus to the Present.* New York: Vintage Books, 1978.

Berlant, Jeffrey L. *Profession and Monopoly: A Study of Medicine in the United States and Great Britain.* Berkeley: University of California Press, 1975.

Berman, Alex. "The Heroic Approach in Nineteenth Century Therapeutics." *Bulletin of the American Society of Hospital Pharmacists* (September–October 1954), 11:321–27.

—— "The Impact of the Nineteenth-Century Botanico-Medical Movement on American Pharmacy and Medicine." Ph.D. dissertation, University of Wisconsin, Madison, 1954.

—— "Neo-Thomsonianism in the United States." *Journal of the History of Medicine and Allied Sciences* (April 1956), 11:133–55.

—— "Social Roots of the Nineteenth-Century Botanico-Medical Movement in the United States." *Actes du VIIIᵉ Congres International d'Histoire des Sciences* (1956), 2:561–65.

—— "A Striving for Scientific Respectability: Some American Botanics and the Nineteenth-Century Plant Materia Medica." *Bulletin of the History of Medicine* (January–February 1956), 30:7–31.

—— "The Thomsonian Movement and its Relation to American Pharmacy and Medicine." *Bulletin of the History of Medicine* (September–October 1951), 25:405–28.

Bernard, Richard M., and Maris A. Vinovskis. "The Female School Teacher in Ante-Bellum Massachusetts." *Journal of Social History* (Spring, 1977), 10:332–45.

Berzon, Judith. *Neither White Nor Black: The Mulatto Character in American Fiction.* New York: New York University Press, 1978.

Bettmann, Otto L. *The Good Old Days—They Were Terrible!* New York: Random House, 1974.

Betts, John R. "American Medical Thought on Exercise, 1820–60." *Bulletin of the History of Medicine* (March–April 1971), 45:138–52.

—— "Mind and Body in Early American Thought." *Journal of American History* (March 1968), 54:787–805.

Blake, John B. *Benjamin Waterhouse and the Introduction of Vaccination.* Philadelphia: University of Pennsylvania Press, 1957.

—— "The Development of American Anatomy Acts." *Journal of Medical Education* (August 1955), 30:431–39.

—— "From Buchan to Fishbein: The Literature of Domestic Medicine." *Medicine Without Doctors: Home Health Care in American History*, pp. 11–30. Edited by Guenter B. Risse, Ronald L. Numbers, and Judith Walzer Leavitt. New York: Science History Publications, 1977.

—— *Safeguarding the Public: Historical Aspects of Medicinal Drug Control.* Baltimore: Johns Hopkins Press, 1970.

—— "Women and Medicine in Ante-Bellum America." *Bulletin of the History of Medicine* (March–April 1965), 39:99–123.

Blalock, Hubert M., Jr. *Social Statistics.* New York: McGraw-Hill, 1960.

Blassingame, John W. *The Slave Community: Plantation Life in the Antebellum South.* New York: Oxford University Press, 1972.

Bledstein, Burton. *The Culture of Professionalism: The Middle Class and the Development of Higher Education in America.* New York: W. W. Norton, 1976.

Blochman, Lawrence G. *Doctor Squibb: The Life and Times of A Rugged Idealist.* New York: Simon and Schuster, 1958.

Bloom, Samuel W. *The Doctor and His Patient: A Sociological Interpretation.* New York: Free Press, 1965, 1963.

Bloomfield, Maxwell. *American Lawyers in a Changing Society, 1776–1876.* Cambridge: Harvard University Press, 1976.

Bockoven, J. Sanbourne. *Moral Treatment in Community Mental Health.* New York: Springer, 1972.

Bodo, John R. *The Protestant Clergy and Public Issues, 1812–1848.* Princeton: Princeton University Press, 1954.

Boland, Frank K. *The First Anesthetic: The Story of Crawford Long.* Athens: University of Georgia Press, 1950.

Boller, Paul F., Jr. *American Transcendentalism 1830–1860: An Intellectual Inquiry.* New York: G. P. Putnam, 1974.

Bonner, Thomas N. "The Social and Political Attitudes of Midwestern Physicians 1840–1940: Chicago as a Case History," *Journal of the History of Medicine and Allied Sciences* (April 1953), 8:133–64.

Boorstin, Daniel J. *The Americans: The National Experience.* New York: Vintage Books, Random House, 1967, 1965.

Boring, Edwin G. *Sensation and Perception in the History of Experimental Psychology.* New York: Appleton-Century-Crofts, 1942.

Borrowman, Merle. *The Liberal and the Technical in Teacher Education.* New York: Teachers College, Columbia University Press, 1956.

Bousfield, M. O. "An Account of Physicians of Color in the United States." *Bulletin of the History of Medicine* (January 1945), 17:61–84.

Bowker, John. *Problems of Suffering in the Religions of the World*. Cambridge: Cambridge University Press, 1970.

Bozeman, Theodore Dwight. "Inductive and Deductive Politics: Science and Society in Antebellum Presbyterian Thought." *Journal of American History* (December 1977), 64:704–22.

Brace, C. Loring. "The 'Ethnology' of Josiah Clark Nott." *Bulletin of the New York Academy of Medicine* (April 1974), 50:509–28.

Branch, E. Douglas. *The Sentimental Years, 1836–1860*. American Century Series. New York: Hill and Wang, 1965. New York: D. Appleton-Century, 1934.

Breeden, James O. "States-Rights Medicine in the Old South." *Bulletin of the New York Academy of Medicine* (March–April 1976), 52:348–72.

Bremner, Robert H. "The Impact of the Civil War on Philanthropy and Social Welfare." *Civil War History* (December 1966), 12:293–303.

Brena, Steven. *Pain and Religion*. Springfield, Ill.: Charles C Thomas, 1972.

Bridges, William E. "Warm Hearth, Cold World: Social Perspectives on the Household Poets." *American Quarterly* (Winter, 1969), 21:764–79.

Brieger, Gert H. "Therapeutic Conflicts and the American Medical Profession in the 1860s." *Bulletin of the History of Medicine* (May–June 1967), 41:215–22.

Brodeur, Paul. "Annals of Chemistry." *The New Yorker*, November 24, 1975, pp. 122–48.

Brooks, Stewart. *Civil War Medicine*. Springfield, Ill.: Charles C Thomas, Publisher, 1966.

Brown, Richard D. "The Emergence of Voluntary Associations in Massachusetts, 1760–1830." *Journal of Voluntary Action Research* (April 7, 1973), 2:64–73.

—— *Modernization: The Transformation of American Life, 1600–1865*. American Century Series. New York: Hill and Wang, 1976.

Bryan, Leon S., Jr. "Blood-Letting in American Medicine, 1830–1892." *Bulletin of the History of Medicine* (November–December 1964), 38:516–29.

Bullough, Vern, and Martha Voight. "Women, Menstruation, and Nineteenth Century Medicine." *Bulletin of the History of Medicine* (January–February 1973), 47:66–82.

Burns, Chester R., ed. *Legacies in Ethics and Medicine*. New York: Science History Publications, 1977.

—— ed. *Legacies in Law and Medicine*. New York: Science History Publications, 1977.

—— "Professional Ethics and the Development of American Law as Applied to Medicine." *Legacies in Law and Medicine*, pp. 299–310. New York: Science History Publications, 1977.

Burnum, John F. "The Physician as a Double Agent." *New England Journal of Medicine*, (August 4, 1977), 297:278–79.

Burrage, Walter L. *History of the Massachusetts Medical Society, with Brief Biographies . . . 1791–1922*. Norwood, Mass.: privately printed, Plimpton Press, 1923.

Burrow, James G. *AMA: Voice of American Medicine*. Baltimore: Johns Hopkins Press, 1963.

Burstyn, Joan N. "Catharine Beecher and the Education of American Women." *New England Quarterly* (September 1974), 47:386–403.

—— "Education and Sex: The Medical Case Against Higher Education for Women in England, 1870–1900." *Proceedings of the American Philosopical Society* (1973), 117(2):79–84.

Bushman, Richard. *From Puritan to Yankee: Character and the Social Order in Connecticut, 1690–1765.* New York: W. W. Norton, 1970.

Caldwell, Anne E. "The History of Psychopharmacology: Its Relation to Anesthesiology." *Diseases of the Nervous System* (December 1967), 28:816–20.

Calhoun, Daniel H. *The American Civil Engineer: Origins and Conflict.* Cambridge: Technology Press, 1960.

—— *The Intelligence of a People.* Princeton, N.J.: Princeton University Press, 1973.

—— *Professional Lives in America: Structure and Aspiration, 1750–1850.* Cambridge: Harvard University Press, 1965.

Calvert, Monte A. *The Mechanical Engineer in America, 1830–1910: Professional Cultures in Conflict.* Baltimore: Johns Hopkins Press, 1967.

Cameron, Rondo. "The Diffusion of Technology as a Problem in Economic History." *Economic Geography* (July 1975), 51:217–30.

Carlson, Eric T. "Benjamin Rush on Revolutionary War Hygiene." *Bulletin of the New York Academy of Medicine* (July–August 1979), 55:614–35.

Carlton, Wendy. *"In Our Professional Opinion": The Primacy of Clinical Judgement Over Moral Choice.* Notre Dame: University of Notre Dame Press, 1978.

Carr-Saunders, A. M., and P. A. Wilson. *The Professions.* Oxford, England: The Clarendon Press, 1933.

Carson, Joseph. *A History of the Medical Department of the University of Pennsylvania, from its Foundation in 1765.* Philadelphia: Lindsay and Blakiston, 1869.

Cartwright, F. F. "Antiseptic Surgery." *Medicine and Science in the 1860s,* pp. 77–103. Edited by F. N. L. Poynter. London: Wellcome Institute, 1968.

Cassedy, James H. *American Medicine and Statistical Thinking, 1800–1860.* Cambridge: Harvard University Press, 1984.

Cipolla, Carlo M. "The Professions: The Long View." *Journal of European Economic History* (1973), 2:37–52.

Clouser, K. Danner. "Allowing or Causing: Another Look." *Annals of Internal Medicine* (1977), 87:622–24.

Clouser, K. Danner and Arthur Zucker, compilers. *Abortion & Euthanasia: An Annotated Bibliography.* Philadelphia: Society for Health and Human Values, 1974.

Cohen, Patricia C. "A Calculating People: The Origins of a Quantitative Mentality in America." Ph.D. dissertation, University of California, Berkeley, 1977.

Coleman, James S., Elihu Katz, and Herbert Menzel. *Medical Innovation: A Diffusion Study.* Indianapolis: Bobbs-Merrill, 1966.

Colp, Ralph Jr. " 'I was born a naturalist': Charles Darwin's 1838 Notes about Himself." *Journal of the History of Medicine and Allied Sciences* (January 1980), 35:8–39.

Cominos, Peter T. "Late Victorian Sexual Respectability and the Social System." *International Review of Social History* (1963), 8(1,2):18–48, 216–50.

Conforti, Joseph A. "Samuel Hopkins and the New Divinity: Theology, Ethics, and

Social Reform in Eighteenth-Century New England." *William and Mary Quarterly*, (October 1977), 3d Ser., 34:572–89.

Connor, H. "Anesthesia and the British Public 1846–56." *Anaesthesia* (1970), 25:115–20.

Conway, Jill Ker. "Perspectives on the History of Women's Education in the United States." *History of Education Quarterly* (Spring, 1974), 14:1–12.

—— "Women Reformers and American Culture, 1870–1930." *Journal of Social History* (1971–1972), 5:164–77.

Coombs, Robert H. *Mastering Medicine: Professional Socialization in Medical School.* New York: Free Press, Macmillan, 1978.

Corner, George W. *Two Centuries of Medicine: A History of the School of Medicine of the University of Pennsylvania.* Philadelphia: J. B. Lippincott, 1965.

Cott, Nancy F. *The Bonds of Womanhood: "Woman's Sphere" in New England, 1780–1835.* New Haven: Yale University Press, 1977.

Coulter, Harris L. *Divided Legacy: A History of the Schism in Medical Thought.* Vol. 1, *The Patterns Emerge; Hippocrates to Paracelsus.* Washington, D.C.: Wehawken Publishing Co., 1975. Vol. 3, *Science and Ethics in American Medicine, 1800–1914.* Washington, D.C.: McGrath Publishing Company, 1973.

—— "Orthodox and Sectarian Medicine in the United States: The Struggle of the American Medical Association with the Homoeopathic and Eclectic Physicians." A longer manuscript version of his *Science and Ethics in American Medicine, 1800–1914.*

Courtwright, David T. *Dark Paradise: Opiate Addiction in America before 1940.* Cambridge, Mass.: Harvard University Press, 1982.

Cowan, J. L. *Pleasure and Pain: A Study in Philosophical Psychology.* New York: St. Martin's Press, 1968.

Crane, Diana. *Invisible Colleges: Diffusion of Knowledge in Scientific Communities.* Chicago: University of Chicago Press, 1972.

Crawford, Rob. "Sickness as Sin." *Health/PAC Bulletin* (January–February 1978), No. 80, 10–16.

Crosby, Alfred. "Virgin Soil Epidemics as a Factor in the Aboriginal Depopulation in America." *William and Mary Quarterly* (April 1976), 3d Ser., 33:289–99.

Cross, Whitney R. *The Burned-Over District: The Social and Intellectual History of Enthusiastic Religion in Western New York, 1800–1850.* Ithaca, N.Y.: Cornell University Press, 1950.

Cunningham, H. H. *Doctors in Gray: The Confederate Medical Service.* 2d ed. Baton Rouge: Louisiana State University Press, 1960, 1958.

Czoniczer, Gabor. "The Role of the Patient in Modern Medicine." *Man and Medicine* (1978), 3(1):17–28.

Dain, Norman. *Disordered Minds: The First Century of Eastern State Hospital in Williamsburg, Virginia, 1766–1866.* Charlottesville: University Press of Virginia, 1971.

Dallenbach, K. M. "Pain: History and Present Status." *American Journal of Psychology* (1939), 52:331–47.

Daniels, George H. *American Science in the Age of Jackson.* New York: Columbia University Press, 1968.

—— "The Process of Professionalization in American Science: The Emergent Period, 1820–1860." *Isis* (Summer, 1967), 58:151–66.

Darnton, Robert. *Mesmerism and the End of the Enlightenment in France.* Cambridge: Harvard University Press, 1968.

Davidson, Lynn R. "Sex Roles, Affect, and the Woman Physician: A Comparative Study of the Impact of Latent Social Identity Upon the Role of Women and Men Professionals." Ph.D. dissertation, New York University, 1975.

Davies, John D. *Phrenology: Fad and Science, A Nineteenth Century Crusade.* New Haven: Yale University Press, 1955.

Demos, John. "The Anti-slavery Movement and the Problem of Violent 'Means.' " *New England Quarterly* (December 1964), 37:501–26.

Devereux, Daniel T. "Courage and Wisdom in Plato's *Laches.*" *Journal of the History of Philosophy* (April 1977), 15:129–41.

Dictionary of American Biography. New York: Scribner, 1959 (1927–36).

Dittrick, Howard. "The Introduction of Anesthesia into Ohio." *Ohio Archaeological and Historical Quarterly* (1941), 50:338–50.

Douglas, Ann. *The Feminization of American Culture.* New York: Knopf, 1977.

—— "Heaven Our Home: Consolation Literature in the Northern United States, 1830–1880." *American Quarterly* (December 1974), 26:496–515.

Downie, R. W. "Pennsylvania Hospital Admissions, 1751–1850." *Transactions and Studies of the College of Physicians of Philadelphia* (1964), 32:20–35.

Drachman, Virginia. "Women Doctors and the Women's Medical Movement: Feminism and Medicine 1850–1895." Ph.D. dissertation, State University of New York at Buffalo, 1976.

Dubos, René. *Mirage of Health: Utopias, Progress, and Biological Change.* New York: Harper & Row, 1959.

Dubos, René and Jean Dubos. *The White Plague: Tuberculosis, Man, and Society.* Boston: Little, Brown & Co., 1952.

Duffy, John. "Anglo-American Reaction to Obstetrical Anesthesia." *Bulletin of the History of Medicine* (January–February 1964), 38:32–44.

—— *A History of Public Health in New York City, 1625–1866.* New York: Russell Sage Foundation, 1968.

—— "Medical Practice in the Ante Bellum South." *Journal of Southern History* (February 1959), 25:53–72.

—— "Mental Strain and 'Overpressure' in the Schools: a Nineteenth-Century Viewpoint." *Journal of the History of Medicine and Allied Sciences* (January 1968), 23:63–79.

—— "A Note on Ante Bellum Southern Nationalism and Medical Practice." *Journal of Southern History* (May 1968), 34:266–76.

—— "Science and Medicine." *Science and Society in the United States,* pp. 107–34. Edited by David D. Van Tassel and Michael G. Hall. Homewood, Ill.: Dorsey Press, 1966.

—— "Sectional Conflict and Medical Education in Louisiana." *Journal of Southern History* (August 1957), 23:289–306.

Duncum, Barbara M. *The Development of Inhalation Anaesthesia.* London: Geoffrey Cumberlege, Oxford University Press, 1947.

Duns, John. *Memoir of Sir James Y. Simpson, Bart.* Edinburgh: Edmunston Douglas, 1873.

Dupree, A. Hunter. *Science in the Federal Government: A History of Policies and Activities to 1940.* New York: Harper & Row, 1957.

Durden, Robert F. "Ambiguities in the Antislavery Crusade of the Republican Party." *The Antislavery Vanguard: New Essays on the Abolitionists,* pp. 362–94. Edited by Martin Duberman. Princeton, N.J.: Princeton University Press, 1965.

Dykstra, David L. "The Medical Profession and Patent and Proprietary Medicines During the Nineteenth Century." *Bulletin of the History of Medicine* (September–October 1955), 29:401–19.

Eaton, Clement. *A History of the Southern Confederacy.* New York: Free Press, 1954.

Eaton, Leonard K. "Medicine in Philadelphia and Boston, 1805–1830." *Pennsylvania Magazine of History and Biography* (January 1951), 75:66–75.

—— *New England Hospitals, 1790–1833.* Ann Arbor: University of Michigan Press, 1957.

Eckenhoff, James E. *Anesthesia from Colonial Times: A History of Anesthesia at the University of Pennsylvania.* Philadelphia: J. B. Lippincott, 1966.

Eckman, James. "Anglo-American Hostility in American Medical Literature of the Nineteenth Century." *Bulletin of the History of Medicine* (January 1941), 9:31–71.

Edel, Abraham. "Happiness and Pleasure." *Dictionary of the History of Ideas.* New York: Scribner, 1973, 2:374–87.

Edelstein, Ludwig. *The Hippocratic Oath.* Baltimore: Johns Hopkins Press, 1964, 1943.

Edwards, Linden F. "Resurrection Riots During the Heroic Age of Anatomy in America." *Bulletin of the History of Medicine* (March–April 1951), 178–84.

Ehrenreich, Barbara, and Deirdre English. *Complaints and Disorders: The Sexual Politics of Sickness.* Glass Mountain Pamphlet No. 2. Old Westbury, N.Y.: Feminist Press, 1973.

—— *For Her Own Good: 150 Years of the Experts' Advice to Women.* Garden City, N.Y.: Anchor Press/Doubleday, 1978.

Elkins, Stanley M. *Slavery: A Problem in American Institutional and Intellectual Life.* 2d ed. Chicago: University of Chicago Press, 1968.

Elliott, Philip. *The Sociology of the Professions.* New York: Herder & Herder, 1972.

Engelhardt, H. Tristram, Jr. "John Hughlings Jackson and the Mind-Body Relation." *Bulletin of the History of Medicine* (Summer, 1975), 49:137–51.

English, Peter. *Shock, Physiological Surgery, and George Washington Crile: Medical Innovation in the Progressive Era.* Westport, Conn.: Greenwood Press, 1980.

Estes, J. Worth. *Hall Jackson and the Purple Foxglove: Medical Practice and Research in Revolutionary America, 1760–1820.* Hanover, N.H.: University Press of New England, 1980.

Evans, Daniel E. N. "Anaesthesia and the Epileptic Patient: A Review." *Anaesthesia* (1975), 30:34–45.

"Eye Color and Pain Sensitivity." *Science News,* May 31, 1975, p. 350.

Eyler, John M. *Victorian Social Medicine: The Ideas and Methods of William Farr.* Baltimore: Johns Hopkins University Press, 1979.

Farr, A. D. "Early Opposition to Obstetric Anaesthesia." *Anaesthesia* (1980), 35:896–907.

Feigl, Herbert, Michael Scriven, and Grover Maxwell, eds. *Concepts, Theories, and the Mind-Body Problem*. Minnesota Studies in the Philosophy of Science. Vol. 2. Minneapolis: University of Minnesota Press, 1958.

Ferguson, John. *The Place of Suffering*. Greenwood, S.C.: Attic Press, 1972.

Filene, Peter G. *Him-Her-Self: Sex Roles in Modern America*. New York: Harcourt, Brace, Jovanovich, 1975.

Fischer, David Hackett. *Growing Old in America: The Bland-Lee Lectures Delivered at Clark University*. New York: Oxford University Press, 1977.

—— *The Revolution of American Conservatism: The Federalist Party in the Era of Jeffersonian Democracy*. New York: Harper & Row, 1965.

Fishbein, Morris. *A History of the American Medical Association, 1847–1947*. Philadelphia: W. B. Saunders, 1947.

Fitz, Reginald H. "The Rise and Fall of the Licensed Physician in Massachusetts, 1781–1860." *Transactions of the Association of American Physicians* (1894), 9:1–18.

Fleming, Donald. "Charles Darwin, the Anaesthetic Man." *Victorian Studies*, (March 1961), 4:219–36.

Fletcher, Robert S. "Bread and Doctrine at Oberlin." *Ohio State Archeological and Historical Quarterly* (January 1940), 49:58–67.

Flexner, Eleanor. *Century of Struggle: The Woman's Rights Movement in the United States*. New York: Atheneum, 1970, 1959.

Flexner, James Thomas. *Doctors on Horseback: Pioneers of American Medicine*. New York: Dover, 1969. New York: Viking Press, 1937.

Flood, Dom Peter, ed. *New Problems in Medical Ethics, 3d Ser.* Westminster, Md.: Newman Press, 1956.

Foucalt, Michel. *The Birth of the Clinic: An Archaeology of Medical Perception*. New York: Pantheon Books, Random House, 1973.

—— *Madness and Civilization: A History of Insanity in the Age of Reason*. New York: Mentor Books, 1965.

Fox, Renée C. "The Evolution of Medical Uncertainty." *Milbank Memorial Fund Quarterly* (Winter, 1980), 58:1–49.

Fredrickson, George M. *The Black Image in the White Mind: The Debate on Afro-American Character and Destiny, 1817–1914*. New York: Harper & Row, 1971.

—— *The Inner Civil War: Northern Intellectuals and the Crisis of the Union*. New York: Harper & Row, 1965.

Freidson, Eliot. *Profession of Medicine: A Study of the Sociology of Applied Knowledge*. New York: Dodd, Mead, 1970.

—— *Professional Dominance: The Social Structure of Medical Care*. New York: Atherton Press, 1970.

French, Richard D. *Antivivisection and Medical Science in Victorian Society*. Princeton, N.J., and London: Princeton University Press, 1975.

Fülöp-Miller, René. *Triumph Over Pain*. Translated by Eden and Cedar Paul. New York: Literary Guild of America, 1938.

Fulton, John F. *A Century of Surgical Anesthesia: An Annotated Catalog of Books and Pamphlets Bearing on the Early History of Surgical Anesthesia.* New York: Henry Schuman, 1946.

Fye, W. Bruce. "Active Euthanasia: An Historical Survey of Its Conceptual Origins and Introduction to Medical Thought." *Bulletin of the History of Medicine* (1979), 52:492–502.

Garrison, Fielding H. *Garrison's History of Neurology.* Revised by Lawrence C. McHenry, Jr. Springfield, Ill.: Charles C Thomas, 1969.

Gastineau, Jane. "Healing the Sick and Suffering Sisterhood: Dr. Rachel Brooks Gleason and the Care of Female Patients, 1852–98." Paper presented at North of 40 Midwest Historians of Medicine Conference, March 27, 1982, Bloomington, Indiana.

Gaustad, Edwin Scott. *A Religious History of America.* New York: Harper & Row, 1974, 1966.

—— ed. *The Rise of Adventism: Religion and Society in Mid-Nineteenth Century America.* New York: Harper & Row, 1974.

Gawalt, Gerard W. *The Promise of Power: The Emergence of the Legal Profession in Massachusetts, 1760–1840.* Westport, Conn.: Greenwood Press, 1979.

Gaylin, Willard. *Partial Justice: A Study of Bias in Sentencing.* New York: Vintage Books, Random House, 1975, 1974.

Gelfand, Toby. *Professionalizing Modern Medicine: Paris Surgeons and Medical Science and Institutions in the Eighteenth Century.* Westport, Conn.: Greenwood Press, 1980.

"General Anesthesia by Dentists Unacceptable." *Anesthesiology* (1978), 48:384–85.

Genovese, Eugene D. *In Red and Black: Marxian Explorations of Southern and Afro-American History.* New York: Pantheon, 1971.

—— *Roll, Jordan, Roll: The World the Slaves Made.* New York: Pantheon Books, 1974.

Gibson, Mary. "On the Insensitivity of Women: Criminological Experiments in Pre-World War I Italy." Paper presented at Fifth Berkshire Conference on the History of Women, Vassar College, June 18, 1981.

Gilbert, James B. "Anthropometrics in the U.S. Bureau of Education: The Case of Arthur MacDonald's 'Laboratory.' " *History of Education Quarterly* (Summer, 1977), 17:169–95.

Gladstone, Francis, producer. "Nova: Strange Sleep." Public Broadcasting System, WGBH, Boston.

Glaser, Frederick B. "Inhalation Psychosis and Related States." *Archives of General Psychiatry* (1966), 17:315–22.

Glenn, Myra. *Campaigns against Corporal Punishment: Prisoners, Sailors, Women, and Children in Antebellum America.* Albany: State University of New York Press, forthcoming.

Gloyne, S. Roodhouse. *John Hunter.* Edinburgh: E. & S. Livingstone, 1950.

Goode, William J. "The Theoretical Limits of Professionalization." *The Semi-Professions and their Organization,* pp. 266–313. Edited by Amitai Etzioni. New York: Free Press, 1969.

Goodman, Nathan G. *Benjamin Rush, Physician and Citizen.* Philadelphia: University of Pennsylvania Press, 1934.

Gordon Jones, R. G. "A Short History of Anaesthesia for Hare-Lip and Cleft Palate Repair." *British Journal of Anaesthesia* (1971), 43:796–802.

Gorovitz, Samuel, and Alasdair MacIntryre. "Toward a Theory of Medical Fallibility." *Journal of Medicine and Philosophy* (March 1976), 1:51–71.

Gossett, Thomas F. *Race: The History of an Idea in America.* Dallas: Southern Methodist University Press, 1963.

Green, Fletcher M. *The Role of the Yankee in the Old South.* Athens: University of Georgia Press, 1972.

Green, Samuel A. *The History of Medicine in Massachusetts: A Centennial Address Before the Massachusetts Medical Society at Cambridge, June 7, 1881.* Boston: A. Williams, 1881.

Greene, Nicholas M. "Anesthesia and the Development of Surgery, 1846–1896." *Anesthesia and Analgesia* (1979), 58:5–12.

—— *Anesthesiology and the University.* Philadelphia: J. B. Lippincott, 1975.

—— "A Consideration of Factors in the Discovery of Anesthesia and their Effects on its Development." *Anesthesiology* (1971), 35:515–22.

Greenwood, Ernest. "Attributes of a Profession." *Social Work* (July 1957), 2:45–55.

Griffin, C. S. *The Ferment of Reform, 1830–1860.* The Crowell American History Series. New York: Thomas Y. Crowell, 1967.

—— *Their Brothers' Keepers: Moral Stewardship in the United States, 1800–1865.* New Brunswick, N.J.: Rutgers University Press, 1960.

Grob, Gerald N. *Edward Jarvis and the Medical World of Nineteenth-Century America.* Knoxville: University of Tennessee Press, 1978.

—— *Mental Institutions in America: Social Policy to 1875.* New York: Free Press, 1973.

—— "Modernization and Traditionalism in Jacksonian Social Reform: Horace Mann, Dorothea L. Dix, Orestes A. Brownson." *Men, Women, and Issues in American History,* pp. 192–214. Edited by Howard H. Quint and Milton Cantor. Vol. 1. Homewood, Ill.: The Dorsey Press, 1974.

—— "Rediscovering Asylums: The Unhistorical History of the Mental Hospital." *Hastings Center Report* (August 1977), 7:33–41.

—— *The State and the Mentally Ill: A History of Worcester State Hospital in Massachusetts, 1830–1920.* Chapel Hill: University of North Carolina Press, 1966.

Gruman, Gerald. "An Historical Introduction to Ideas About Voluntary Euthanasia: With a Bibliographic Survey and Guide for Interdisciplinary Studies." *Omega* (Summer, 1973), 4:87–138.

Gusfield, Joseph R. *Symbolic Crusade: Status Politics and the American Temperance Movement.* Urbana: University of Illinois Press, 1963.

Haber, Samuel. "The Professions and Higher Education in America: A Historical View." *Higher Education and the Labor Market,* pp. 237–80. Edited by Margaret S. Gordon. New York: McGraw-Hill, 1974.

Haggard, Howard. *Devils, Drugs, and Doctors: The Story of the Science of Healing from Medicine-Man to Doctor.* New York and Evanston: Harper & Row, 1929.

Haller, John S. "Acupuncture in Nineteenth Century Western Medicine." *New York State Journal of Medicine,* May 15, 1973, pp. 1213–21.

—— "The Negro and the Southern Physician: A Study of Medical and Racial Attitudes, 1800–1860." *Medical History* (July 1972), 16:238–53.

Haller, John S. and Robin M. Haller. *The Physician and Sexuality in Victorian America.* Urbana: University of Illinois Press, 1974.

Hamilton, David. "The Nineteenth-Century Surgical Revolution—Antisepsis or Better Nutrition?" *Bulletin of the History of Medicine* (Spring, 1982), 56:30–40.

Handlin, Oscar. *Boston's Immigrants: A Study in Acculturation.* Revised and enlarged ed. New York: Atheneum, 1971.

Handlin, Oscar and Mary Flug Handlin. *Commonwealth: A Study of the Role of Government in the American Economy, Massachusetts, 1774–1861.* Revised ed. Cambridge, Mass.: Belknap Press of Harvard University Press, 1969.

Hardy, T. K., and I. W. Jones. "Early Experiences of Ether Anaesthesia in North Wales." *Anaesthesia* (1978), 31:264–67.

Hare, R. M. "Pain and Evil." *Proceedings of the Aristotelian Society* (1964), Supplement 38:91–106.

Harries-Jenkins, G. "Professionals in Organizations." *Professions and Professionalization,* pp. 53–107. Edited by J. A. Jackson. Cambridge, England: At the University Press, 1970.

Harrington, Thomas F. *Harvard Medical School, A History.* Vol. 2. New York: Lewis, 1905.

Harris, Seale. *Woman's Surgeon: The Life Story of J. Marion Sims.* New York: Macmillan, 1950.

Hartman, Mary S., and Lois Banner, eds. *Clio's Consciousness Raised: New Perspectives on the History of Women.* New York: Harper & Row, 1974.

Harvey, Samuel D. "Effect of the Introduction of Anesthesia Upon Surgery." *Journal of the American Dental Association* (November 1945), 32:1351–57.

Haskell, Thomas L. *The Emergence of Professional Social Science: The American Social Science Association and the Nineteenth-Century Crisis of Authority.* Urbana: University of Illinois Press, 1977.

—— "Power to the Experts." *New York Review of Books* (October 13, 1977), 24(16):28–33.

The Hastings Center. "Values, Ethics, and C.B.A. in Health Care." *The Implications of Cost-Effectiveness Analysis of Medical Technology,* pp. 168–82. Washington, D.C.: Congressional Office of Technology Assessment, 1980.

Hawke, David Freeman. *Benjamin Rush: Revolutionary Gadfly.* Indianapolis: Bobbs-Merrill, 1971.

Heale, M. J. "From City Fathers to Social Critics: Humanitarianism and Government." *Journal of American History* (June 1976), 63:21–41.

Hemminki, Elina. "Review of the Literature on the Factors Affecting Drug Prescribing." *Social Science and Medicine* (1975), 9:111–15.

Henry, F. P. *Standard History of the Medical Profession of Philadelphia.* Chicago: Goodspeed, 1897.

Higham, John. *From Boundlessness to Consolidation: The Transformation of American Culture 1848–1860.* Ann Arbor: University of Michigan Press, 1969.

—— "Hanging Together: Divergent Unities in American History." *Journal of American History* (June 1974), 61:5–28.

Hindle, Brooke. *Emulation and Invention*. New York: New York University Press, 1981.

Hofstadter, Richard. *The Idea of a Party System: The Rise of Legitimate Opposition in the United States, 1780–1840*. Berkeley: University of California Press, 1969.

—— *Social Darwinism in American Thought*. Revised ed. New York: George Braziller, 1959, 1955.

Hogarth, John. *Sentencing as a Human Process*. Toronto: University of Toronto Press, 1971.

Hogeland, Ronald W. " 'The Female Appendage': Feminine Life-Styles in America 1820–1860." *Civil War History* (June 1971), 17:101–14.

Holbrook, Stewart H. *The Golden Age of Quackery*. New York: Collier Books, 1962, 1959.

Hollon, W. Eugene. *Frontier Violence*. New York: Oxford University Press, 1974.

Holmfeld, John. "From Amateurs to Professionals in American Science: The Controversy Over the Proceedings of an 1853 Meeting." *Proceedings of the American Philosophical Society* (February 1970), 114:22–36.

Hoover, Suzanne. "Coleridge, Humphry Davy, and Some Early Experiments with a Consciousness-altering Drug." *Bulletin of Research in the Humanities* (Spring, 1978), 81:9–27.

Howe, Mark De Wolfe. *Justice Oliver Wendell Holmes: The Shaping Years, 1841–1870*. Vol. 1. Cambridge: Belknap Press of Harvard University Press, 1957.

Hughes, Everett C. "Professions." *The Professions in America*, pp. 1–14. Edited by Kenneth S. Lynn and the editors of *Daedalus*. Boston: Houghton Mifflin, 1965.

Hugins, Walter. *Jacksonian Democracy and the Working Class: A Study of the New York Workingmen's Movement, 1829–1837*. Stanford: Stanford University Press, 1960.

Humphrey, David C. "Dissection and Discrimination: Social Origin of Cadavers in America, 1760–1915." *Bulletin of the New York Academy of Medicine* (September 1973), 49:819–27.

—— "The King's College Medical School and the Professionalization of Medicine in Pre-Revolutionary New York." *Bulletin of the History of Medicine* (Summer, 1975), 49:206–34.

Huston, K. G. *Resuscitation—An Historical Perspective*. Park Ridge, Ill.: Wood Library Museum, 1976.

Ignatieff, Michael. *A Just Measure of Pain: The Penitentiary in the Industrial Revolution, 1750–1850*. New York: Pantheon, 1978.

Illich, Ivan. *Medical Nemesis: The Expropriation of Health*. New York: Pantheon Books, Random House, 1976.

Ingelfinger, Franz J. "Decision in Medicine." *New England Journal of Medicine* (July 31, 1975), 293:254–55.

Jackson, J. A., ed. *Professions and Professionalization*. Cambridge, England: At the University Press, 1970.

James, Sidney V. *A People Among Peoples: Quaker Benevolence in Eighteenth-Century America*. Cambridge, Mass.: Harvard University Press, 1963.

Jeffrey, Kirk. "The Family as Utopian Retreat from the City." *Soundings* (Spring, 1972), 55:21–41.

Johnson, Terence J. *Professions and Power.* London: Macmillan, 1972.

Johnson, William R. "Education and Professional Life Styles: Law and Medicine in the Nineteenth Century." *History of Education Quarterly* (Summer, 1974), 14:185–207.

—— "Professions in Process: Doctors and Teachers in American Culture." *History of Education Quarterly* (Summer, 1975), 15:185–99.

—— *Schooled Lawyers: A Study in the Clash of Professional Cultures.* New York: New York University Press, 1978.

Jones, Gordon W. "Wartime Surgery." *Civil War Times Illustrated* (1963), 2(2):7–8, 28–30.

Jones, Howard Mumford. *The Pursuit of Happiness.* Ithaca, N.Y.: Cornell University Press, 1966, 1953.

Jones, Russell M. "American Doctors and the Parisian Medical World, 1830–40." Parts 1 and 3. *Bulletin of the History of Medicine* (January–February 1973), 47:40–65, (May–June 1973), 47:177–204.

Jonsen, Albert. "Do No Harm: Axiom of Medical Ethics." *Philosophical Medical Ethics.* Edited by Stuart F. Spicker and H. Tristram Engelhardt, Jr. Philosophy and Medicine, Vol. 3. Dordrecht and Boston: D. Reidel, 1977, pp. 27–42.

Jordan, Winthrop. *White Over Black, American Attitudes Toward the Negro, 1550–1812.* Baltimore: Penguin Books, 1969, 1968.

Journal of the History of Medicine and Allied Sciences (October 1946), Vol. 1.

Kaestle, Carl F. *The Evolution of an Urban School System: New York City, 1750–1850.* Cambridge: Harvard University Press, 1973.

—— "Social Change, Discipline, and the Common School in Early Nineteenth-Century America." *Journal of Interdisciplinary History* (Summer, 1978), 9:1–17.

Kalisch, Philip A., and Beatrice J. Kalisch, *The Advance of American Nursing.* Boston: Little, Brown, 1978.

Kaplan, Fred. "The Mesmeric Mania: The Early Victorians and Animal Magnetism." *Journal of the History of Ideas* (October–December 1974), 35:691–702.

Karcher, Carolyn L. "Melville's 'The 'Gees': A Forgotten Satire on Scientific Racism." *American Quarterly* (October 1975), 27:421–42.

Katz, Elihu, and Paul Lazarsfeld. *Personal Influence: The Part Played by People in the Flow of Mass Communication.* New York: Free Press, 1955.

Katz, Elihu, Martin L. Levin, and Herbert Hamilton. "Traditions of Research on the Diffusion of Innovation." *American Sociological Review* (April 1963), 28:237–52.

Katz, Jay, ed. *Experimentation with Human Beings.* New York: Russell Sage Foundation, 1972.

Katz, Michael. *Class, Bureaucracy, and Schools: The Illusion of Educational Change in America.* New York: Praeger, 1971.

—— *The Irony of Early School Reform: Educational Innovation in Mid-Nineteenth Century Massachusetts.* Cambridge: Harvard University Press, 1968.

—— "The Origins of Public Education: A Reassessment." *History of Education Quarterly* (Winter, 1976), 16:381–408.

Kaufman, Martin. "The Admission of Women to Nineteenth-Century American Medical Societies." *Bulletin of the History of Medicine* (Summer, 1976), 50:251–60.

—— "The American Anti-Vaccinationists and Their Arguments." *Bulletin of the History of Medicine* (September–October 1967), 41:463–78.

—— *American Medical Education: The Formative Years, 1765–1910.* Westport, Conn. and London: Greenwood Press, 1976.

—— *Homeopathy in America: The Rise and Fall of a Medical Heresy.* Baltimore and London: Johns Hopkins Press, 1971.

Kaufmann, Walter. "Suffering and the Bible." *The Faith of a Heretic*, pp. 137–69. Garden City, N.Y.: Doubleday, 1961.

Kelly, Howard A., and Walter L. Burrage. *American Medical Biographies.* Baltimore: Norman, Remington, 1920.

Kelly, William A. "The Physician, The Patient, and the Consent." *University of Kansas Law Review* (March 1960), 8:405–34.

Kennard, June A. "Review Essay: The History of [Women's] Physical Education." *Signs* (Summer, 1977), 2:835–42.

Kerber, Linda K. "The Abolitionist Perception of the Indian." *Journal of American History* (September 1975), 62:271–95.

—— *Federalists in Dissent: Imagery and Ideology in Jeffersonian America.* Ithaca, N.Y. and London: Cornell University Press, 1970.

Kern, Stephen. *Anatomy and Destiny: A Cultural History of the Human Body.* Indianapolis: Bobbs-Merrill, 1975.

Kett, Joseph F. *The Formation of the American Medical Profession: The Role of Institutions, 1780–1860.* New Haven: Yale University Press, 1968.

Keys, Thomas E. *The History of Surgical Anesthesia.* New York: Dover Publications, 1963, 1945.

—— "John Snow, M.D.: Anesthetist." *Journal of the History of Medicine and Allied Sciences* (Fall, 1946), 1:551–66.

King, William Harvey. *History of Homeopathy and its Institutions in America.* New York: Lewis Publishing Company, 1905.

Klaits, Joseph, and Barrie Klaits, eds. *Animals and Man in Historical Perspective.* New York: Harper & Row, 1974.

Koch, Charles R. E., ed. *History of Dental Surgery.* Vol. 2. Chicago: National Art Publishing Company, 1909.

Kohlstedt, Sally Gregory. *The Formation of the American Scientific Community.* Urbana: University of Illinois Press, 1975.

—— "Physiological Lectures for Women: Sarah Coates in Ohio, 1850." *Journal of the History of Medicine and Allied Sciences* (January 1978), 33:75–81.

Kolata, Gina Bari. "Clinical Trials: Methods and Ethics are Debated." *Science* (1977), 198:1127–31.

—— "Scientists Attack Report That Obstetric Medications Endanger Children." *Science* (1979), 204:391–92.

Kraditor, Aileen S. *Means and Ends in American Abolitionism: Garrison and His Critics on Strategy and Tactics, 1834–1850.* New York: Pantheon Books, Random House, 1969, 1967.

Kramer, Howard D. "Early Municipal and State Boards of Health." *Bulletin of the History of Medicine* (November–December 1950), 24:503–29.
—— "Effect of the Civil War Upon the Public Health Movement." *Mississippi Valley Historical Review* (1948–49), 35:449–62.
Kudlien, Fridolf. "Medicine as a 'Liberal Art' and the Question of the Physician's Income." *Journal of the History of Medicine and Allied Sciences* (October 1976), 31:448–59.
Kuhn, Anne L. *The Mother's Role in Childhood Education: New England Concepts, 1830–1860.* New Haven: Yale University Press, 1947.
Kuhn, Thomas. *The Essential Tension: Selected Studies in Scientific Tradition and Change.* Chicago: University of Chicago Press, 1977.
Lain Entralgo, P. *Doctor and Patient.* Translated by Frances Partridge. New York: World University Library, McGraw-Hill, 1969.
Lally, John J., and Bernard Barber. "The 'Compassionate Physician': Frequency and Social Determinants of Physician-Investigator Concern for Human Subjects." *Social Forces* (December 1974), 53:289–96.
Lambert, Wallace E., Eva Libman, and Ernest G. Poser. "The Effect of Increased Salience of a Membership Group on Pain Tolerance." *Journal of Personality* (1960), 28:350–57.
Lane, Roger. *Violent Death in the City: Suicide, Accident, and Murder in Nineteenth-Century Philadelphia.* Cambridge: Harvard University Press, 1979.
Langley, Harold. *Social Reform in the United States Navy, 1798–1862.* Urbana: University of Illinois Press, 1967.
Larkey, Sanford V., and Janet B. Koudelka. "Medical Societies and Civil War Politics." *Bulletin of the History of Medicine* (January–February 1962), 36:1–12.
Larson, Margali Sarfatti. *The Rise of Professionalism: A Sociological Analysis.* Berkeley: University of California Press, 1977.
Lasagna, Louis. "The Conflict of Interest Between Physician as Therapist and As Experimenter." Philadelphia: Society for Health and Human Values, 1975, 26 pp.
Lasch, Christopher. *The World of Nations: Reflections on American History, Politics, and Culture.* New York: Vintage Books, Random House, 1974.
Lawrence, Christopher. "The Nervous System and Society in the Scottish Enlightenment." *Natural Order: Historical Studies of Scientific Culture*, pp. 19–40. Edited by Barry Barnes and Steven Shapin. Beverley Hills: Sage Publications, 1979.
Layton, Edwin T., Jr. *The Revolt of the Engineers: Social Responsibility and the Engineering Profession.* Cleveland: Press of Case Western Reserve University, 1971.
Lazerson, Marvin. *Origins of the Urban School: Public Education in Massachusetts, 1870–1915.* Cambridge, Mass.: Harvard University Press, 1971.
Leach, Maria, ed. *Dictionary of Folklore, Mythology and Legend.* New York: Funk & Wagnalls, 1949.
Leavitt, Judith Walzer. "Birthing and Anesthesia: The Debate Over Twilight Sleep." *Signs* (Autumn, 1980), 6:147–64.
—— and Ronald L. Numbers. "Sickness and Health in America: An Overview."

Sickness and Health in America, pp. 3–10. Madison: University of Wisconsin Press, 1978.

Le Duc, Thomas H. [ed.]. "Grahamites and Garrisonites." *New York History* (April 1939), 20:189–91.

Legan, Marshall Scott, "Hydropathy in America: A Nineteenth Century Panacea." *Bulletin of the History of Medicine* (May–June 1971), 45:267–80.

Leonard, Thomas C. "Red, White and Army Blue: Empathy and Anger in the American West." *American Quarterly* (May 1974), 26:176–90.

Lerner, Ralph. "Commerce and Character: The Anglo-American as New-Model Man." *William and Mary Quarterly* (January 1979), 36:3–26.

Lewis, C. S. *The Problem of Pain*. New York: Macmillan, 1962.

Lewis, Carl P., Jr. "The Baltimore College of Dental Surgery and the Birth of Professional Dentistry, 1840." *Maryland Historical Magazine* (September 1964), 59:268–85.

Lewis, Gilbert. "The Place of Pain in Human Experience." *Journal of Medical Ethics* (1976), 4:122–25.

Lewis, Sir Thomas. *Pain*. New York: Macmillan, 1942.

Lilienfeld, Abraham. "Ceteris Paribus: The Evolution of the Clinical Trial." *Bulletin of the History of Medicine* (Spring, 1982), 56:1–18.

Livingston, W. K. "What Is Pain?" *Scientific American*, March 1953. Reprint No. 407. San Francisco: W. H. Freeman 1953.

Longo, Lawrence D. "The Rise and Fall of Battey's Operation: A Fashion in Surgery." *Bulletin of the History of Medicine* (Summer, 1979), 53:244–67.

Lovejoy, David B., Jr. "The Hospital and Society: Growth of Hospitals in Rochester, New York, in the Nineteenth Century." *Bulletin of the History of Medicine* (Winter, 1975), 49:536–55.

Lowenfels, Walter. *Walt Whitman's Civil War*. New York: Knopf, 1961.

Lowrance, William W. *Of Acceptable Risk: Science and the Determination of Safety*. Los Altos, Calif.: Wm. Kaufmann, 1976.

Lucid, Robert F. "The Influence of *Two Years Before the Mast* on Herman Melville." *American Literature* (November 1959), 31:243–56.

——— "*Two Years Before the Mast* as Propaganda." *American Quarterly* (Fall, 1960), 12:392–403.

Lynn, Kenneth S. and the Editors of *Daedalus*, eds. *The Professions in America*. Boston: Houghton Mifflin, 1965.

McCluggage, Robert W. *A History of the American Dental Association*. Chicago: American Dental Association, 1959.

McCullough, Laurence B. "Historical Perspectives on the Ethical Dimensions of the Patient-Physician Relationship: The Medical Ethics of Dr. John Gregory." *Ethics in Science & Medicine* (1978), 5(1):47–53.

McLachlan, James. *American Boarding Schools: A Historical Study*. New York: Scribner, 1970.

MacLeod, Laurie. "The Dyspepsia Generation: An Investigation into the Causes and Cures of Sickness in the Early Nineteenth Century. . . ." Senior honors thesis, Hampshire College, 1977.

McPherson, James M. *The Struggle for Equality: Abolitionists and the Negro in the Civil War and Reconstruction*. Princeton, N.J.: Princeton University Press, 1964.

MacQuitty, Betty. *The Battle for Oblivion: The Discovery of Anaesthesia*. London: George G. Harrap, 1969.

Majno, Guido. *The Healing Hand: Man and Wound in the Ancient World*. Cambridge: Harvard University Press, 1975.

Maltby, J. R. "Francis Sibson, 1814–1876." *Anaesthesia* (1977), 32:53–62.

Mann, Arthur. *The One and the Many: Reflections on American Identity*. Chicago: University of Chicago Press, 1979.

Marcuse, Herbert. *Eros and Civilization*. Boston: Beacon Press, 1955.

Marsden, George M. *The Evangelical Mind and the New School Presbyterian Experience*. New Haven: Yale University Press, 1970.

Marsh, Frank H. "An Ethical Approach to Paternalism in the Physician-Patient Relationship." *Ethics in Science & Medicine* (1977), 4(3–4):135–38.

Marshall, Helen E. *Mary Adelaide Nutting: Pioneer of Modern Nursing*. Baltimore: Johns Hopkins Press, 1972.

Mathews, Mitford M. *A Dictionary of Americanisms*. Chicago: University of Chicago Press, 1951.

Matthiessen, F. O. *American Renaissance: Art and Expression in the Age of Emerson and Whitman*. London: Oxford University Press, 1941.

Mattingly, Paul H. *The Classless Profession: American Schoolmen in the Nineteenth Century*. New York: New York University Press, 1975.

Marx, Leo. *The Machine in the Garden: Technology and the Pastoral Ideal in America*. London, Oxford, New York: Oxford University Press, 1964.

Maurits, Reuben. "Individualized Anesthesia." *Journal of the Michigan State Medical Society* (August 1935), 34:463–68.

Maxwell, William Quentin. *Lincoln's Fifth Wheel: The Political History of the United States Sanitary Commission*. New York: Longmans, Green, 1956.

Melder, Keith E. "Ladies Bountiful: Organized Women's Benevolence in Early Nineteenth Century America." *New York History* (July 1967), 48:231–54.

—— "Woman's High Calling: The Teaching Profession in America, 1830–1860." *American Studies* (Fall, 1972), 13:19–32.

Melzack, Ronald. *The Puzzle of Pain*. New York: Basic Books, 1973.

Mendelsohn, Everett, Judith P. Swazey, and Irene Taviss, eds. *Human Aspects of Biomedical Innovation*. Cambridge: Harvard University Press, 1971.

Menninger, W. Walter. "Caring as Part of Health Care Quality." *Journal of the American Medical Association* (November 24, 1975), 238:836–37.

Mersky, Harold. "The Perception and Measurement of Pain." *Journal of Psychosomatic Research* (1973), 17:251–55.

Merton, Robert King, George C. Reader, and Patricia L. Kendall. *The Student-Physician: Introductory Studies in the Sociology of Medical Education*. Cambridge: Commonwealth Fund, Harvard University Press, 1957.

Metzger, Walter P. "What is a Profession?" Columbia University Program of General and Continuing Education in the Humanities. *Seminar Reports* (1975), 3(1):1–12.

Meyers, Marvin. *The Jacksonian Persuasion: Politics and Belief.* New York: Vintage Books, Random House, 1960, 1957.

Michler, Markwart. "Medical Ethics in Hippocratic Bone Surgery." *Bulletin of the History of Medicine* (July–August 1968), 42:297–311.

Milgram, Stanley. *Obedience to Authority.* New York: Harper & Row, 1974.

Miller, Lawrence G. "Pain, Parturition, and the Profession: Twilight Sleep in America." *Health Care in America: Essays in Social History,* pp. 19–44. Edited by Susan Reverby and David Rosner. Philadelphia: Temple University Press, 1979.

Miller, Perry. *The Life of the Mind in America from the Revolution to the Civil War.* New York: Harcourt, Brace & World, 1965.

—— *Nature's Nation.* Cambridge: Belknap Press of Harvard University Press, 1967.

—— *The New England Mind: The Seventeenth Century.* Boston: Beacon Press, 1961, 1939.

Mitchell, Martha Carolyn. "Health and the Medical Profession in the Lower South, 1845–1860." *Journal of Southern History* (November 1944), 10:424–46.

Mitscherlich, Alexander, and Fred Mielke. *Doctors of Infamy: The Story of the Nazi Medical Crimes.* Translated by Heinz Norden. New York: H. Schuman, 1949.

Mohl, Raymond A. *Poverty in New York, 1783–1825.* New York: Oxford University Press, 1971.

Mohr, James C. *Abortion in America: The Origins and Evolution of National Policy.* New York: Oxford University Press, 1978.

—— *The Radical Republicans and Reform in New York during Reconstruction.* Ithaca, N.Y., and London: Cornell University Press, 1973.

Moore, Wilbert E. *The Professions: Roles and Rules.* New York: Russell Sage Foundation, 1970.

Morais, Herbert M. *The History of the Negro in Medicine.* New York: Publishers Co., 1967.

Morantz, Regina Markell, "The 'Connecting Link': The Case for the Woman Doctor." *Sickness and Health in America: Readings in the History of Medicine and Public Health,* pp. 117–28. Edited by Judith Walzer Leavitt and Ronald L. Numbers. Madison: University of Wisconsin Press, 1978.

—— "The Lady and Her Physician." *Clio's Consciousness Raised: New Perspectives on the History of Women,* pp. 38–53. Edited by Mary S. Hartman and Lois Banner. New York: Harper & Row, 1974.

Morantz, Regina Markell and Sue Zschoche. "Professionalism, Feminism, and Gender Roles: A Comparative Study of Nineteenth-Century Medical Therapeutics." *Journal of American History* (December 1980), 67:568–88.

Morgan, H. Wayne. *Drugs in America: A Social History 1800–1980.* Syracuse, N.Y.: Syracuse University Press, 1981.

Morton, Thomas G. and Frank Woodbury. *A History of the Pennsylvania Hospital, 1751–1895.* Philadelphia: Times Printing House, 1897.

Mosedale, Susan Sleeth. "Science Corrupted: Victorian Biologists Consider 'The Woman Question.' " *Journal of the History of Biology* (Spring, 1978), 11:1–56.

Mostert, Jacobus W. "States of Awareness During General Anesthesia." *Perspectives in Biology and Medicine* (Autumn, 1975), 19:68–76.

Moulin, Daniel de. "A Historical-Phenomenological Study of Bodily Pain in Western Man." *Bulletin of the History of Medicine* (Winter, 1974), 48:540–70.

Muldoon, James. "The Indian as Irishman." *Essex Institute Historical Collections,* (October 1975), 111:267–89.

Mumford, James Thomas. *Memoir of Samuel Joseph May.* Boston: Roberts Brothers, 1873.

Musto, David F. *The American Disease: Origins of Narcotic Control.* New Haven: Yale University Press, 1973.

Neal, Helen. *The Politics of Pain.* New York: McGraw-Hill, 1978.

Neufeldt, Leonard N. "The Science of Power: Emerson's Views on Science and Technology in America." *Journal of the History of Ideas* (April–June 1977), 38:329–44.

Niebyl, Peter H. "The English Bloodletting Revolution, or Modern Medicine Before 1850." *Bulletin of the History of Medicine* (Fall, 1977), 51:464–83.

Nissenbaum, Stephen. *Sex, Diet, and Debility in Jacksonian America: Sylvester Graham and Health Reform.* Westport, Conn.: Greenwood Press, 1980.

Northrup, Jack. "Letters of a Frontier Doctor." *Bulletin of the History of Medicine* (January–February 1973), 47:83–90.

Notable American Women 1607–1950: A Biographical Dictionary. Edited by Edward T. James, Janet Wilson James, and Paul S. Boyer. Cambridge: Belknap Press of Harvard University Press, 1971. 3 Vols.

Novak, Steven J. "Professionalism and Bureaucracy: English Doctors and the Victorian Public Health Administration." *Journal of Social History* (Summer, 1973), 6:440–62.

Numbers, Ronald L. "The Making of an Eclectic Physician." *Bulletin of the History of Medicine* (March–April 1973), 47:155–66.

—— *Prophetess of Health: A Study of Ellen G. White.* New York: Harper & Row, 1976.

Numbers, Ronald L. and John Harley Warner. "The Maturation of American Medical Science." *Scientific Colonialism, 1800–1930: A Cross-Cultural Comparison.* Edited by Nathan Reingold and Marc Rothenberg. Washington, D.C.: Smithsonian Institution Press, forthcoming.

Nye, Russel Blaine. *Society and Culture in America, 1830–1860.* New American Nation Series. New York: Harper & Row, 1974.

Olmsted, J. M. D. *François Magendie.* New York: Schuman's, 1944.

Osler, William. "The Influence of Louis on American Medicine." *An Alabama Student and Other Essays,* pp. 189–210. New York: Oxford University Press, 1908.

Oxford English Dictionary. The Compact Edition. Oxford, England: Oxford University Press, 1971.

Packard, Francis R. *Guy Patin and the Medical Profession in Paris in the Seventeenth Century.* New York: Paul B. Hoeber, 1925.

—— *A History of Medicine in the United States.* Vol. 1. Philadelphia: J. B. Lippincott, 1901. Vol. 2. New York: Paul B. Hoeber, Inc., 1931.

—— *The Pennsylvania Hospital of Philadelphia.* Philadelphia: Engle Press, 1938.

Palfreman, Jon. "Mesmerism and the English Medical Profession: A Study of a Conflict." *Ethics in Science & Medicine* (1977), 4, (1–2):51–66.

Palmer, Paul A. "Benthamism in England and America." *American Political Science Review* (October 1941), 35:855–71.

Palumbo, Dennis J. and Richard A. Styskal. "Professionalism and Receptivity to Change." *American Journal of Political Science* (May 1974), 18:385–94.

Parry, Noel, and José Parry. *The Rise of the Medical Profession: A Study of Collective Social Mobility.* London: Croom, Helm, 1976

Parry-Jones, William L. *The Trade in Lunacy: A Study of Private Madhouses in England in the Eighteenth and Nineteenth Centuries.* Toronto: University of Toronto Press, 1972.

Parsons, Gail Pat. "Equal Treatment for All: American Medical Remedies for Male Sexual Problems, 1850–1900." *Journal of the History of Medicine and Allied Sciences* (January 1977), 32:55–71.

Parsons, Talcott. "The Professions and Social Structure." *Essays in Sociological Theory,* pp. 34–39. Revised ed. Glencoe, Ill..: Free Press, 1954.

—— "Social Structure and Dynamic Process: The Case of Modern Medical Practice." *The Social System,* pp. 428–79. Glencoe, Ill.: Free Press, 1951.

Pauly, Mark V. "What is Unnecessary Surgery." *Milbank Memorial Fund Quarterly* (Winter, 1979), 57:95–117.

Pearce, Roy Harvey. *The Savages of America: A Study of the Indian and the Idea of Civilization.* Baltimore: Johns Hopkins Press, 1953.

Pellegrino, Edmund D. "The Sociocultural Impact of Twentieth-Century Therapeutics." *The Therapeutic Revolution,* pp. 245–66. Edited by Morris J. Vogel and Charles E. Rosenberg. Philadelphia: University of Pennsylvania Press, 1979.

Pernick, Martin S. "Medical Professionalism." *Encyclopedia of Bioethics,* 3:1028–34. Edited by Warren T. Reich. New York: Free Press, Macmillan, 1978.

—— "The Patient's Role in Medical Decisionmaking: A Social History of Informed Consent in Medical Therapy." *Making Health Care Decisions: A Report on the Ethical and Legal Implications of Informed Consent in the Patient-Practitioner Relationship.* Vol. 3, *Studies on the Foundations of Informed Consent.* President's Commission for the Study of Ethical Problems in Medicine. Washington, D.C.: GPO, 1982, pp. 1–35.

—— "Politics, Parties, and Pestilence: Epidemic Yellow Fever in Philadelphia and the Rise of the First Party System." *William and Mary Quarterly* (October 1972), 3d Ser., 29:559–86.

—— "Women and the Infliction of Pain in the Practice of 19th Century Professions: The Case of Surgical Anesthesia." Paper given at the Berkshire Conference of Women Historians, Conference on the History of Women, June 1976, Bryn Mawr.

Pessen, Edward. "Egalitarian Myth and American Social Reality: Wealth, Mobility, and Equality in the 'Era of the Common Man.' " *American Historical Review* (October 1971), 76:989–1034.

Peterson, M. Jeanne. *The Medical Profession in Mid-Victorian London.* Berkeley: University of California Press, 1978.

Petrie, Asenath. *Individuality in Pain and Suffering*. Chicago: University of Chicago Press, 1967.

Pitcher, George. "The Awfulness of Pain." *Journal of Philosophy* (July 23, 1970), 67:481–92.

Pitcock, Cynthia De Haven. "Doctors in Controversy: An Ethical Dispute Between Joseph Nash McDowell and William Beaumont." *Missouri Valley Historical Review* (1966), 60(3):336–49.

Pleck, Elizabeth. "Two Worlds in One: Work and Family." *Journal of Social History* (Winter, 1976), 10:178–95.

Pole, J. R. *American Individualism and the Promise of Progress*. New York: Oxford University Press, 1980.

Pool, Eugene H., and Frank J. McGowan. *Surgery at the New York Hospital One Hundred Years Ago*. New York: Paul B. Hoeber, 1930.

Posey, William Campbell, and Samuel Horton Brown. *The Wills Hospital of Philadelphia*. Philadelphia: J. B. Lippincott, 1931.

Pred, Allan. "Large City Interdependence and the Preelectronic Diffusion of Innovation in the United States." *Geographical Analysis* (April 1971), 3:165–81.

Quen, Jacques M. "Acupuncture and Western Medicine." *Bulletin of the History of Medicine* (Summer, 1975), 49:196–205.

—— "Case Studies in Nineteenth Century Scientific Rejection: Mesmerism, Perkinsism, and Acupuncture." *Journal of the History of the Behavioral Sciences* (April 1975), 11:149–56.

Radbill, Samuel X. "Hospitals and Pediatrics, 1776–1976." *Bulletin of the History of Medicine* (Summer, 1979), 53:286–91.

Raichle, Donald R. "The Abolition of Corporal Punishment in New Jersey Schools." *History of Childhood Quarterly* (Summer, 1974), 2:53–78.

Ramsey, Matthew. "The Politics of Professional Monopoly in Nineteenth-Century Medicine: The French Model and Its Rivals." *Professions and the French State*, pp. 225–305. Edited by Gerald L. Geison. Philadelphia: University of Pennsylvania Press, 1984.

Ransom, John E. "The Beginnings of Hospitals in the United States." *Bulletin of the History of Medicine* (May 1943), 13:514–39.

Raper, Howard Riley. *Man Against Pain: The Epic of Anesthesia*. New York: Prentice-Hall, 1945.

Rayack, Elton. *Professional Power and American Medicine: The Economics of the American Medical Association*. Cleveland: World, 1967.

Reader, William Joseph. *Professional Men: The Rise of the Professional Classes in Nineteenth-Century England*. New York: Basic Books, 1966.

Redding, Joseph Stafford and John Carter Matthews. "Anesthesia During the American Civil War." *Clinical Anesthesia* (1968), No. 2, 1–18.

Reingold, Nathan. "Definitions and Speculations: The Professionalization of Science in America in the Nineteenth Century." *The Pursuit of Knowledge in the Early American Republic*, pp. 33–69. Edited by Alexandra Oleson and Sanborn C. Brown. Baltimore: Johns Hopkins University Press, 1976.

Reiser, Stanley Joel. *Medicine and the Reign of Technology*. Cambridge: Cambridge University Press, 1978.

Reverby, Susan and David Rosner, eds. *Health Care in America: Essays in Social History*. Philadelphia: Temple University Press, 1979.

Rezneck, Samuel. "A Course of Medical Education in New York City in 1828–29: The Journal of Asa Fitch." *Bulletin of the History of Medicine* (November–December 1968), 42:555–68.

Richman, Irwin. *The Brightest Ornament: A Biography of Nathaniel Chapman, M.D.* Bellefonte, Pa.: Pennsylvania Heritage, Inc., 1967.

Risse, Guenter B. "Epidemics and Medicine: The Influence of Disease on Medical Thought and Practice." *Bulletin of the History of Medicine* (Winter, 1979), 53:505–19.

Robinson, Victor. *Victory Over Pain*. New York: Henry Schuman, 1946.

Rogers, Everett M., and George M. Beal. "The Importance of Personal Influence in the Adoption of Technological Change." *Social Forces* (May 1958), 36:329–35.

Ronda, James P. " 'We Are Well As We Are': An Indian Critique of Seventeenth-Century Christian Missions." *William and Mary Quarterly* (January 1977), 3d Ser., 34:66–82.

Rook, A. "The First Experience with Ether Anaesthesia in Cambridgeshire and West Suffolk." *Anaesthesia* (1975), 30:677.

Rorabaugh, W. J. *The Alcoholic Republic: An American Tradition*. New York: Oxford University Press, 1979.

Rosen, George. *Fees and Fee Bills: Some Economic Aspects of Medical Practice in Nineteenth Century America. Bulletin of the History of Medicine*. Supplement No. 6. Baltimore: Johns Hopkins Press, 1946.

—— "The Hospital: Historical Sociology of a Community Institution." *The Hospital in Modern Society*, pp. 1–36. Edited by Eliot Freidson. New York: Free Press, 1963.

—— "Mesmerism and Surgery: A Strange Chapter in the History of Anesthesia." *Journal of the History of Medicine and Allied Sciences* (October 1946), 1:527–50.

—— "Political Order and Human Health in Jeffersonian Thought." *Bulletin of the History of Medicine* (January–February 1952), 26:32–44.

—— "Social Stress and Mental Disease in the Eighteenth to Twentieth Centuries." *Milbank Memorial Fund Quarterly* (January 1959), 37:5–32.

—— *The Specialization of Medicine, with Particular Reference to Ophthalmology*. New York: Froben Press, 1944.

Rosenberg, Charles E. "The American Medical Profession: Mid-Nineteenth Century." *Mid-America* (July 1962), 44:163–71.

—— "And Heal the Sick: The Hospital and the Patient in the 19th Century America [sic]." *Journal of Social History* (June 1977), 20:428–47.

—— "The Bitter Fruit: Heredity, Disease, and Social Thought in Nineteenth-Century America." *Perspectives in American History* (1974), 8:189–235.

—— *The Cholera Years: The United States in 1832, 1849, and 1866*. Chicago and London: University of Chicago Press, 1962.

—— "Florence Nightingale on Contagion: The Hospital as Moral Universe." *Healing and History*, pp. 116–36. New York: Science History Publications, 1979.

—— "The Hospital in America: A Century's Perspective." *Medicine and Society: Contemporary Medical Problems in Historical Perspective,* pp. 181–94. Library Publication No. 4. Philadelphia: American Philosophical Society Library, 1971.

—— "Science and American Social Thought." *Science and Society in the United States,* pp. 135–62. Edited by David D. Van Tassel and Michael G. Hall. Homewood, Ill.: Dorsey Press, 1966.

—— "Sexuality, Class, and Role in Nineteenth Century America." *American Quarterly* (1973), 25(2):131–53.

—— "Social Class and Medical Care in Nineteenth Century America: The Rise and Fall of the Dispensary." *Journal of the History of Medicine and Allied Sciences* (January 1974), 29:32–54.

—— "The Therapeutic Revolution: Medicine, Meaning, and Social Change in Nineteenth-Century America." *Perspectives in Biology and Medicine* (Summer, 1977), 20:485–506.

Rosenberg, Charles E. and Carroll Smith-Rosenberg. "Pietism and the Origins of the American Public Health Movement: A Note on John H. Griscom and Robert M. Hartley." *Journal of the History of Medicine and Allied Sciences* (January 1968), 23:16–35.

Rosenkrantz, Barbara Gutmann. "Causal Thinking in Erewhon and Elsewhere." *Journal of Medicine and Philosophy* (December 1976), 1:372–84.

—— *Public Health and the State: Changing Views in Massachusetts, 1842–1936.* Cambridge: Harvard University Press, 1972.

—— "The Search for Professional Order in 19th Century American Medicine." *Proceedings of the XIVth International Congress of the History of Science.* Tokyo: Science Council of Japan, 1975, No. 4, pp. 113–24.

Rosner, David. *A Once Charitable Enterprise: Hospitals and Health Care in Brooklyn and New York, 1885–1915.* Cambridge: Cambridge University Press, 1982.

Roth, Julius A. "Care of the Sick: Professionalism vs. Love." *Science, Medicine, and Man* (April 1974), 1:173–80.

Rothman, David J. *The Discovery of the Asylum: Social Order and Disorder in the New Republic.* Boston and Toronto: Little, Brown, 1971.

—— Review of *Children and Youth in America: A Documentary History,* by Robert H. Bremner et al. *Journal of Interdisciplinary History* (Autumn, 1971), 2:377.

Rothman, Sheila M. *Woman's Proper Place: A History of Changing Ideals and Practices, 1870 to the Present.* New York: Basic Books, 1978.

Rothstein, William G. *American Physicians in the Nineteenth Century: From Sects to Science.* Baltimore and London: Johns Hopkins University Press, 1972.

Saum, Lewis O. "Death in the Popular Mind of Pre-Civil War America." *American Quarterly* (December 1974), 26:477–95.

Savitt, Todd L. *Medicine and Slavery: The Health Care of Blacks in Antebellum Virginia.* Urbana: University of Illinois Press, 1978.

—— "The Use of Blacks for Medical Experimentation and Demonstration in the Old South." *Journal of Southern History* (August 1982), 48:331–48.

Scholten, Catherine M. " 'On the Importance of the Obstetrick Art': Changing Customs of Childbirth in America, 1760–1825.'' *William and Mary Quarterly* (July 1977), 3d Ser., 34:426–45.

Schultz, Stanley K. *The Culture Factory: Boston Public Schools, 1789–1860*. New York: Oxford University Press, 1973.

Schwartz, Harold. *Samuel Gridley Howe: Social Reformer, 1801–1876*. Cambridge, Mass.: Harvard University Press, 1956.

Schwartz, L. Laszlo. ''Historical Relations of American Dentistry and Medicine.'' *Bulletin of the History of Medicine* (November–December 1954), 28:542–49.

Schwarz, Richard W. *John Harvey Kellogg, M.D.* Nashville: Southern Publishing Association, 1970.

Scott, Anne Firor. *The Southern Lady: From Pedestal to Politics, 1830–1930*. Chicago: University of Chicago Press, 1970.

Scull, Andrew, ed. *Madhouses, Mad-Doctors, and Madmen: The Social History of Psychiatry in the Victorian Era*. Philadelphia: University of Pennsylvania Press, 1981.

Seeman, Bernard. *Man Against Pain: 3,000 Years of Effort to Understand and Relieve Physical Suffering*. Philadelphia and New York: Chilton Books, 1962.

Shafer, Henry Burnell. *The American Medical Profession, 1783–1850*. New York: Columbia University Press, 1936.

Shaw, Wilfred B., ed. *The University of Michigan: An Encyclopedic Survey*. Ann Arbor: University of Michigan Press, 1951.

Shedlin, Michael, and David Wallechinsky. [The East Bay Chemical Philosophy Symposium], eds. *Laughing Gas: Nitrous Oxide*. [New York and San Francisco]: And /Or Press, 1973.

Shelton, Stephanie. ''CBS Evening News.'' Radio Broadcast of January 3, 1978, 8:00 P.M., E.S.T.

Shklar, Judith. ''Putting Cruelty First.'' *Daedalus* (Summer, 1982), 111(3):17–27.

Shortt, S. E. D. ''Physicians, Science, and Status: Issues in the Professionalization of Anglo-American Medicine in the Nineteenth Century, *Medical History* (1983), 27:51–68.

Shryock, Richard Harrison. *American Medical Research: Past and Present*. New York: Commonwealth Fund, 1947.

—— *The Development of Modern Medicine: An Interpretation of the Social and Scientific Factors Involved*. New York: Knopf, 1947.

—— ''The History of Quantification in Medical Science.'' (Isis (June 1961), 52:215–37.

—— *Medical Licensing in America, 1650–1965*. Baltimore: Johns Hopkins Press, 1967.

—— *Medicine in America: Historical Essays*. Baltimore: Johns Hopkins Press, 1966.

—— *Medicine and Society in America, 1660–1860*. Ithaca, N.Y.: Cornell University Press, 1962. New York: New York University Press, 1960.

—— ''Nursing Emerges as a Profession: The American Experience.'' *Clio Medica* (1968), 3:131–47.

Sicherman, Barbara. ''The Paradox of Prudence: Mental Health in the Gilded Age.'' *Journal of American History* (March 1976), 62:890–912.

Siddall, A. Clair. "Bloodletting in American Obstetric Practice, 1800–1945." *Bulletin of the History of Medicine* (Spring, 1980), 54:101–110.

Siegel, Rudolph E. *Galen's System of Physiology and Medicine.* Basel, Switzerland, and New York: S. Karger, 1968.

Sigerest, Henry E. *Civilization and Disease.* Chicago: University of Chicago Press, 1962, 1943.

—— "An Outline of the Development of the Hospital." *Bulletin of the History of Medicine* (July 1936), 4:573–81.

Skinner, B. F. *Science and Human Behavior.* New York: Macmillan, 1953.

Sklar, Kathryn Kish. *Catharine Beecher: A Study in American Domesticity.* New Haven, Conn.: Yale University Press, 1973.

Slotkin, Richard. *Regeneration Through Violence: The Mythology of the American Frontier, 1600–1860.* Middletown, Conn.: Wesleyan University Press, 1973.

Smith, Dale C. "Quinine and Fever: The Development of the Effective Dosage." *Journal of the History of Medicine and Allied Sciences* (July 1976), 31:343–67.

Smith, Daniel Scott. "Family Limitation, Sexual Control, and Domestic Feminism in Victorian America." *Clio's Consciousness Raised: New Perspectives on the History of Women,* pp. 119–36. Edited by Mary S. Hartman and Lois W. Banner. New York: Harper & Row, 1974.

Smith, George Winston, and Charles Judan, eds. *Chronicles of the Gringos: The U.S. Army in the Mexican War, 1846–1848.* Albuquerque: University of New Mexico Press, 1968.

Smithcors, J. F. "History of Veterinary Anesthesia." *Textbook of Veterinary Anesthesia,* pp. 1–23. Edited by Lawrence R. Soma. Baltimore: Williams & Wilkins, 1971.

Smith-Rosenberg, Carroll. "The Hysterical Woman: Sex Roles and Role Conflict in Nineteenth-Century America." *Social Research* (1972), 39:652–78.

—— *Religion and the Rise of the American City: The New York City Mission Movement, 1812–1870.* Ithaca, N.Y.: Cornell University Press, 1971.

Smith-Rosenberg, Carroll, and Charles E. Rosenberg. "The Female Animal: Medical and Biological Views of Woman and Her Role in Nineteenth-Century America." *Journal of American History* (September 1973), 60:332–56.

Soelle, Dorothee. *Suffering.* Translated by Everett Kalin. Philadelphia: Fortress Press, 1975.

Sontag, Susan. *Illness as Metaphor.* New York: Farrar, Straus, Giroux, 1978.

Stampp, Kenneth M. *The Peculiar Institution: Slavery in the Ante-Bellum South.* New York: Vintage Books, Random House, 1956.

Stannard, David E. "Death and Dying in Puritan New England." *American Historical Review* (December 1973), 78:1305–30.

—— *The Puritan Way of Death.* New York: Oxford University Press, 1977.

Stanton, William. *The Leopard's Spots: Scientific Attitudes Toward Race in America, 1815–1859.* Chicago: University of Chicago Press, 1960.

Starr, Paul. "Medicine, Economy and Society in Nineteenth-Century America." *Journal of Social History* (June 1977), 10:588–607.

Staum, Martin S. *Cabanis: Enlightenment and Medical Philosophy in the French Revolution.* Princeton, N.J.: Princeton University Press, 1980.

Stern, Bernhard J. *Society and Medical Progress*. Princeton, N.J.: Princeton University Press, 1941.

Sternbach, Richard A. and Bernard Tursky. "Ethnic Differences Among Housewives in Psychophysical and Skin Potential Responses to Electric Shock." *Psychophysiology* (January 1965) 1:241–46.

Stevens, Rosemary. *American Medicine and the Public Interest*. New Haven: Yale University Press, 1971.

Stevenson, Lloyd G. "Emergence of American Medicine in the Nineteenth Century." *Cahiers d'Histoire Mondiale* (1968), 11(3):455–66.

—— "Suspended Animation and the History of Anesthesia." *Bulletin of the History of Medicine* (Winter, 1975), 49:482–511.

Stevenson, Lloyd G. and Robert P. Multhauf, eds. *Medicine, Science, and Culture: Historical Essays in Honor of Owsei Temkin*. Baltimore: Johns Hopkins Press, 1968.

Stookey, Byron. "Origins of the First National Medical Convention: 1826–1846." *Journal of the American Medical Association* (July 15, 1961), 177:123–30.

Storms, William O. "Chloroform Parties." *Journal of the American Medical Association* (July 9, 1973), 225:160.

Strauss, Maurice B., ed. *Familiar Medical Quotations*. Boston: Little, Brown, 1968.

Struik, Dirk J. *Yankee Science in the Making*. New, revised ed. New York: Collier Books, 1962.

"Sufficient Treatment for Pain." *Annals of Internal Medicine* (June, 1973), 78:974–75.

Sykes, W. Stanley. *Essays on the First Hundred Years of Anaesthesia*. Edinburgh: E. & S. Livingstone, 1960, 2 Vols.

Taylor, J. A. *History of Dentistry*. Philadelphia: Lea and Febiger, 1922.

Taylor, William Rogers. *Cavalier and Yankee: The Old South and the American National Character*. New York: George Braziller, 1961.

Temkin, Owsei. *The Double Face of Janus and Other Essays in the History of Medicine*. Baltimore: Johns Hopkins Press, 1977.

—— *Galenism: The Rise and Decline of a Medical Philosophy*. Ithaca, N.Y.: Cornell University Press, 1973.

Tesson, E., S.J. "Analgesics and Christian Perfection." *New Problems in Medical Ethics , 3d Series*, pp. 244–50. Edited by Dom Peter Flood. Westminster, Md.: Newman Press, 1956.

Thatcher, Virginia Sarah. *The History of Anesthesia, With Emphasis on the Nurse Specialist*. Philadelphia: J. B. Lippincott, 1953.

Thomas, John L. "Romantic Reform in America, 1815–1865." *American Quarterly* (Winter, 1965), Vol. 17. Reprinted in *Intellectual History in America*, 1:192–217. Edited by Cushing Strout. New York: Harper & Row, 1968.

Thomas, K. Bryn. "Chloroform or Ether—A Literary Question." *Anaesthesia* (1975), 30:88–89.

Thomas, Robert D. *The Man Who Would Be Perfect: John Humphrey Noyes and the Utopian Impulse*. Philadelphia: University of Pennsylvania Press, 1977.

Thompson, E. P. "Time, Work Discipline, and Industrial Capitalism." *Past & Present* (December 1967), 37:56–97.

Thompson, John D., and Grace Goldin. *The Hospital: A Social and Architectural History.* New Haven: Yale University Press, 1975.

Thompson, Stith. *Motif-Index of Folk-Literature.* Bloomington: Indiana University Press, 1966.

Thorwald, Jürgen. *The Century of the Surgeon.* New York: Pantheon Books, 1957.

Tilton, Eleanor M. *Amiable Autocrat: A Biography of Dr. Oliver Wendell Holmes.* New York: Henry Schuman, 1947.

Tomkins, Silvan S. "The Psychology of Commitment: The Constructive Role of Violence and Suffering for the Individual and His Society." *The Antislavery Vanguard: New Essays on the Abolitionists,* pp. 270–98. Edited by Martin Duberman. Princeton: Princeton University Press, 1965.

Toulmin, Stephen. "The Meaning of Professionalism: Doctors' Ethics and Biomedical Science." *Knowledge, Value and Belief,* pp. 254–78. Edited by H. Tristram Engelhardt, Jr. and Daniel Callahan. Hastings-on-Hudson, N.Y.: The Hastings Center, 1977.

Trautmann, Joanne, and Carol Pollard. *Literature and Medicine: Topics, Titles & Notes.* Philadelphia: Society for Health and Human Values, 1975.

Trent, Josiah Charles. "Surgical Anesthesia, 1846–1946." *Journal of the History of Medicine and Allied Sciences* (October 1946), 1:505–14.

Trigg, Roger. *Pain and Emotion.* Oxford, England: Clarendon Press, 1970.

Troen, Selwyn K. *The Public and the Schools: Shaping the St. Louis System, 1838–1920.* Columbia: University of Missouri Press, 1975.

Trowell, Hugh. *The Unfinished Debate on Euthanasia.* London: SCL Press, 1973.

Truax, Rhoda. *The Doctors Warren of Boston.* Boston: Houghton-Mifflin, 1968.

Turner, E. S. *All Heaven in a Rage.* New York: St. Martin's Press, 1965.

Turner, Frank M. "The Victorian Conflict between Science and Religion: A Professional Dimension." *Isis* (September 1978), 69:356–76.

Turner, James Crewdson. "The Emergence of a Modern Sensibility: Love for Animals and the Anglo-American Mind." A longer draft version of his *Reckoning with the Beast.* 1977.

—— *Reckoning with the Beast: Animals, Pain, and Humanity in the Victorian Mind.* Baltimore: Johns Hopkins University Press, 1980.

Tyack, David B. *The One Best System: A History of American Urban Education.* Cambridge: Harvard University Press, 1974.

Tyler, Alice Felt. *Freedom's Ferment: Phases of American Social History from the Colonial Period to the Outbreak of the Civil War.* New York: The Academy Library, Harper & Row, 1962, 1944.

Tyrell, Ian R. *Sobering Up: From Temperance to Prohibition in Antebellum America, 1800–1860.* Westport, Conn.: Greenwood Press, 1979.

"University of Pennsylvania Alumni in the Civil War." *Medical Affairs,* Vol. 2 (Spring 1961).

Vandam, L. D. "Early American Anesthetists: The Origins of Professionalism in Anesthesia." *Anesthesiology* (1973), 38:264–74.

Van Ingen, Philip. *The New York Academy of Medicine: Its First Hundred Years.* New York: Columbia University Press, 1949.

Veith, Ilza. *Hysteria: The History of a Disease.* Chicago: University of Chicago Press, 1965.

Verbrugge, L. M. and R. P. Steiner. "Physician Treatment of Men and Women Patients: Sex Bias or Appropriate Care?" *Medical Care* (1981), 19:609–32.

Verbrugge, Martha. "Historical Complaints and Political Disorders." *International Journal of Health Services* (1975), 5:323–33.

—— "Women and Medicine in Nineteenth-Century America." *Signs* (Summer, 1976), 1:957–72.

Viets, Henry R. *A Brief History of Medicine in Massachusetts.* Boston: Houghton-Mifflin, 1930.

Vinovskis, Maris A. "Angels' Heads and Weeping Willows: Death in Early America." *Proceedings of the American Antiquarian Society* (1977), 86:273–302.

—— "Trends in Massachusetts Education, 1826–1860." *History of Education Quarterly* (Winter, 1972), 12:501–29.

Vogel, Joan and Richard Delgado. "To Tell the Truth: Physicians' Duty to Disclose Medical Mistakes." *UCLA Law Review* (1980), 28:52–94.

Vogel, Morris J. "The Civil War and the Hospital." Graduate seminar paper, University of Chicago, 1969.

—— *The Invention of the Modern Hospital: Boston, 1870–1930.* Chicago: University of Chicago Press, 1980.

—— "Patrons, Practitioners, and Patients: The Voluntary Hospital in Mid-Victorian Boston." *Victorian America,* pp. 120–38. Edited by Daniel Walker Howe. Philadelphia: University of Pennsylvania Press, 1976.

Vollmer, Howard M., and Donald Mills, eds. *Professionalization.* Englewood Cliffs, N.J.: Prentice-Hall, 1966.

Walsh, Mary Roth. *"Doctors Wanted: No Women Need Apply": Sexual Barriers in the Medical Profession, 1835–1975.* New Haven, Conn., and London: Yale University Press, 1977.

Walters, Ronald G. *American Reformers, 1815–1860.* American Century Series. New York: Hill and Wang, 1978.

—— *The Antislavery Appeal: American Abolitionism after 1830.* Baltimore & London: Johns Hopkins University Press, 1977.

—— "The Erotic South: Civilization and Sexuality in American Abolition." *American Quarterly* (May 1973), 25:177–201.

—— "The Family and Ante-bellum Reform: An Interpretation." *Societas* (Summer, 1973), 3:221–32.

Ward, David. *Cities and Immigrants: The Geography of Change in Nineteenth Century America.* New York: Oxford University Press, 1971.

Ward, John William. *Andrew Jackson, Symbol for an Age.* New York: Oxford University Press, 1955.

Warner, John Harley. "Physiological Theory and Therapeutic Explanation in the 1860s: The British Debate on the Medical Use of Alcohol." *Bulletin of the History of Medicine* (Summer, 1980), 54:235–57.

—— " 'The Nature-Trusting Heresy': American Physicians and the Concept of the Healing Power of Nature." *Perspectives in American History* (1977–78), 11:291–324.

Warren, Edward. *The Life of John Collins Warren.* Boston: Ticknor and Fields, 1860, 2 Vols.

Wasserman, Manfred J. "Benjamin Rush on Government and the Harmony and Derangement of the Mind.'' *Journal of the History of Ideas* (October–December 1972), 33:639–42.

Weber, Max. *From Max Weber: Essays in Sociology.* Translated by H. H. Gerth and C. Wright Mills. New York: Oxford University Press, 1946.

Weller, R. M. ''Death in Bristol: An Exchange of Views Between Augustin Prichard and John Snow.'' *Anaesthesia* (1976), 31:90–96.

—— ''*Punch,* On Anesthesia.'' *Anaesthesia* (1976), 31:1267–72.

Welter, Barbara. ''The Cult of True Womanhood, 1820–1860.'' *American Quarterly* (Summer, 1966), 18:151–74.

—— ''The Feminization of American Religion, 1800–1860.'' *Clio's Consciousness Raised: New Perspectives on the History of Women,* pp. 137–57. Edited by Mary S. Hartman and Lois W. Banner. New York: Harper & Row, 1974.

Welter, Rush. *The Mind of America, 1820–1860.* New York: Columbia University Press, 1975.

Wertz, Richard W., and Dorothy C. Wertz. *Lying-In: A History of Childbirth in America.* New York: Free Press, Macmillan, 1977.

Whipple, Allen O. *The Evolution of Surgery in the United States.* Springfield, Ill.: Charles C Thomas, 1963.

Whitehouse, Walter M., and Frank Whitehouse, Jr. ''The Daily Register of Dr. Cyrus Bacon, Jr.: Care of the Wounded at the Battle of Gettysburg.'' *Michigan Academician* (Spring, 1976), 8:373–86.

Whorton, James C. ''Christian Physiology: William Alcott's Prescription for the Millenium.'' *Bulletin of the History of Medicine* (Winter, 1975), 49:466–81.

—— ''Tempest in a Flesh-Pot: The Formulation of a Physiological Rationale for Vegetarianism.'' *Journal of the History of Medicine and Allied Sciences* (April 1977), 32:115–39.

Wiebe, Robert H. *The Search for Order; 1877–1920.* The Making of America. New York: Hill & Wang, 1967.

—— *The Segmented Society: An Historical Preface to the Meaning of America.* London: Oxford University Press, 1975.

Wiley, Bell Irvin. *The Life of Johnny Reb, The Common Soldier of the Confederacy.* Indianapolis: Bobbs-Merrill, 1943.

—— ''The Movement to Humanize the Institution of Slavery During the Confederacy.'' *Emory University Quarterly* (December 1949), 5:207–20.

Williams, William H. *America's First Hospital: The Pennsylvania Hospital 1751–1841.* Wayne, Pa.: Haverford House, 1976.

Wills, Garry. *Inventing America: Jefferson's Declaration of Independence.* Garden City, N.Y.: Doubleday, 1978.

Wilson, Edmund. *Patriotic Gore: Studies in the Literature of the American Civil War.* New York: Farrar, Straus and Giroux, 1977, 1962.

Wishy, Bernard. *The Child and the Republic: The Dawn of Modern American Child Nurture.* Philadelphia: University of Pennsylvania Press, 1968.

Wolff, B. Berthold. ''Factor Analysis of Human Pain Responses: Pain Endurance as a Specific Pain Factor.'' *Journal of Abnormal Psychology* (1971) 78:292–98.

Wood, Ann Douglas. '' 'The Fashionable Diseases': Women's Complaints and their Treatment in Nineteenth-Century America.'' *Journal of Interdisciplinary History* (Summer, 1973), 4:25–52.

Woodward, Grace S. *The Man Who Conquered Surgical Pain: A Biography of William Thomas Green Morton.* Boston: Beacon Press, 1962.

Woodward, John. *To Do the Sick No Harm: A Study of the British Voluntary Hospital System to 1875.* London and Boston: Routledge and Kegan Paul, 1974.

Woolmer, Ronald. *The Conquest of Pain: Achievements of Modern Anaesthesia.* New York: Knopf, 1961.

Wyatt, Philip R. "John Humphrey Noyes and the Stirpicultural Experiment." *Journal of the History of Medicine and Allied Sciences* (January 1976), 31:55–66.

Young, James Harvey. *The Toadstool Millionaires: A Social History of Patent Medicines in America before Federal Regulation.* Princeton, N.J.: Princeton University Press, 1961.

Youngson, A. J. *The Scientific Revolution in Victorian Medicine.* New York: Holmes & Meier, 1979.

Zborowski, Mark. *People in Pain.* San Francisco: Jossey-Bass, 1969.

INDEX

Massachusetts General Hospital: ether demonstration at, 3, 42; anesthesia usage data,
4, 189-192, 196, 201-202, 249-251; discriminatory treatment at, 18; and female
suffering, 164; and debility, 179; nonanesthetic operations, cases, 179, 229,
264*n*7, 331*n*4; anesthesia usage and surgeon's age, 199, 333*n*9; postanesthetic increase in surgery at, 208-223, 255-262,
337*n*11, 339*n*29; and regional rivalries, 203-
204; ovariotomy at, 213-214; involuntary
anesthetization at, 229-231; outpatients at,
222; records of, 264*n*7-265*n*8, 330*n*2; surgery as last resort of, 300*n*57
Massachusetts Medical Society, 67, 288*n*153
Massachusetts State Prison, 57
Massachusetts Teachers Association, 269*n*29,
312*n*108
Masturbation, 18, 178
Materialism, 145, 236, 345*n*106. *See also* Vitalism
Mather, Cotton, 79, 282*n*90
May, Jonathan Frederick, 83
"Mean," 315*n*15
Medical and surgical records: hospital vs. private, 4; and particularization, 142; confidentiality of, 263*n*1; completeness of,
264*n*6-265*n*8, 330*n*2, 332*n*14; errors in,
297*n*32, 337*n*7, 340*n*39; modern, 341*n*41.
See also Quantification; Statistics
Medical education, *see* Apprenticeship; Medical schools; Medical students
Medical ethics and values: behind technical
controversies, 19-22, 28-29, 58, 97-98, 101,
121, 137, 238-242; and evaluation of anesthesia, 94-98, 101, 104, 109, 112, 122-124.
See also Consent; Conservative professionalism; Experimentation; Heroic professionalism; Individuality vs. uniformity; Medical etiquette; Natural healing; Omission vs.
commission; Professionalism; Utilitarianism
Medical etiquette: and ethics codes, 22, 26,
113; and anesthesia, 66-76, 89. *See also*
Medical ethics; Professionalism
Medical schools, 13, 27-28, 145-146, 203-204,
273*n*69. *See also* Medical students; names
of specific schools
Medical societies, *see* Individual vs. professional unity; Professional organization;
Medical societies, *see* Individual vs. profes-

sional unity; Professional organization;
names of specific societies
Medical students: and suffering, 106-107,
300*n*51-*n*52; learn detachment, 107, 115,
300*n*52; defer to professors, 199, 205;
challenge professors, 199, 207; and regionalism, 203-204
Medical therapy: theory vs. practice, 12-15,
67-69, 146, 289*n*155; specificity of, 12-13,
29, 83, 128-129, 137, 238; tonics and
stimulation, 13, 15, 96, 135, 298*n*36; efficacy of, 13, 123; depletion, 13, 132-134;
humoral, 12-13, 132, 308*n*36; counterirritation, 44, 57-58, 90, 96-97, 108,
279*n*56,*n*58, 284*n*110, 296*n*9, 300*n*61,
317*n*36; as punishment, 56-58, 102, 107,
134-135, 284*n*110,*n*112, 296*n*17, 298*n*35-
299*n*41; anesthesia as, 83, 325*n*27, 326*n*42;
safety of, 95, 98-101; vs. relief of suffering, 105-117; individualized vs. uniform,
124-147. *See also* Conservative professionalism; Disease; Drugs; Environmental-moral;
Heroic therapy; Natural healing; Nihilism;
Surgery
Meigs, Charles: and obstetric anesthesia, 48,
98, 221; and surgical anesthesia, 48, 281*n*76;
antiutilitarianism of, 98, 122, 123, 221; and
Simpson, 98, 131; and patient variability,
144; and paternalism, 145; and female sensitivity, 161; vs. Oliver Wendell Holmes,
203-204
Melville, Herman, 114-115, 119, 156-157,
161, 235
Memory: and suffering, 37, 150, 172; and
anesthesia, 37-38, 275*n*16
Men: anesthesia as unmanly, 46-47; endurance and masculinity, 46-47, 108-109, 118-
119; anesthesia and dominance of, 61, 86-
87, 294*n*44; cruelty of, 117, 225-226; traditional vs. modern roles of, 118-119; Walt
Whitman on, 119-120; sensitivity of, 150,
160-161, 176, 181-182, 327*n*63; and female suffering, 165; indications for anesthesia in, 175-176, 181-183, 325*n*23; anesthesia usage on, 191-195, 250-253,
332*n*15,*n*17; postanesthetic rate of surgery
on, 211, 256. *See also* Courage; Military;
Sex
Men medical practitioners: and suffering, 114,
224-227; and use of anesthesia, 225, 342*n*64
Menstruation, 151-152, 175